Principles of
Neurobiological
Signal
Analysis

Principles of Neurobiological Signal Analysis

Edmund M. Glaser
Daniel S. Ruchkin

School of Medicine
University of Maryland
Baltimore, Maryland

ACADEMIC PRESS   New York   San Francisco   London   1976
A Subsidiary of Harcourt Brace Jovanovich, Publishers

ACADEMIC PRESS, INC.
111 Fifth Avenue, New York, New York 10003

United Kingdom Edition published by
ACADEMIC PRESS, INC. (LONDON) LTD.
24/28 Oval Road, London NW1

Library of Congress Cataloging in Publication Data

Glaser, Edmund M
  Principles of neurobiological signal analysis.

    Bibliography: p.
    Includes index.
    1.   Neural analyzers—Mathematical models.   I.   Ruch-
kin, Daniel S., joint author.   II.   Title.   III.   Title:
Signal analysis.
QP363.G58   591.1'88   76-42267
ISBN 0-12-285950-2

CONTENTS

CHAPTER 3 POWER SPECTRA AND COVARIANCE FUNCTIONS

CHAPTER 4   EVOKED POTENTIALS: AVERAGING AND DISCRIMINANT ANALYSIS

CHAPTER 5   EVOKED POTENTIALS: PRINCIPAL COMPONENTS AND VARIMAX ANALYSIS

CHAPTER 6   SPONTANEOUS AND DRIVEN SINGLE UNIT ACTIVITY

PREFACE

More years ago than we care to think of or mention, we convinced ourselves of the need for a monograph on the principles of signal analysis as applied to the electrical activity of the nervous system. This book is the result. Our premise in organizing it has been simple: that neurobiologists are generally uneasy in their use of signal analysis simply because they have had little formal training in the mathematics underlying its framework and that therefore they have little intuitive feel for what signal analysis procedures mean. Our goal, consequently, is to provide neurobiologists with a reasonably detailed discussion of signal analysis as it has been variously applied to neuronal signals. We wish to make them more aware of what these analyses can and cannot do, their implications, and limitations. We have used mathematics where it is essential, but in doing so we have tried to avoid unnecessary rigor. We have assumed that mathematically the reader is equipped with a hazy recollection of calculus. Our hope is that we can dispel most of this haze in the early going. On another front, we have consciously refrained from treating the cuisine of signal analysis. Recipes or programs for signal analysis are readily available for a variety of computers. We do not feel they provide much elucidation of the basic issues.

The first three chapters establish the theoretical groundwork of signal analysis. Chapter 1 presents an introductory discussion of the properties of signal and noise, especially as they apply to the nervous system. It reflects our judgment that the essential ingredients of neurobiological signal analysis are the related concepts of signal spectra and covariance functions. They are likely to remain so even as the present, predominantly linear methods of signal analysis are broadened to encompass nonlinear techniques. Chapter 2 discusses the methods of sampling and converting biological signals into sequences of digital numbers readily digestible by a computer. Chapter 3 then develops more thoroughly the concepts of spectrum and covariance analysis. This chapter is mathematically somewhat more demanding than the first two. Those who find it too trying should not feel distressed since much of what appears subsequently will still be comprehensible. The loss is in the appreciation of some of the analytic details.

Chapters 4 and 5 deal with techniques for extracting evoked responses from background noise and with multivariate statistical procedures for treating evoked response waveshapes as variables dependent upon the experimental manipulations performed upon a subject. Chapters 6 and 7 deal with the analysis of spike (action potential) activity generated by individual neurons and small groups of neurons. Chapter 8 presents methods for studying how such spike activity may be related to the concurrently observed slow wave (EEG-like) activity of the nervous system.

A number of individuals have contributed to the completion of this work. It was Dr. José del Castillo who provided us with facilities at the Laboratory of Neurobiology of the University of Puerto Rico. It was there that this book had its inception. Drs. Donald Childers, Emanuel Donchin, and George Gerstein reviewed various chapters and provided much helpful criticism. A special note of thanks goes to Drs. José Negrete and Guillermina Yankelevich de Negrete who lent much encouragement during the initial tribulations of writing. Finally, we would like to express our special appreciation to Mrs. Frances Pridgen who, equipped with an extensive background as a legal secretary, typed the manuscript and suffered with us in guiding it to completion. In a moment of relaxation, when all was done, we asked her opinion of the work. She flipped slowly through its pages, smiled and said, "Naturally, this is taxable." We wonder.

Chapter 1

SOME PROPERTIES
OF BIOLOGICAL SIGNALS

1.1. INTRODUCTION

Speaking in a somewhat general way, we say that all biological data can be considered to be signals. Obviously, however, some data are more signallike than others. The dividing line between data that can be profitably considered to be signallike and data that cannot depends upon both the origin of the data and how we propose to process it and analyze it conceptually. A discussion of the many facets of this idea in the light of modern computer data processing methods is one of the major purposes of this book. Embarking in this direction requires that we first establish some of the major concepts and properties of signals insofar as they relate to biological processes. The properties of these signals influence, guide, and sometimes determine the ways in which computer programs are developed to perform signal analysis.

Signal: A variation in the amplitude and polarity of an observed physical quantity produced by a process whose mechanisms we desire to understand by experimental investigation.

The requirement that the variation be produced by a mechanism we are interested in is of basic importance and brings us to consider at once, noise, the inseparable companion of signal.

Noise: A variation in the size of an observed physical quantity we are investigating produced by a process or an aspect of a process that we have no present interest in.

Data: Some combination, often additive, of signal and noise. The additive situations are easiest to deal with in terms of analysis and interpretation of results. In much of what follows we will assume it applies. In general, however, additivity should not be taken for granted.

1

The errant course of scientific progress is such that often what is considered to be a signal in one investigation turns out to be noise in another. Or more colloquially, one man's signal is another man's noise.

The variations in the size of a physical quantity are often time-dependent. When they are, the data is said to be a function of time and written $x(t)$. Temporal data variation is most convenient for us to consider and also most appropriate since a real-time computer generally accepts data in time sequential form. However, we may also profitably consider data which are functions of such variables as distances or angle, for it is usually a simple matter to convert them into functions of time by a signal transducer. As an example, a scanning densitometer converts the spatially varying density of a translucent object into a function of time as the densitometer is moved over the scanned object. An oscilloscope screen is an example of the process in reverse for there the time-varying data is converted into a function of distance along the horizontal axis of the oscilloscope screen. Hereafter, when we mention data signals and noise, we will consider them to be temporally varying.

We are interested in establishing the basic principles of a wide assortment of procedures by which we analyze the signallike data of neurobiological investigations. Temporally generated signals and noises exhibit a wide variety of waveform features or parameters, and it is essential to classify them according to such features, for the validity of much of the subsequent data processing depends upon the presence or magnitude of these features. The following pages contain a discussion of some of the properties of signals to serve as the basis of understanding the signal analysis procedures and techniques to be described in later chapters.

1.2. CONTINUOUS SIGNALS AND THEIR DISCRETE COUNTERPARTS

Let us begin with data which consist only of signals. A

2

signal is said to be continuous if it is defined at all instants of time during which it occurs. A continuous signal may, however, possess discontinuities or sudden changes in amplitude at certain instants of time. At these instants the slope of the signal is infinite. At other times the signal amplitude changes gradually so that by choosing an interval short enough, the corresponding change in amplitude can be made as small as we like. While continuous signals without discontinuities are the rule in such biological phenomena as the EEG, deliberately generated discontinuous signals may be generated by the instrumentation associated with neurobiological investigations. As an example, the signal produced by a rat when it pushes a switch to obtain food is discontinuous. This type of signal is referred to as a step function. Illustrations of continuous and discontinuous signals are shown in Fig. 1.1. It is also to be noted that whether continuous or not, the signals are always single valued: they have only one value at any particular instant in time. A particularly interesting and important discontinuous signal is the unit step signal of Fig. 1.1(c):

$$u(t) = \begin{cases} 0 \text{ when } t \leq t_d, \\ 1 \text{ when } t > t_d \end{cases} \tag{1.1}$$

t_d is the instant of discontinuity. The equation indicates that the signal jumps to 1 as soon as t becomes greater than t_d. The unit step is used, among other purposes, to describe a stimulus that has a sudden onset.

Besides speaking of a continuous signal, $x(t)$, we will also have occasion to speak of its time derivatives, the first derivative being written $dx(t)/dt$ or, alternatively, $x'(t)$. The first derivative is, of course, the time rate of change of the variable. When it is zero, the variable itself is at a local maximum or minimum value or, less frequently, at an inflection point. (The derivative of a constant signal is always zero.) This property is often used in determining when a spikelike waveform reaches a maximum or minimum. A peak detection device which essentially

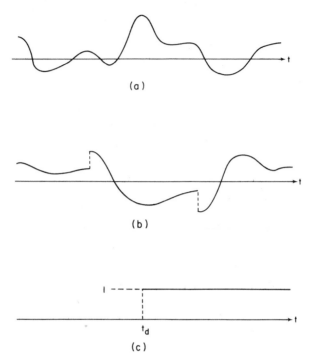

Fig. 1.1. (a) A continuous signal; (b) a discontinuous
signal; (c) the unit step $\mu(t)$, *showing step onset at* $t = t_d$.

takes the time derivative of the waveform is commonly employed for
this. When its output, the waveform time derivative, goes through
zero in a negative direction, a positive maximum has occurred;
when it goes through zero in a positive direction, a negative
maximum has occurred. Figure 1.2(a) illustrates the situation
for the former case. The first derivative is also important in
indicating when the signal is changing most rapidly because it has
its greatest value at that time. A positive maximum in the first
derivative indicates the time when the signal is increasing most
rapidly; a negative maximum, when it is decreasing most rapidly.
Just as a continuous signal may exhibit discontinuities, so may
its derivatives. A discontinuity in the first derivative occurs
when there is a cusp in the original signal. An example is the
sawtooth signal of Fig. 1.2(b). When it is at its maximum and

4

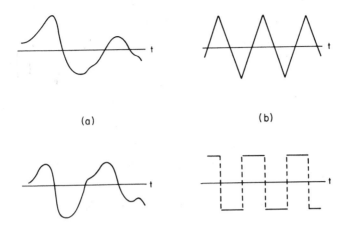

(a)   (b)

Fig. 1.2. (a) Above, a continuous signal; below, its time derivative. The negative and positive going zero crossings of the derivative correspond to positive and negative peaks in the signal. (b) Above, a periodic sawtooth signal; below, its time derivative which is a periodic discontinuous square wave.

minimum values, discontinuities occur in its first derivative, a square wave.

The derivative operation is not without practical difficulties since noise contributions tend to corrupt the derivative measurement. In computer analysis of data, the derivative operation is approximated by comparing successive sampled values of the signal with one another to see when maximum and minimum rates of change occur. Although this is an approximation, the results are often more than adequate. It is worth noting here that approximation is different from estimation, the latter being a statistical procedure whose meaning will be made clear in the subsequent pages.

In contrast to temporally continuous (T-continuous) signals are the temporally discrete (T-discrete) signals. These are signals which exist only at discrete instants in time. For our purposes the most important discrete signals are those which occur when a continuous signal has its amplitude measured or sampled at discrete instants of time that are usually equally spaced. A T-discrete signal is thus a sequence of measurements $x_1, x_2, \cdots,$

x_T lasting for the duration of the time the signal is observed. In digital data processing it is furthermore usually quantized in amplitude by an analog-to-digital converter. This gives it the property of being amplitude discrete (A-discrete). The result is a signal, T- and A-discrete, which provides the basic data thereafter for all subsequent computer analyses of the original signal.

Having introduced the continuous signal and its sampled T-discrete representation, it is useful to establish here a form of notation which permits us to distinguish between them with a minimum amount of confusion. We will use the symbol ° to distinguish a sampled T-discrete signal from its continuous source signal. We will drop the ° when no confusion seems possible. Similarly, we will use t to represent continuous time and $t°\Delta$ to represent those instants that a signal is sampled at a uniform rate. Δ is the interval between neighboring samples, and $t°$ is an integer-valued index: 1, 2, 3, ..., etc. Signal analyses are often most easy to describe when $\Delta = 1$. This results in no loss of generality. When there is no possibility of confusion, the Δ will be dropped.

The signals or data handled by a digital computer are discrete not only in time but also in amplitude. This arises from the fact that the amplitude of a signal at a particular sampling instant is represented as a number within the computer, a number containing a limited number of digits or bits depending upon the computer's structure. To arrive at this numeric representation a continuous signal is first transformed into its A-discrete amplitude version by quantization in an analog-to-digital (A-D) converter. At each sampling time the quantization procedure assigns to the signal amplitude one of a finite number of levels. This level has a numeric value which represents the sample in subsequent data analysis computations. The subject of A-D conversion, or quantization, is discussed more thoroughly in Chapter 2.

Perhaps the simplest way of reconstructing a continuous signal from a set of its samples is shown in Fig. 1.3. Here the signal is assumed to remain constant at its sampled value for the

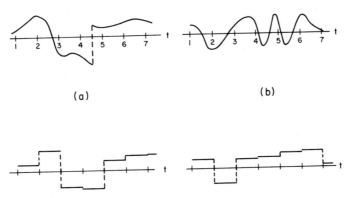

Fig. 1.3. (a) Above, a signal with a discontinuity between t = 4 and 5; below, a reconstruction of that signal by interpolation with a constant value between sampling instants. (b) Above, another continuous signal fluctuating rapidly between the 4th and 5th sampling instants. Note how the same type of sampling reconstruction totally lacks evidence of the rapid fluctuation of the original.

time interval between the present and the next sample time. It is important to recognize that the sampling and interpolation process can produce severe alterations of the signal depending upon the interrelationships between signal and sampling parameters. Two of the simplest errors are seen in Fig. 1.3 where in (a) a discontinuity is lost and in (b) a rapidly fluctuating component is suppressed because the sampling rate is too low. This type of error occurs regardless of how the interpolation between sampling instants is performed. A more thorough discussion of sampling problems is also presented in Chapter 3.

In some cases a signal is intrinsically T-discrete as for example is the count of the number of events occurring within an interval of time, such as the number of times an EEG waveform has a zero-crossing (a transition through zero amplitude) in one second. A second example is a list of measurements characterizing the structure of an object. It is important to note, however, that in the latter example the order in which the measurements are placed into a sequence may be of little or no importance. In temporal measurements or in measurements that are functions of a scanning process, the measurements follow one another in an order which must not be tampered with. The T-discrete or sampled version of a continuous signal is often used to construct estimates of parameters of the original continuous waveform, while an inherently discrete signal can, of course, never be meaningfully analyzed in this way.

Thus far we have spoken of a signal as a one-dimensional quantity or variable. This is unduly restricting to many biological variables that can rightfully be called signals. For example, the amplitude of the EEG as measured at three different locations on the scalp is described by three coordinates. The net signal describing the observed EEG is therefore three-dimensional. If there were six recording locations, the observed EEG would be a six-dimensional signal. Each of the components of a multidimensional signal is distinguishable from a unidimensional signal and can be processed as such. There is an unavoidable burden placed upon a data processor employed to handle rapidly fluctuating multidimensional signals and keep up with these fluctuations, a burden that increases with the dimensionality of the signal. Basically, the data processor must be able to sample each signal coordinate sequentially at a rate which preserves the information content in the signal as it is being processed. We will have more to say about this in Chapter 2.

1.3. REPETITIVE AND PERIODIC SIGNALS

Of considerable importance to biological signal analysis are repetition and periodicity. A signal is said to be repetitive if it has a particular waveform which recurs for as long as the signal persists. If, furthermore, this repetition occurs at uniformly spaced intervals in time, the signal is said to be periodic. Exact periodicity does not exist in biological signals unless external periodic stimulation is supplied to the preparation as is frequently done in the study of evoked responses from the nervous system. The periodicity of the stimulus is then looked for in the biological response. The EKG is an example of a biological signal which comes close to being periodic. Periodicity is important not only because it lends itself to relatively easily analyzable data, but also because it leads to the spectral concept of a signal. In this concept, to be discussed later in this chapter and throughout the book, the signal is represented as the sum of sine waves of different frequencies and amplitudes.

The periodic signal of duration T is of greatest interest to us here. It is represented by the equation

$$x(t) = x(t + mT), \quad m = 0, \pm1, \pm2, \ldots \qquad (1.2)$$

with T being the period of the signal. The sawtooth wave of Fig. 1.2 is an example of such a signal. Note that the signal persists from the infinite past to the infinite future.

1.4. SAMPLED REPRESENTATION OF A SIGNAL

Let us assume that we sample a signal $x(t)$ without error once every Δ seconds throughout all time. We represent the signal by the discrete sequence of its sampled values, ignoring the behavior of the signal between sample times. The important question that arises is, how useful a representation of the signal is this set of ordered samples? We shall show here that the goodness of the discrete representation depends upon what is called the spectrum of the signal and its relation to the sampling rate. If sampling is done at the proper rate, it happens that this representation contains all the structure of the original signal. First, let us re-examine the signal reconstruction illustrated in Fig. 1.3(b), where the signal amplitude is assumed to stay constant during the interval between successive samples. Such a reconstruction is useful when data are being inspected as they are received although, obviously, it almost always distorts the signal. The signal reconstruction that we shall discuss now is one that cannot be performed until all the signal data has been obtained. It therefore is not of practical value in the same sense that the previous method is;

but it does demonstrate the degree to which the sampled data
represent the original process.

The sequence of data samples obtained by the sampling process
is: ..., $x(-\Delta)$, $x(0)$, $x(\Delta)$, $x(2\Delta)$, ... We now multiply each
sample value $x(t°\Delta)$ by the so-called 'sinc' function,

$$\text{sinc}\left(\frac{t - t°\Delta}{\Delta}\right) = \frac{\sin[\pi(t - t°\Delta)/\Delta]}{\pi(t - t°\Delta)/\Delta} \tag{1.3}$$

This function is shown in Fig. 1.4. It has the value of unity at

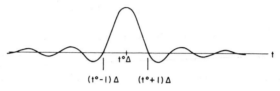

$$(t°-1)\Delta \qquad (t°+1)\Delta$$

*Fig. 1.4. The sinc function. The function is unity
at t = t Δ and 0 at all other integer multiples of Δ.*

$t = t°\Delta$ and zero whenever t is any other integer multiple of Δ,
$t°$ being, as before, an integer. (It has the further important
property that its Fourier transform, to be discussed later, has
amplitude Δ when f is between $- 1/2\Delta$ and $1/2\Delta$ and is zero for all
other values of f.) The sinc function whose amplitude is $x(t°\Delta)$
at $t = t°\Delta$, and is zero at all other integer multiples of Δ, $u°\Delta$.
That is,

$$x(t°\Delta) \; \text{sinc}\left(\frac{t - t°\Delta}{\Delta}\right) = \begin{cases} x(t°\Delta), & t = t°\Delta \\ \\ 0, & t = u°\Delta \end{cases} \tag{1.4}$$

Because of this, when all the sinc functions representing the
signal at integer multiples of Δ are added together, we obtain
the sum

$$x_s(t) = \sum_{t°=-\infty}^{\infty} x(t°\Delta) \; \text{sinc}\left(\frac{t - t°\Delta}{\Delta}\right) \tag{1.5}$$

The value of $x_s(t)$ at each sample time $t°\Delta$ is just the amplitude
of the original sample obtained at that time, i.e., there is no
interaction of samples at the sampling points. There is interaction, however, at all times between the sample points. In a

10

sense, the sinc function provides a method of interpolating a smooth curve between the sample points $x(t°\Delta)$. Now, it is possible to prove that if $x(t)$, the original function, has what is called its spectral bandwidth, F, smaller than $1/2\Delta$, the sum of the individual weighted sinc functions of Eq. (1.5) will yield exactly $x(t)$ *at all points in time*, not just at the sample points. On the other hand, if the spectral bandwidth of $x(t)$ exceeds $1/2\Delta$, the reconstruction will not be perfect, the amount of error between $x(t)$ and $x_s(t)$ being related to the amount by which the bandwidth F exceeds $1/2\Delta$. When the sampling rate $1/\Delta$ is related to the bandwidth by $F = 1/2\Delta$, the rate is said to be the Nyquist sampling rate, a rate that is twice the signal bandwidth.

1.5. FOURIER SERIES REPRESENTATION OF A SIGNAL

Having pointed out the adequacy of sample values as a representation of a signal in terms of the relationship between sample rate and bandwidth, we must now put meaning into the term bandwidth. This can be done in the following way. Let us consider that we only know the behavior of $x(t)$ over a T second interval of time starting at $t = 0$. This is typical of what occurs in real situations. Since we have no knowledge of what $x(t)$ has done earlier than 0 or later than T, we assume that it repeats itself periodically with period T indefinitely. This is an artifice, but a valid one as long as our interest in confined only to what $x(t)$ does between 0 and T. $x(t)$ can be represented by the sum of a set of sine and cosine waves of different amplitudes and harmonically related frequencies infinite in number. This is its Fourier series representation which is given by

$$x(t) = \frac{A_T(0)}{2} + \sum_{n=1}^{\infty} \left[A_T(n) \cos \frac{2\pi n t}{T} + B_T(n) \sin \frac{2\pi n t}{T} \right] \qquad (1.6)$$

The lowest or fundamental frequency of the series is $1/T$. The amplitudes $A_T(n)$ and $B_T(n)$ of the components of this series are obtained from $x(t)$ by the equations and

$$A_T(n) = \frac{2}{T} \int_0^T x(t) \cos \frac{2\pi n t}{T} \, dt$$

(1.7)

$$B_T(n) = \frac{2}{T} \int_0^T x(t) \sin \frac{2\pi n t}{T} \, dt$$

The frequency of the nth component is n/T Hz. The nth frequency component of $x(t)$ is defined by the two coefficients $A_T(n)$ and $B_T(n)$. If the amplitudes $A_T(n)$ and $B_T(n)$ are 0 whenever $f > F$, $x(t)$ is said to be bandlimited to the frequencies extending from 0 to F Hz.

From Eq. (1.7) it can be seen that the waveform of the observed segment of the signal determines the values of the Fourier coefficients uniquely. To obtain these coefficients, the amplitude of $x(t)$ must be processed at all values of time within the observation interval. When this is done the complete Fourier series so obtained will reconstruct the original waveform, if it is continuous, without error. Continuity generally prevails in biological signals although there are signals, such as those representing neuronal spike sequences, where continuity does not apply. These will be discussed later. Here we ignore continuous signals with discontinuities in them. For any signal, we can construct a curve relating the amplitudes of its $A_T(n)$ and $B_T(n)$ to the frequency $f_n = n/T$. Moreover, since $A_T(n)$ and $B_T(n)$ both pertain to the same frequency, we shall see that a more economical and significant plot is that of $|X_T(n)| = |A_T^2(n) + B_T^2(n)|^{1/2}$ against frequency. An example of such a plot is shown in Fig. 1.5 for the sawtooth wave of Fig. 1.2(b). The period T of the wave is taken to be 1 sec. The value of the spectral coefficient $|X_T(n)| = 8/(\pi^2 n^2)$ for n even, and is 0 when n is odd or zero. Vertical lines are drawn with a height equal to the magnitude of $X_T(n)$. The existence of terms out to indefinitely large values of n is caused principally by the sudden changes (discontinuities) in the slope of the sawtooth at its peaks. $|X_T(n)|$ is referred to as the amplitude spectrum of $x(t)$, and $|X_T(n)|^2$ as the power spectrum, often shortened to spectrum. They are usually plotted as a function of frequency, n/T

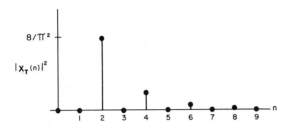

Fig. 1.5. The spectrum $\left|X_T(n)\right|^2$ of the sawtooth wave from Fig. 1.2(b) when the peak-peak amplitude is 2. The special coefficients are 0 for all odd values of n = 0.

or n. The term power is employed because it is the square of an amplitude related to force (often voltage) and this is proportional to power. Because $\left|X_T(n)\right|^2$ is defined only for discrete frequencies corresponding to integer values of n, it is also called a line spectrum. More will be said of the power spectrum later.

Although we have thus far restricted the lower frequency limit of the spectrum to 0 Hz, it is useful to talk about the negative frequencies of a spectrum. Doing so introduces some simplifications into our dealings with signal spectra. Negative frequencies can be introduced by an alternative way of writing a Fourier series for $x(t)$, one that employs complex notation:

$$x(t) = \sum_{n=-\infty}^{\infty} X_T(n) \, \exp \frac{j2\pi nt}{T} \tag{1.8}$$

where the $X_T(n)$ are complex numbers given by

$$X_T(n) = \frac{1}{T} \int_0^T x(t) \, \exp \frac{-j2\pi nt}{T} \, dt \tag{1.9}$$

That this series is equivalent to the original expression is seen by considering the sum of the pair of terms corresponding to the integers $-n$ and n:

$$X_T(-n) \, \exp(-j2\pi nt/T) + X_T(n) \, \exp(j2\pi nt/T) \tag{1.10}$$

By employing the Euler formula, $\exp j\theta = \cos \theta + j \sin \theta$, we obtain for this pair of terms,

$$[X_T(n) + X_T(-n)] \cos(2\pi nt/T)$$

$$+ j [X_T(n) - X_T(-n)] \sin(2\pi nt/T) \qquad (1.11)$$

This has the same form as the right-hand side of Eq. (1.6). If $x(t)$ is real, as it is for the kinds of signals we consider, Eq. (1.11) must be real regardless of the integer value of n. Then, by algebraic manipulation of the real and imaginary quantities we find that

$$X_T(n) = [A_T(n) - jB_T(n)]/2 = X_T^*(-n), \qquad n = 1, 2, \ldots$$

and $\qquad (1.12)$

$$X_T(0) = A_T(0)/2$$

The asterisk denotes the conjugate complex value. Thus the complex series is a simple rearrangement of the real Fourier series. It has the advantage of introducing negative frequencies, those frequencies in the expansion corresponding to negative values of n. Although it is not necessary to employ negative frequencies in dealing with spectral properties of signals, a certain amount of simplicity and overall clarity results when this is done. This becomes even more apparent when extended to the more general Fourier integral treatment of signals. The complex series has also justified more fully our use of $X_T(n)$ to indicate the magnitude of the spectral component corresponding to frequency n/T. We call the frequencies associated with the Fourier series of Eq. (1.6) real frequencies. They are always positive. We call the frequencies associated with the complex Fourier series of Eq. (1.8) complex frequencies. The average power of a unit amplitude cosine wave of real frequency n/T is $1/2$, since $A_T(n) = 1$, $B_T(n) = 0$. This is equally divided between the component at complex frequencies $-n/T$ and n/T. Generally, from Eq. (1.12)

$$\left| X_T(n) \right|^2 = A_T^2(n) + B_T^2(n) = \left| X_T(-n) \right|^2 \qquad (1.13)$$

The amplitude spectrum of a real $x(t)$ is the plot of $\left| X_T(n) \right|$ as a function frequency n/T and it is symmetric about the origin.

Each frequency component of the signal contributes a power equal
to the square of its magnitude, $|X_T(n)|^2$. The sum of all these
powers is the total power in the signal. There is also information
about signal structure in the phase of $X_T(n)$. This is given by

$$\theta_x(n) = \arctan[-B_T(n)/A_T(n)] \tag{1.14}$$

$\theta(n)$, when plotted as a function of n or frequency n/T, yields the
phase spectrum of the signal.

1.6 BANDWIDTH LIMITED SIGNALS

Consider now the special case where the signal is bandwidth
(or band) limited to frequencies between 0 and $1/2\Delta$. The total
time of observation of the signal is T seconds and is such that
$T = N\Delta$. Starting at time 0, N samples of the signal are taken at
Δ second intervals yielding the values $x(0)$, $x(\Delta)$, ... $x(t°\Delta)$,
... $x[(N - 1)\Delta]$. This is sampling at the Nyquist rate. For simplicity, let N be even; it is not a confining restriction. Because
of the bandwidth limitation, the Fourier series representation for
the continuous $x(t)$ during this time span is given by

$$x(t) = \frac{A_T(0)}{2} + \sum_{n=1}^{N/2} \left[A_T(n) \cos \frac{2\pi nt}{T} + B_T(n) \sin \frac{2\pi nt}{T} \right] \tag{1.15}$$

which is the same as Eq. (1.6) except that the upper limit for the
index n is now $N/2$ instead of infinity. The integer $N/2$ is associated with frequency $N/2T = 1/2\Delta = F$, the highest frequency present
in $x(t)$. It is also true that when $x(t)$ is bandlimited and periodic,
the coefficient $B_T(N/2) = 0$ (cf., Hamming, 1973). We can thus see
from Eq. (1.15) that we need to evaluate a total of N coefficients
for a complete representation of $x(t)$. These can be evaluated by
means of Eq. (1.7) or they can be obtained from the N sample values
in a manner to be discussed in Chapter 3. What should be emphasized
here is that sampling at the Nyquist rate provides just as many
time samples as are necessary to evaluate the Fourier coefficients
uniquely. That is, the sample values in themselves contain all
the information necessary to completely reconstruct $x(t)$

provided its band limit is related to the sampling interval Δ by the equation $F = 1/2\Delta$. Restating this in a slightly different way, as long as the T sec sample of signal $x(t)$ can be represented by a Fourier series, all of whose coefficients are 0 for the terms higher in frequency than $1/2\Delta$, the sampling process is guaranteed to represent all the information or structure in the signal.

When the signal bandwidth is larger than $1/2\Delta$, a number of difficulties ensue in the processing of the data. These we discuss in more detail in Chapters 2 and 3. Briefly however, the data processing proceeds just as though the signal were band limited. But when the Fourier coefficients are determined from the sample values, each may suffer an error whose size depends upon the amount by which the signal bandwidth F exceeds $1/(2\Delta)$. The greater this excess is, the greater the errors and the less adequate are the samples as a representation of the signal. Many rather serious misinterpretations are likely to arise if this situation goes unrecognized. It is up to the investigator to see to it that the bandwidth of the signal is suitable for the sampling rate employed. Caution is required. Preliminary spectrum analysis performed by instruments specifically designed for this is often called for.

Thus far we have not been concerned with whether the T sec signal segment would periodically recur during an arbitrarily long observation time, or whether the segment is one glimpse of an infinite number of possible manifestations of signal activity, none of which ever recur. The sampling process is indifferent to these alternatives. Nonetheless, there is a distinction to be made in the kinds of spectra associated with each. When the signal is band limited and truly periodic with period T, doubling the time of observation to $2T$ would yield a Fourier series in which the $A_T(n)$, $B_T(n)$ and $X_T(n)$ are different from 0 only when $n/2$ is an integer, where now $0 \leq n \leq T/\Delta$. If a $3T$ segment of signal were used and a Fourier series obtained from it, the nonzero terms would correspond to integer values of $n/3$, etc. That is, the frequency spectrum would exhibit components only at a discrete set of fre-

quencies corresponding to harmonics of the basic period T.
Periodic signals thus possess discrete or line spectra, related
to the repetition period, not the time of observation.

1.7. AUTOCOVARIANCE FUNCTIONS
AND POWER SPECTRA OF PERIODIC SIGNALS

The nature of a signal's temporal structure is often investigated by means of autocovariance function analysis. It is a method
of comparing or correlating the signal with a replica of itself
delayed in time. The autocovariance function takes on a continuous
form for continuous signals and a discrete form for discrete signals. It provides an indication of the degree to which a signal's
amplitude at one time relates to or can be inferred from its amplitude at another time. There are other measures of signal temporal
variability but correlation thus far has proved to be the most useful though it is not without flaws. The autocovariance function
receives its name by being an extension of the statistical covariance measures for random variables x and y. From statistics, the
covariance of x and y, written cov $[x, y]$, is the average value of
the product $(x - \mu_x) \cdot (y - \mu_y)$ where μ_x and μ_y are the average
values of x and y. Suppose now that $x = x(t)$ and $y = x(t + \tau)$.
The covariance of $x(t)$ and $x(t + \tau)$ is seen to be a function of
their time separation, τ. Because the covariance is that of an
individual signal, it is called an autocovariance. If, in addition, $x(t)$ is periodic with period T and has zero mean, we can
define the autocovariance function (acvf) for $x(t)$ as the average
of $x(t)x^*(t + \tau)$:

$$c_{xx}(\tau) = \frac{1}{T} \int_0^T x(t)x^*(t + \tau) \, dt \qquad (1.16)$$

Though $x(t)$ is real, its complex conjugate is used here to facili-
tate later consideration of the power spectrum associated with
$x(t)$. If the mean of $x(t)$ is not zero, the right hand side of
Eq. (1.16) is referred to as an autocorrelation function. It can

17

be converted to an acvf by subtracting out the mean, μ_x. The product being averaged would then be $[x(t) - \mu] \cdot [x^*(t + \tau) - \mu]$. Unless otherwise stated, the time functions we deal with will be considered to have zero mean or to have had their nonzero means removed first. Because the signal here is periodic, averaging needs to be carried out only over the time interval T. A longer averaging time than this is of no value since it only repeats measurements of amplitude products already obtained. For this reason $c_{xx}(\tau)$ is itself periodic with the same period T as that of the signal. The time required to measure the acvf for one value of time separation is the period T. This means that as T increases, so does the computation time.

The data processing operation called for in Eq. (1.16) is a continuous one utilizing the signal amplitudes at all times during one of its periods. The computation must also be carried out for all possible time lags up to T and so it can be seen that unless some type of sampling procedure involving τ is possible, the total time required to estimate the acvf is infinite. Fortunately, when the signal is band limited, there is a valid sampling procedure that makes the computation feasible. It uses the sequence of signal samples Δ seconds apart that were shown to fully represent a band limited signal. The acvf of the sampled signal T sec in duration is formed by the products of each sample and a second sample delayed in time from it by τ° sample intervals. The $N(= T/\Delta)$ individual products are then summed and divided by the total number of sample products to obtain

$$c_{xx}(\tau^\circ\Delta) = \frac{1}{N} \sum_{t^\circ=0}^{N-1} x(t^\circ\Delta) \; x^*[(t^\circ + \tau^\circ)\Delta] \tag{1.17}$$

If we now substitute for $x(t^\circ\Delta)$ and $x^*[(t^\circ + \tau^\circ)\Delta]$ their Fourier series representations as given by Eq. (1.8) and then interchange the order of summations, we find that

$$c_{xx}(\tau^\circ\Delta) = \sum_{n=-N/2}^{N/2-1} \left| X_T(n) \right|^2 \exp \frac{j2\pi n\tau^\circ\Delta}{T} \tag{1.18}$$

Here, in substituting for $x*[(t° + τ°)\Delta]$ we have used the complex conjugate of the series in Eq. (1.8). This shows that the acvf of the sampled signal can be expressed by a Fourier series whose coefficients $|X_T(n)|^2$ are completely determined by those of the original signal. Henceforth we represent $|X_T(n)|^2$ by $C_{xx}(n)$. On occasion we will also use the notation $C_{xx}(f_n)$ where $f_n = n/T$, so as to relate this more easily to the spectrum of aperiodic signals. $C_{xx}(f_n)$ is the power spectrum of $x(t)$, the distribution of signal power or variance at the harmonically related frequencies f_n. Now let us return to the definition of the acvf of a continuous periodic signal as given in Eq. (1.16). Here we also substitute the Fourier series representation of Eq. (1.8) for $x(t)$. Performance of integration and then summation yields

$$c_{xx}(\tau) = \sum_{n=-N/2}^{N/2-1} C_{xx}(n) \exp \frac{j2\pi n\tau}{T} \qquad (1.19)$$

When $\tau = \tau°\Delta$, this is the same as Eq. (1.18). This shows that the acvf of the sampled band limited signal has the same values at the sample times as the acvf of the original signal. It can be shown further that $c_{xx}(\tau)$ is itself a band limited signal in the τ domain and therefore that it can be completely reconstructed at all values of τ by using the coefficients $C_{xx}(n)$. Thus the acvf of the sampled signal completely represents the acvf of the continuous signal. Note that $C_{xx}(n)$ is the previously defined power spectrum of $x(t)$ and is given by the inverse relationship

$$C_{xx}(n) = \frac{1}{T} \int_0^T c_{xx}(\tau) \exp \frac{-j2\pi n\tau}{T} \, d\tau \qquad (1.20)$$

This is an important relationship between the acvf and the power spectral density of the signal. We also point out that $C_{xx}(n) = C_{xx}(-n)$ and consequently that $c_{xx}(\tau) = c_{xx}(-\tau)$. Another important relation that applies to band limited periodic signals is

$$C_{xx}(n) = \frac{1}{N} \sum_{\tau°=0}^{N-1} c_{xx}(\tau°\Delta) \exp \frac{-j2\pi n\tau°}{N} \qquad (1.21)$$

This shows how the Fourier coefficients are related to the N values of the acvf at the times $\tau°\Delta$. It will be discussed in more detail in Chapter 3.

Since $C_{xx}(n) = C_{xx}(-n)$, the true autocovariance function is defined by $N/2$ parameters in distinction to the N required for $x(t)$. What has happened is that the autocovariance procedure has removed the phase structure properties given by the $A_T(n)$ and $B_T(n)$ and left only the $C_{xx}(n)$ terms measuring the power of the individual frequency components that describe $x(t)$. It is important to note that the absence of phase information in the autocovariance function makes it impossible to deduce from the acvf the waveform of the signal that produced it. Thus an individual autocovariance function or power spectrum can be obtained from an infinite number of signals differing only in their phase structure.

1.8. APERIODIC SIGNALS

In contrast to the periodic signal, the aperiodic signal would, when the observation time is increased to $2T$, then $3T$, etc., yield nonzero values for the $A_T(n)$, $B_T(n)$ and $X_T(n)$ regardless of the value of n. By making the observation time large enough, we can make the frequencies at which we measure the spectral intensity as close as we like. In the limit, as T becomes infinite, the lines merge to a continuous spectrum that is characteristic of aperiodic signals. Aperiodic signals are treated by means of a generalization of the Fourier spectrum, the Fourier transform,

$$X(f) = \int_{-\infty}^{\infty} x(t) \exp j2\pi ft \, dt \qquad (1.22)$$

$X(f)$ is referred to as the Fourier transform of the signal $x(t)$. $x(t)$ can be recovered from its transform by the inverse Fourier transform,

$$x(t) = \int_{-\infty}^{\infty} X(f) \exp j2\pi ft \, df \qquad (1.23)$$

The Fourier transform is useful not only with aperiodic signals, as for example the EEG where we deal with its power spectral density, but also with transitory signals which exist for only a

short period of time, such as the nerve impulse and the impulse
response of signal filters to be discussed in Chapter 2. In this
case the energy of the response is more important than its power
and we deal with the energy spectral density.

1.9. AUTOCOVARIANCE FUNCTIONS AND POWER SPECTRA OF APERIODIC SIGNALS

When we pass from the periodic signal to the aperiodic (by
extending to infinity the period of repetition), the expression
for $c_{xx}(\tau)$ becomes

$$c_{xx}(\tau) = \lim_{T \to \infty} \frac{1}{T} \int_0^T x(t)\ x*(t + \tau)\ dt \tag{1.24}$$

In the situation of the infinite interval, the Fourier power spectral density for the signal passes from a series to an integral
representation similar to that given in Eq. (1.18). As a result,
the relationships between autocovariance function and power spectral
density for the aperiodic signal become (Jenkins and Watts, 1968)

$$C_{xx}(f) = \int_{-\infty}^{\infty} c_{xx}(\tau)\ \exp(-j2\pi f\tau)\ d\tau \tag{1.25}$$

while the inverse relationship is

$$c_{xx}(\tau) = \int_{-\infty}^{\infty} C_{xx}(f)\ \exp(-j2\pi f\tau)\ df \tag{1.26}$$

Both f and τ can range from plus to minus infinity. Here, $C_{xx}(f)$
is the power spectral density of the signal $x(t)$, the amount of
signal power in the small frequency band from f to $f + df$. This
pair of equations is referred to as a Fourier transform pair. The
knowledge of either function permits unique determination of the
other.

An idealized spectrum whose shape is somewhat typical of
continuous signals is shown in Fig. 1.6. It has significant components below F, the cut-off frequency. As the frequency increases
above F, the spectral intensity falls rather sharply. The width
of the region below F in which $C_{xx}(f)$ is near its maximum value is
the bandwidth of the signal. As with periodic signals, if the frequency components of the signal actually vanish at all frequencies

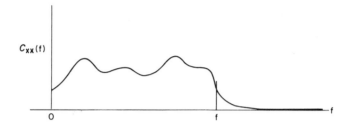

Fig. 1.6. A hypothetical spectrum $C_{xx}(f)$ of an aperiodic signal. F is the cutoff frequency.

quency components of the signal actually vanish at all frequencies above F, the signal is said to be band limited with bandwidth F.

Aperiodic signals that are band limited to $f = 1/2\Delta$ also can be represented exactly by their sample values at times Δ sec apart and these sample amplitudes permit estimation of the covariance function and the spectrum of the signal. The distinction between an estimate of a function and the function itself is made in Section 1.12. Some difficulties are encountered when a T sec segment of an aperiodic signal is considered. These difficulties affect the adequacy of the representation of the signal by its T-discrete version near the beginning and end of the segment. They arise when we consider an aperiodic signal to be one period of a periodic wave that repeats itself continually outside the time of observation. This artifice, commonly employed in the analysis of finite lengths of data, yields a discrete or line spectrum with components at integer multiples of $1/T$. The original signal, of course, has a continuous spectrum. Finally, since we have only a finite time to accumulate data, we can never obtain the precise autocovariance function and spectrum of the aperiodic signal regardless of whether there is noise interference. What we do obtain is estimates of them. The goodness of the estimates varies with the time available for observing the data. These are matters of great importance that are to be discussed in Chapter 3.

1.10. CROSS COVARIANCE FUNCTIONS AND CROSS
SPECTRA FOR A PAIR OF PERIODIC SIGNALS

There are many circumstances in which the data to be analyzed
consist of two or more signals whose interrelationships are interesting. The relationship between an external stimulus and the
several responses it gives rise to is also of considerable interest.
The autocovariance function of a signal cannot cope with these
matters because it deals only with the internal structure of an
isolated signal. The analysis of signal interrelationships is a
more complex affair. One approach to this general problem is via
the use of the cross covariance function. A cross covariance function (ccvf) differs from the autocovariance function only in that
the delayed signal $x(t + \tau)$ is replaced by $y(t + \tau)$, the delayed
version of the second of the two signals being analyzed. The two
signals are now denoted as $x(t)$ and $y(t)$. The cross covariance
function is therefore an indication of the degree to which one
signal's amplitude at one time relates to or can be inferred from
a second signal's amplitude at another time. If both signals
have period T, the cross covariance function also will have the
same period and can be written

$$c_{xy}(\tau) = \frac{1}{T} \int_0^T x(t)\ y^*(t + \tau)\ dt \qquad (1.27)$$

The ccvf is obtained by continuous processing of the two signal
waveforms.

For the ccvf there is a spectral counterpart, the cross
spectrum which has a relationship to the ccvf similar to that which
the spectrum has to the acvf. To see this we express the periodic
$c_{xy}(\tau)$ of Eq. (1.27) in terms of the complex Fourier series:

$$c_{xy}(\tau) = \sum_{n=-N/2}^{N/2-1} C_{xy}(n)\ \exp\frac{j2\pi n\tau}{T} \qquad (1.28)$$

It is the set of coefficients which we call the cross spectrum.
$C_{xy}(n)$ is given by

$$C_{xy}(n) = \frac{1}{T} \int_0^T c_{xy}(\tau) \exp \frac{-j2\pi n\tau}{T} \, d\tau \tag{1.29}$$

If we then substitute for the ccvf the right-hand side of this equation and replace both $x(t)$ and $y*(t + \tau)$ by their Fourier expansions, we obtain, after carrying out the indicated integrations,

$$C_{xy}(n) = X_T(n) \, Y_T^*(n) \tag{1.30}$$

$X_T(n)$ and $Y_T(n)$ are the Fourier coefficients for signals x and y. Thus the cross spectrum is the complex conjugate product of the Fourier series for each of the constituent signals. If we now substitute Eq. (1.30) in Eq. (1.28), we obtain

$$c_{xy}(\tau) = \sum_{n=-N/2}^{N/2-1} X_T(n) Y_T^*(n) \exp \frac{j2\pi n\tau}{T} \tag{1.31}$$

This is to be compared with Eq. (1.21) which relates the ccvf to its spectrum.

The ccvf and cross spectrum can be extended as well to aperiodic signals. This involves the same limiting procedure as T in Eq. (1.27) that was used with the autocovariance function. In this instance we have the Fourier transform pair relating the ccvf and cross spectrum:

$$C_{xy}(f) = \int_{-\infty}^{\infty} c_{xy}(\tau) \exp(-j2\pi f\tau) \, d\tau \tag{1.32}$$

$$c_{xy}(\tau) = \int_{-\infty}^{\infty} C_{xy}(f) \exp j2\pi f\tau \, df \tag{1.33}$$

Cross covariance functions and cross spectra can be defined for sampled signals. The ccvf of two sampled periodic signals is defined by

$$c_{xy}(\tau^\circ \Delta) = \frac{1}{N} \sum_{t^\circ=0}^{N-1} x(t^\circ \Delta) y*[(t^\circ + \tau^\circ)\Delta] \tag{1.34}$$

We can proceed as before to show that

$$c_{xy}(\tau^\circ \Delta) = \sum_{n=-N/2}^{N/2-1} X_T(n) Y_T^*(n) \exp \frac{j2\pi n\tau^\circ \Delta}{T} \tag{1.35}$$

The cross spectrum, $C_{xy}(n)$, originally defined in Eq. (1.29), is also given by

$$C_{xy}(n) = \frac{1}{N} \sum_{\tau°=-N/2}^{N/2-1} c_{xy}(\tau°\Delta) \exp \frac{-j2\pi n\tau°\Delta}{T} \qquad (1.36)$$

This is the cross spectral counterpart of Eq. (1.23). Equation (1.35) shows that the ccvf is defined by N coefficients of the form $X_T(n)Y_T^*(n)$. The original signals each require N coefficients, the set of $X_T(n)$ and $Y_T(n)$ to describe them. Since the coefficients appear together in Eq. (1.35) as products, there is no way of separating them unless either $x(t)$ or $y(t)$ is also known. Thus the ccvf and its companion cross spectral density do not by themselves preserve all of the information in the two signal waveforms. Remember that the same statement was made of the acvf and spectrum of a single signal.

1.11. A SUMMARY OF PROPERTIES OF COVARIANCE FUNCTIONS AND SPECTRA

There are several properties of covariance functions spectra that are worthwhile noting here. They are stated in terms of the continuous covariance functions but, except for A3, apply equally well to covariance functions and spectra of sampled signals. No proof of these properties is given here. They are easy to derive and more will be said of them in Chapter 3.

A. *AUTOCOVARIANCE FUNCTIONS AND POWER SPECTRA*

1. $c_{xx}(\tau)$ is an even function of time, i.e., $c_{xx}(\tau) = c_{xx}(-\tau)$.

2. The maximum value of $c_{xx}(\tau)$ occurs at $\tau = 0$.

3. If $x(t)$ is continuous, $c_{xx}(\tau)$ is continuous also.

4. The power spectral density of $x(t)$ is real and an even function of frequency: $C_{xx}(f) = C_{xx}(-f)$.

B. *CROSS COVARIANCE FUNCTIONS AND CROSS SPECTRA*

1. $c_{xy}(\tau)$ is not necessarily an even function of time. In general, $c_{xy}(\tau) = c_{yx}(-\tau)$.

2. The maximum value of $c_{xy}(\tau)$ does not necessarily occur at $\tau = 0$.

3. If $x(t)$ and $y(t)$ are continuous, $c_{xy}(\tau)$ is continuous also.

4. The cross spectral density of $x(t)$ and $y(t)$ is complex and $C_{xy}(f) = C_{yx}^{*}(-f)$.

Though these by no means exhaust the interesting properties of co-variance functions and spectra, they are the most important in terms of a working knowledge useful for ordinary signal analysis problems.

1.12. RANDOM OR PROBABILISTIC SIGNALS

In the previous section we have considered aperiodic signals and the manner of representing them in terms of their covariance functions and spectral densities. To do this we employed the arti-fice of considering such signals to be an extension of the more simple periodic signals with the period of these signals becoming infinite. This is a useful approach to deterministic but aperiodic signals since it provides a straightforward frequency domain de-scription . A simple example of a deterministic aperiodic signal is

$$x(t) = \sin 2\pi ft + \sin 2\pi\sqrt{2}ft \qquad (1.37)$$

Although it is impossible to find a finite value of t corresponding to a repetition period for this signal, it does possess a power spectrum and an autocovariance function, both of which can be found easily. The signal is bandwidth limited, nonrandom and aperiodic, although its two components individually are periodic. Its behavior for all time is known from its functional form. We can infallibly predict its future behavior and also state how it behaved in the remote past. To see how this can be done, we recall from calculus that an explicit function of time can be described exactly for all time in terms of a Taylor series expansion provided that all its derivatives are known at some arbitrary time. Its past and future history are completely specified by the values of these derivatives at that time. If, on the other hand, not all the higher derivatives exist (in the sense that they "blow up"), or if they cannot be measured, and practically they cannot, then the past and future history of the function or signal cannot possibly be determined infallibly.

Nondeterministic signals, and neurobiological signals are generally in this category, cannot be inherently described by an explicit equation valid for all time either because (a) although it may be possible to determine one, we do not have all the information at hand to permit doing so, or (b) it is inherent in the nature of the signal that it cannot be so described. Both cases are of considerable biological interest, with the latter case being especially so for both theoretical and practical reasons. The principal examples of nondeterministic neurobiological signals are (a) the spike activity of a single neuron or a small group of isolated neurons, and (b) the electroencephalogram (EEG). The signals are nondeterministic because the mechanisms responsible for them are subject to internal and external influences which can never be completely described. Signals that have these properties are spoken of as being random for their behavior follows or seems to follow probabilistic rather than deterministic laws. They are manifestations of random processes, biological or nonbiological, that are themselves governed by probabilistic laws. In describing random signals we speak of their probability density functions, their means, variances, covariance functions, power spectra, and other statistical measures, and not about their functional descriptions except where it is occasionally useful to do so, as with the alpha bursts of the EEG.

The probabilistic nature of a biological signal may not be entirely due to its generating process. Quite often, such a signal is observed in a background of other electrical activity unrelated to it. This activity is considered to be noise and may arise from other sources within the nervous system or it may arise from the measuring instrumentation itself. In either case its presence obscures the signal of interest making it more difficult to detect and analyze. Even though the signal being observed may be deterministic or nearly so, as in the case of the cochlear microphonic, its combination with the interfering noise makes the resulting mixture also qualify as a random signal. The reason is that noise is itself an example of a random process, different from the signal mainly in that the process that gives rise to it is not the one being studied. We exclude from our discussion of noise such phenomena as power line interference and stray electromagnetic emissions from radio sources. Troublesome though these may be, they can be eliminated by careful laboratory practices. The noise which we are considering is an inherent basic constituent of an experiment. It may be minimized to some extent but can never be eliminated. Somewhat different but also noiselike are the data corrupting effects produced by signal quantization and by jitter in the time of sampling of the signal. These effects are inherent in the data processing operations and are treated in Chapter 2.

Random signals are best understood by considering the properties of a collection or ensemble of them as generated by their associated random process. This ensemble of signals characterizes the process. It can be, for example, a collection of all particular samples of signal of some given length T generated by the process. Each member of the collection is a unique function of time different from the others and is referred to generally as a sample function or as a realization. To avoid confusion with the physical sampling process, we will adopt an alternate designation, specimen function. The specimen functions of an ensemble might be, for example, a collection of ten-minute parietal lobe EEGs obtained from awake normal males between the ages of 20 and 30. A wide variety of EEG waveforms may be included in the ensemble, each being a different realization generated by the underlying process. The fact that there can be substantial differences within an observed collection of specimen functions often leads to the question of whether or not there is but a single process responsible for the observations. Sometimes the specimen functions are so different as to make it obvious that they come from different processes; in other cases

the differences are more subtle and considerable uncertainty arises
as to whether more than one process is at work. It is possible to
test the hypothesis of a single process being the source of the
collected specimen functions although we shall not explore this
problem. Some aspects of hypothesis testing are discussed in
Section 1.17.

The existence of an ensemble of specimen functions makes it
possible to describe the generating process in terms of the statistical measures of the ensemble. These measures are taken across
the ensemble, each specimen function being but one member of the
population. This concept of the statistical measure of an ensemble
is to be distinguished from the previously employed time averages
that are performed on a single member of an ensemble. Time averages
tell us only of the properties of the individual ensemble member.
They are rather easy to perform experimentally. When the averaging time is taken to the limit, infinite time, we have the definitions of the mean, variance and covariance function of the signal.
Ensemble averages, in contrast, describe the overall properties of
the process in terms of the ensemble. Thus, we can speak of the
expected value of the ensemble of functions $\{x(t)\}$ at a particular
time, $E[x(t)]$, or the variance $\mathrm{var}[x(t)]$ or the autocovariance
function $E[x(t)x(t + \tau)]$. But they are more difficult to deal with
experimentally because they require measurements of many ensemble
members. However, the value of the ensemble approach is that it
leads to a far more penetrating understanding of the random process.
The concept of a random process and its associated ensemble of
specimen functions also applies not just to continuous signals but
also to the sampled version of a continuous random signal, to a
discrete signal, or to some function derived from originally continuous or discrete signals. An example of the last is the number
of alpha bursts per ten-second interval as observed in each of the
ten-minute EEGs previously described.

Suppose we now consider the value of a specimen function
$x(t)$ at a particular time t'. Each member of the ensemble $x(t)$

will range over a set of permissible values in a probabilistic way
that is determined by the random process itself. $x(t')$ is thus said
to be a random variable. It is in fact a function whose value depends upon the many underlying events associated with the random
process. To illustrate, an observer monitors the EEG tracing of a
normal sleeping adult through the night in order to study its fluctuating patterns. He classifies the sleep status of the individual
at any time into one of six different states: awake, stages 1
through 4, and rapid eye movement (REM) sleep. He does this by
analyzing the fluctuations in the EEG during the minute preceding
each classification. He proceeds to do so for a number of subjects
for each of which he constructs a chart of the type shown in
Fig. 1.7. The sleep states are assigned values 0 to 5. The $x(t)$

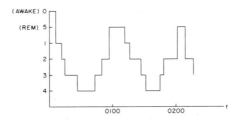

*Fig. 1.7. Sleep as classified by the ongoing EEG into
one of six possible states existing between the hours of
midnight (0) and 2 AM (0200).*

resulting is a specimen function of the sleep process. The value
of $x(t)$, at 1 AM, say, $x(0100)$ is a random variable which can take
on one of six different values for each of the subjects. The frequency with which the different values occur is determined by the
sleep process and the observer's judgments of the EEGs associated
with it. Assuming the validity of the observer's procedures, the
result is a new, A-discrete, T-continuous signal derived (or filtered) from the EEG. Each of the six possible levels of the signal
corresponds to an event, the sleep state of the subject, and the
six possible events cover all the possible states that the subject
can be in at any time. We can refer to these events in terms of
an event or sample space. The sample space we have used here has
a single dimension, depth of sleep, and it has a finite number of

events in it, six. More generally, event spaces can be multidimensional and they can also be continuous with an uncountably infinite number of events possible. An example of a single-dimensional sample space with an infinite number of events in it is the temperature of a particular location of the body. If sleep were defined in terms of the original six states of the EEG and temperature of the hypothalamus, say, the event space of interest would be two-dimensional, one dimension being discrete and the other continuous. An example of a five-dimensional continuous event space is the possible set of EEG voltages from a particular electrode at five instants that are one second apart. Sample spaces are used to describe specimen functions and the processes they arise from, and can be discrete or continuous according to whether the specimen functions are A-discrete or continuous. This is regardless of whether the specimen functions are T-discrete or continuous. In the sleep example the two-hour records of sleep states are A-discrete, T-continuous.

By making a small change in the manner of performing the previous experiment we can obtain a T-discrete specimen function instead. This would be accomplished by periodic examination of one-minute segments of the EEG at fifteen-minute intervals, say, and classification of them into sleep stages at those times. Under these circumstances the number of random variates is equal to the number of samples obtained for each specimen function while the properties of the individual random variables are the same as under the continuous case.

The two kinds of spaces, specimen space for the specimen functions and sample space for the random variables, should not be confused. Since a specimen function is composed of the sequence of particular values assumed by a random variable, it may be useful to note that a point in specimen space can be considered to represent a particular trajectory traveled by the random variable in sample space as the sampling proceeds.

1.13. SOME IMPORTANT PROBABILITY DISTRIBUTIONS

A. PROBABILISTIC DESCRIPTIONS
OF DYNAMIC PROCESSES

Basic to the study of dynamic probabilistic processes is a knowledge of the statistical properties of their random variables. This applies, first of all, to the derivation of the theoretical behavior of these processes, for, in most situations, they can be analyzed only after the probabilistic laws have been specified. It applies, secondly, to the validity of experimental data analyses which are generally dependent upon how the data conform to these laws. In the case of continuous processes, the Gaussian probability distribution has been found to be by far the most applicable to them. Most of the work done on dynamic processes has been centered upon those that have Gaussian properties insofar as the amplitude fluctuations of the random variables are concerned. It is worth noting, moreover, that many of the statistical techniques that have been developed for testing Gaussian processes have also been found applicable to the study of some non-Gaussian processes. Such tests have been labeled "robust" for this reason and in recent years extensive efforts have been devoted to the development of such statistical techniques. Nonetheless, it is the Gaussian probability distribution which is basic to the understanding of continuous processes. We shall, therefore, summarize some of its basic properties.

Another distribution of great importance to both continuous and point process analysis is the chi-squared distribution. It arises not because it is a description of either continuous or point process random variables but because it gives an effective way of dealing with the sums of Gaussian or exponential random variables that are encountered in the statistical analyses of long records of data. The chi-squared distribution offers a compact representation of such data and also is a help in developing insights into the strengths and weaknesses of a variety of statistical tests.

A third probability distribution that is encountered exten-
sively in neurophysiological work is the exponential distribution.
It finds its application in the study of sequences of action potentials generated by individual neurons. These are sequences in
which the times of occurrence of events are the only data of importance. The processes generating the events are referred to as point
processes and we shall have more to say about them in Chapters 6
through 8. In the remaining part of this section we shall briefly
summarize some of the basic properties of the Gaussian, chi-squared
and exponential distributions. A more detailed exposition of them
may be found in such standard texts as Mood (1950) and Cramér (1946).

B. THE GAUSSIAN DISTRIBUTION

A random variable X is said to be Gaussianly or normally
distributed if its probability density function is

$$\frac{\text{prob }\{x<X\leq x+dx\}}{dx} = p(x) = \frac{1}{\sigma\sqrt{2\pi}} \exp\left[\frac{-(x-\mu)^2}{2\sigma^2}\right] \qquad (1.38)$$

where x can take on any positive value or negative value. The mean
of the random variable is μ and its variance is σ^2. These follow
from the definition of the nth moment and nth central moment of a
random variable:

$$E[x^n] = \int_{-\infty}^{\infty} x^n p(x)\ dx$$
$$E[(x-\mu)^n] = \int_{-\infty}^{\infty} (x-\mu)^n p(x)\ dx \qquad (1.39)$$

Also, the second central moment $E[(x-\mu_x)^2] = \text{var}[x]$. The Gaussian
or normal distribution occurs so frequently as to warrant a special
notation. A Gaussian random variable with mean μ and standard
deviation σ is said to be normal (μ, σ).

All the odd order central moments of a normal random variable
are zero. This follows from the fact that the Gaussian density
function is symmetrical about its mean. The even moments of the
normal $(0, \sigma)$ random variable are given by

$$E[x^n] = 1 \cdot 3 \cdot \ldots \cdot (2n - 1)\sigma^{2n} \tag{1.40}$$

If we have a sum of N random variables, x_i, the sum of their means is the mean of their sum. If the random variables are independent, the sum of their variances is the variance of their sum. If the random variables are also normal (μ_{x_i}, σ_{x_i}), then their sum y is also normal with mean and variance given by

$$\mu_y = \sum_{i=1}^{N} \mu_{x_i} \qquad \text{and} \qquad \sigma_y^2 = \sum_{i=1}^{N} \sigma_{y_i}^2$$

When the x_i are normal and identically distributed (μ, σ), then y is normal ($N\mu, N\sigma^2$). Should the x_i not be independent, their sum will still be normal but the sum of their variances will not be equal to the variance of their sum.

A useful characterization of a random variable is its coefficient of variation (cvar), the ratio of its standard deviation to its mean. For the sum of N identically distributed normal random variables we have

$$\text{cvar}[y] = \frac{\sigma_y}{\mu_y} = \frac{\sigma}{N^{1/2}\mu} \tag{1.41}$$

This result will be applied to signal averaging as discussed in Chapter 4.

C. THE CHI-SQUARED DISTRIBUTION

The chi-squared distribution describes a family of probability distributions. The first member of the family is the distribution of the random variable χ^2 which is the square of a normal random variable $(0,1)$. χ^2 is restricted to values that are 0 or greater. In this case we have the probability distribution

$$\frac{\text{prob}\{x < \chi^2 \le x+dx\}}{dx} = p(x) = \frac{x^{-1/2} \exp(-x/2)}{\sqrt{2\pi}} \tag{1.42}$$

The mean and variance of this distribution are $E[\chi^2] = 1$ and $\text{var}[\chi^2] = 2$. More generally, the random variable χ_N^2 is defined as the sum of the squares of N independent and identically distributed normal random variables $(0,1)$. The subscript N, since it represents

34

the number of independent normal random variables composing χ_N^2, is often referred to as the number of degrees of freedom (*d.f.*) of the chi-squared random variable.

$$\chi_N^2 = \sum_{i=1}^{N} x_i^2 \qquad (1.43)$$

The probability density function for χ_N^2 is given by

$$p(x) = \frac{x^{N/2-1} \exp(-x/2)}{2^{N/2}\Gamma(N/2)} \qquad (1.44)$$

where $\Gamma(\ )$ is the well-known gamma function. Since χ_N^2 is just the sum of N random variables, its mean and variance are seen to be given by

$$E\left[\chi_N^2\right] = N$$
$$\qquad (1.45)$$
$$\mathrm{var}\left[\chi_N^2\right] = 2N$$

When the x_i's are independent and normal $(0,\sigma)$, the sum of N of them is distributed according to $\sigma^2\chi_N^2$. Hence, $E\left[\Sigma x_i^2\right] = N\sigma^2$ and $\mathrm{var}\left[\Sigma x_i^2\right] = 2N\sigma^4$. It can be shown that as N becomes large, the distribution of χ_N^2 approaches the normal with mean and variance given by Eq. (1.45). This is often a useful approximation when $N \geq 30$.

The sum S_K of the squares of K independent normally distributed random variables is not distributed according to chi-squared when the random variables do not have identical distributions. Nonetheless, the distribution of this sum is sufficiently close to such a chi-squared distribution as to justify its approximation as such. To arrive at the approximation, one merely finds the hypothetical $\chi_{d.f.}^2$ random variable which has the same mean and variance. Thus one sets

$$E\left[S_K\right] = (d.f.)\sigma^2$$
$$\qquad (1.46)$$
$$\mathrm{var}\left[S_K\right] = 2(d.f.)\sigma^4$$

d.f. here takes the place of N in the preceding paragraph.

This yields

$$d.f. = 2E^2[S_K]/\text{var}[S_K]$$

$$\sigma^2 = \text{var}[S_K]/2E[S_K] \tag{1.47}$$

The sum of the K squared normal random variables is said to possess the number of "equivalent" degrees of freedom given by Eq. (1.47). A similar technique can be used with the sum of $K \simeq \chi_2^2$ random variables that do not have the same mean and variance. If they were identically distributed, their sum would be chi-squared with $2K$ degrees of freedom; if not, the number of equivalent degrees of freedom is always less. Note also from Eq. (1.47) that

$$(d.f.) \, \text{cvar}^2[S_K] = 2 \tag{1.48}$$

These aspects of the chi-squared distribution have important applications to spectral smoothing discussed in Chapter 3.

D. THE EXPONENTIAL DISTRIBUTION

The probability density function for the exponentially distributed random variable is given by

$$p(x) = \begin{cases} \nu \exp(-\nu x), & x \geq 0 \\ 0, & x < 0 \end{cases} \tag{1.49}$$

The mean and variance of the exponential random variable can easily be shown to be

$$E[x] = 1/\nu$$

$$\text{var}[x] = E[x^2] - E^2[x] = 1/\nu^2 \tag{1.50}$$

From this it follows that $\text{cvar}[x] = 1$. The sum of M independently and identically distributed exponential random variables is distributed according to what is known as a gamma distribution:

$$p(x) = \frac{\nu(\nu x)^{N-1}}{(N-1)!} \exp(-\nu x) \tag{1.51}$$

The mean and variance of this sum are, as might be anticipated

$$E[x] = N/\nu$$

$$\text{var}[x] = N^2/\nu^2 \tag{1.52}$$

We show the form of the gamma distribution because it is closely related to the chi-squared distribution. If we consider a random variable which is 2ν times the random variable in Eq. (1.49), i.e., a random variable whose mean is 2, we find that the sum of N such random variables has a χ^2_{2N} distribution. This property of sums of exponentially distributed random variables will be discussed more in Chapter 6. It is also true that as N becomes large, the sum of N exponentially distributed random variables becomes nearly normal with mean $2N$ and variance $4N$.

1.14. ENSEMBLE AUTOCOVARIANCE FUNCTIONS

Statistical measures of ensembles of signals generated by random processes are defined in terms of the probability density functions (PDFs) or cumulative distribution functions (CDFs) of the ensemble. The mean of the ensemble $\{x(t)\}$ is given by

$$E[x_t] = \int x_t p(x_t) \, dx_t \qquad (1.53)$$

where for convenience we have written $x(t)$ as x_t. $p(x_t)$ is the PDF of the ensemble of signals at time t and the integration is over all values of x_t. Here x_t represents either a continuous or a sampled random variable. $p(x_t) \, dt$ is the probability that at time t a member of the signal ensemble will take on some value between x_t and $x_t + dx_t$. Similarly, the variance of x_t is defined by

$$\text{var}[x_t] = E[x_t - \mu_{x_t}] = \int (x_t - \mu_{x_t})^2 p(x_t) \, dx_t \qquad (1.54)$$

where $\mu_{x_t} = E[x_t]$. The ensemble autocovariance function (acvf) is defined in terms of the expected value of the product of the amplitudes of the signal at times t and u:

$$\text{cov}[x_t, x_u] = c_{xx}(t,u) = E[(x_t - \mu_{x_t})(x_u - \mu_{x_u})^*] \qquad (1.55)$$

The asterisk denotes the complex conjugate. Even though x is real (making $x* = x$), its presence facilitates later consideration of the spectrum of the process. In most cases the average value of x_t is of no interest and can be subtracted from the data. This makes $\mu_{x_t} = 0$ for all t. The covariance function is then just the product $E[x_t x_u^*]$. Determination of the ensemble acvf requires knowledge of the second order joint probability density function of the ensemble at times t and u:

$$c_{xx}(t,\ u) = \int (x_t - \mu_{x_t})(x_u - \mu_{x_u})^* p(x_t,\ x_u)\ dx_t\ dx_u \qquad (1.56)$$

The integration is over all values of x_t and x_u. While the ensemble acvf superficially bears little resemblance to the time acvf of an individual signal, Eq. (1.24), it will be shown later that the two are in fact closely related and in many important instances are equal. The acvf is a measure of how the fluctuations of the signal amplitude at two different times are related to one another. A positive covariance indicates that when one is greater (or less) than its mean value, the other tends to be also. A negative covariance, on the other hand, indicates that when one is greater than its mean, the other tends to be lower than its mean. The normalized autocovariance function is

$$\rho_x(t,\ u) = \frac{\text{cov}[x_t,\ x_u^*]}{\text{var}[x_t]\,\text{var}[x_u]} \qquad (1.57)$$

It ranges in value from -1 to $+1$.

If a pair of variables, here x_t and x_u, are statistically independent, it is generally true that

$$E[x_t,\ x_u] = E[x_t]E[x_u] \qquad (1.58)$$

It follows that there is 0 covariance between statistically independent random variables. Random variables which have 0 covariance are said to be uncorrelated. However, it is not necessary for a pair of random variables to be independent in order for the mean of their product to be equal to the product of their means. Thus, lack of correlation does not imply statistical independence except in special instances. Gaussianly distributed random variables are particularly interesting in this regard. If x_t and x_u are Gaussian random variables and uncorrelated, then they are also statistically independent. This is the most commonly encountered case in which zero correlation implies statistical independence. Serious errors can often result if one assumes statistical independence only on the basis of lack of correlation. An example of two random variables that are uncorrelated but statistically independent is $x = \sin \theta$ and $y = \sin 2\theta$, where θ is some arbitrary random variable.

1.15. ENSEMBLE AUTOCOVARIANCE AND CROSS COVARIANCE FUNCTIONS, AND STATIONARITY

Some basic properties of the ensemble autocovariance function deserve special mention.

(1) It is an even function of time:

$$c_{xx}(t, u) = c_{xx}(u, t) \qquad (1.59)$$

(2) Its maximum value occurs when $t = u$ and is the variance of the random variable:

$$c_{xx}(t, t) = \text{var}[x_t] \geq c_{xx}(t, u) \qquad (1.60)$$

If a process possesses an autocovariance function in which times t and u always appear in the form of a time difference $t - u = \tau$, the process is said to be covariance stationary. The covariance properties are then dependent only upon relative times, not upon any absolute value of time. Thus, in terms of covariance properties, the process is the same throughout all time. The covariance function notation for a stationary process can be written as $c_{xx}(\tau)$ and we shall generally do so. For covariance stationary processes $c_{xx}(0) = \text{var}[x_t] = \sigma_x^2$ is the average power of the process contributed by the fluctuations. An example of a covariance stationary process is the white noise $n(t)$ generated in electrical resistors. The amplitude of white noise at any one time is statistically independent from its value at any other time. Its covariance function can be shown to be

$$c_{nn}(t, u) = c_{nn}(\tau) = \sigma_n^2 \rho(\tau) \tag{1.61}$$

This means the noise amplitudes at two different times are without correlation.

When we are interested in correlating the behavior of specimen functions belonging to two different ensembles, we employ the ensemble cross-covariance function (ccvf). Thus, for specimen functions $x(t)$ and $y(t)$

$$c_{xy}(t, u) = E[(x_t - \mu_{x_t})(y_u - \mu_{y_u})^*] \tag{1.62}$$

As with the autocovariance function, average values are often of little interest and can be removed from the data. This makes the ccvf equal to $E[x_t y_u^*]$. In contrast to the autocovariance function, the cross-covariance function is not an even function of time nor does it always have a maximum at $t = u$ or at $\tau = 0$ when the processes are stationary.

An example of the dependency of the autocovariance function upon the times t and u is the autocovariance function that would be obtained from the membrane potentials of a population of cells that have been damaged in exactly the same way at $t = 0$ and then gradually healed. First there is a sudden depolarization in membrane potential at the instant of injury. Then, during the healing process there is a slow recovery of the resting membrane potential to its preinjury level. Different cells have different initial changes in membrane potential and different rates of recovery or healing. For extreme but useful simplicity, let the membrane voltage during early stages of recovery be represented by the equation

$$v(t) = V_0 + kt \tag{1.63}$$

V_0 is the initial value of membrane potential immediately after injury and k is the initial rate of recovery. Both are assumed independent random variables with means $\overline{V}_0$ and $\overline{k}$ respectively. The autocovariance function for v is given by

$$c_{vv}(t, u) = E[(v_t - \overline{v}_t)(v_u - \overline{v}_u)^*] \tag{1.64}$$

After some straightforward manipulations, this becomes

$$c_{vv}(t, u) = \text{var}[V_0] + tu \, \text{var}[k] \qquad (1.65)$$

This is a reasonable approximation to the covariance function in the
the early stages of recovery where linear Eq. (1.63) is a valid
representation of the membrane potential. Notice (a) that the covariance function was obtained from the variances and without the
knowledge of the probability distributions of the variables; and
(b) that the covariance function is a function of both t and u.
Only variances were required. A process of this type is said to
be evolutionary.

Covariance stationary processes form a broad class of stationary random processes, processes in which the underlying probabilistic mechanisms up to the second order joint density function
do not change with the passage of time. If the nth order joint
distribution function of some ensemble were obtained at times
$t_1, \ldots, t_m$ and compared with a similar joint distribution function
obtained at later times, $t_1 + \tau, \ldots, t_m + \tau$ and found to be the
same regardless of how high m is or how large τ was chosen, the
process would be said to be strictly stationary. This is a rather
stringent condition for stationarity, if for no other reason than
that it is seldom feasible to measure joint statistics beyond second or third order. Covariance stationarity, also called wide
sense or second order stationarity, is more practical to deal with.
Only the second order joint distributions need be independent of
time. Many of the random signals involved in the study of biological processes are, or can effectively be considered to be, covariance stationary. Unless there is possibility for confusion, hence-
forth we abbreviate covariance stationary to stationary.

In the stationary situation, it is possible to show (Davenport and Root, 1958) that the ensemble autocovariance function and
the power spectrum of a random process are related to each other by
the Fourier transform pair:

$$C_{xx}(f) = \int_{-\infty}^{\infty} c_{xx}(\tau) \, \exp(-j2\pi f\tau) \, d\tau \tag{1.66}$$

$$c_{xx}(\tau) = \int_{-\infty}^{\infty} C_{xx}(f) \, \exp j2\pi f\tau \, df \tag{1.67}$$

This relation was spoken of previously in terms of individual signals; here it is stated in terms of the ensemble autocovariance function and power spectrum of a process.

Some indication of how this relation arises can be obtained by representing the zero mean random periodic signal $x(t)$ and its delayed complex conjugate $x^*(t + \tau)$ by their complex Fourier series. The Fourier coefficients $X_T(n)$ and $X_T(m)$ are uncorrelated (Jenkins and Watts, 1968). That is, $E[X_T(n)X_T^*(m)] = |X_T(n)|^2$ when $m = n$ and 0 otherwise. The Fourier transform of $E[x(t)x^*(t + \tau)]$, the acvf of $x(t)$, is then found to be given by the expression $\sum_{n=-\infty}^{\infty} |X_T(n)|^2 \delta(f - k/T)$. This is the power spectrum of the random periodic signal. Of particular interest is the situation when $\tau = 0$. Here we have

$$c_{xx}(0) = \int_{-\infty}^{\infty} C_{xx}(f) \, df \tag{1.68}$$

That is, the average power in the process is the sum of the powers of all the frequency components in the spectrum. We can also define a cross power spectral density in terms of the cross-covariance function. For this we have the Fourier transform pair:

$$C_{xy}(f) = \int_{-\infty}^{\infty} c_{xy}(\tau) \, \exp(-j2\pi f\tau) \, d\tau \tag{1.69}$$

$$c_{xy}(\tau) = \int_{-\infty}^{\infty} C_{xy}(f) \, \exp j2\pi f\tau \, df \tag{1.70}$$

This is important in that it expresses a general relationship between processes and not just particular specimens of the processes. Unfortunately, the interpretation of the shape of a ccvf can be difficult and there is no simple interpretation to be attached to the relation between $c_{xy}(0)$ and the integral of the cross power spectral density.

1.16. THE RELATIONSHIP BETWEEN ENSEMBLE AND TIME STATISTICS

In biological work directed toward the study of dynamic processes, one is often restricted to studying relatively few ensemble members and for only limited amounts of time. A question then arises as to whether one may legitimately infer the statistical properties of the ensemble from the behavior of just a few, or even one, of its members. This can be done if the stationary process satisfies what is called the ergodic hypothesis. According to it the behavior of one member of an ergodic process, if observed long enough, will be characteristic of all other members. Another way of stating this is that a stationary process is ergodic if time averaging of a single specimen function is equivalent to averaging over the entire ensemble. The frequency of occurrence of events in a single realization or specimen function converges to the ensemble distribution. Furthermore, if a process is ergodic, there is zero probability of getting "stuck" on a particular realization which does not have the long run property. Let us consider the relationship between time and ensemble statistics.

For a continuous random process the time average of a (real) specimen function $x(t)$ is given by

$$<x(t)> = \lim_{T \to \infty} \frac{1}{T} \int_0^T x(t)\ dt \tag{1.71}$$

and its autocovariance function by

$$<x(t)x(t + \tau)> = \lim_{T \to \infty} \frac{1}{T} \int_0^T x(t)x(t + \tau)\ dt \tag{1.72}$$

As indicated, the duration of the averaging interval T is made arbitrarily long. The brackets on the left hand side of the equations indicate temporal averaging. Ergodicity then implies that

$$<x(t)> = E[x(t)] \qquad (1.73)$$

$$<x(t)x(t + \tau)> = c_{xx}(\tau) \qquad (1.74)$$

Equations similar to (1.71) and (1.72) can be written for discrete random processes:

$$<x(t°\Delta)> = \lim_{N\to\infty} \frac{1}{N} \sum_{t°=0}^{N-1} x(t°\Delta) \qquad (1.75)$$

and

$$<x(t°\Delta)x[(t° + \tau°)\Delta]> = c_{xx}(\tau°\Delta)$$

$$= \lim_{N\to\infty} \frac{1}{N} \sum_{t°=0}^{N-1} x(t°\Delta)x[(t° + \tau°)\Delta] \qquad (1.76)$$

The ergodicity relations (1.73) and (1.74) hold here as well. Eq. (1.76) differs from Eq. (1.17) only in that it indicates a limiting process with N becoming indefinitely large. When N is finite and $x(t)$ is a specimen function of an aperiodic process, Eq. (1.76) is an estimate of the autocovariance function of the process. The goodness of this estimate improves as N increases. Estimation problems are considered more fully in Chapter 3.

Another property of ergodic processes is that the joint probability distributions estimated from a single ensemble member approach those of the ensemble as the length of time the specimen is observed increases. Thus a long and detailed enough examination of one member of the ensemble can reveal all the statistical properties of the process, not just the second order ones.

The problem in biology, and neurobiology in particular, is that it is difficult to define at the outset of an investigation whether the process being studied is ergodic. It is often taken for granted, but such a definition can require an extensive examination of many specimen functions and even then there may be no clear-cut indication of the process's ergodicity. It is not possible to demonstrate conclusively that a biological process is ergodic since to do so one needs to observe all members of the ensemble for all time. At best we can only examine the available

specimen functions and infer from them that the process is ergodic.
Stationarity and ergodicity are often appealed to, sometimes implicitly, as justifications for studying but a few specimen functions of a process. They are assumptions that need to be considered
carefully. For example, it is clear that the EEG process observed
at any time by an electrode located anywhere on the scalp of a normal human is not ergodic because there are numerous differences
between the EEGs recorded from anterior and posterior sites. The
relative prevalence of the alpha rhythm is one particular instance
of these differences. On the other hand, if only a single recording location is employed, then a particular specimen function of
the EEG may quite possibly arise from an ergodic process describing
activity over an ensemble of individuals. This can be more precisely defined by restricting the conditions of observation to normal
alert adults. Similar illustrations can also be made for the spontaneous spike activity of individual neurons. When properly defined, their activity can be described as arising from ergodic
processes.

1.17. MIXTURES OF SIGNAL AND NOISE

We have now come to the point where we must deal with mixtures of signals and noise. To rephrase our original definition
at the beginning of the chapter, a signal is that constituent of
the data which we are interested in and noise is whatever else is
present. It is inherent in the observation of electrophysiological
phenomena that some noise be present. What we are concerned with
is the means to extract the signal from the noise. And since one
or both of these data constituents is random in nature, it follows
that the two must be separated by statistical means. Here we give
a brief introduction to this problem.

The simplest method for representing the structure of observed
electrophysiological data is as an additive mixture of signal and
noise. If the observed data is $x(t)$, then

$$x(t) = s(t) + n(t) \qquad\qquad (1.77)$$

where $n(t)$ is the noise. It is in part biological and partly instrumentational in origin. Often in what follows, the signal $s(t)$
will be synonymous with a response. In the latter usage we refer
to the electrophysiological response elicited by a stimulus. The
response process, as already noted, may be random in structure.
We always distinguish the signal or response from the net observed
data $x(t)$. The additive nature of signal and noise is an assumption which, while valid in many situations, is frequently open to
question. The alternative assumption is that the signal and noise
interact in some nonlinear fashion, especially where the biological
component of $n(t)$ is concerned.

The ease with which signal and noise can be separated depends
in large part upon how large the signal is with respect to the
noise. Obviously, the stronger the signal is, the easier it is to
detect and analyze. When signal and noise are comparable in
strength, problems in the reliability of signal detection and
analysis procedures arise. Generally then, the goodness of signal
analysis depends upon the ratio of signal to noise strength, the
signal-to-noise ratio (SNR). The higher this ratio is, the more
reliable are the estimates of signal structure. Several measures
of SNR are in use. We mention two of them. (a) Rms signal-to-rms
noise ratio. When the signal component of the data originates from
a continuous ongoing process, its rms level is a useful characterization of its strength. In this situation we measure SNR in terms
of the rms values of signal and noise. The rms is a time measure
of the standard deviation of a process. It is the square root of
average power. (b) Peak signal-to-rms noise ratio. When the signal
has a pulse or spikelike waveform of limited duration, the most
distinguishing feature of the waveform is its peak amplitude. In
this case the convenient measure of SNR is the peak value of the
signal to the rms value of the noise.

1.18. RESPONSE DETECTION AND CLASSIFICATION--
   HYPOTHESIS TESTING

The randomness of neurobiological signals coupled with the background noise they are immersed in causes signal analysis procedures to involve statistical decision making in uncertain situations. For example, we may desire to ascertain whether a particular stimulus is effective in evoking a response from the test subject. Does the observed data contain a response, however obscure, or does it contain only noise? A related problem is when we know that a stimulus evokes a response and are interested in determining how changes in the stimulus parameters affect the response. To what extent are the observed differences in the data due to stimulus changes and to what extent to the interfering noise? The first of these problems is the signal detection problem and the second the signal classification problem. The signal here is the response to the stimulus. They possess considerable similarity in their theoretical formulations and in their solutions. Detection involves only the determination that the data do or do not have signals in them. Classification involves a quantitative description of what is already accepted to be a response in the data. This description is given in terms of such signal defining parameters as, for example, the amplitude, frequency, and phase of a sine wave. These parameters are estimated from the data with their goodness being affected by the amount of noise present. From these estimates signal classification is performed. Different segments of the data are judged to contain the same or different responses. according to how similar or different the corresponding parameter estimates are. The classification can involve as many groupings as one has reason to suspect exist in the data, perhaps one for each type of stimulus employed.

Solutions to detection and classification problems involve the concepts of hypothesis testing. In detection there are two mutually exclusive hypotheses: H_1, that a signal is present and H_0, that it is absent. In classification there are as many

mutually exclusive hypotheses as there are signal classes to distinguish among. In either detection or classification the data
are processed according to an algorithm determined by the experimental design and by the properties of the signals and noise, insofar as they are known. The algorithm yields a number whose magnitude then determines which of the hypotheses to accept. Associated
with the acceptance or rejection of a hypothesis is the fact that
decision errors are inevitable. Minimization of these errors is
in fact a critical ingredient that goes into the choice of the data
processing algorithm.

Two types of errors can occur in signal detection. If H_1 is
the hypothesis that a signal is present and H_0 is the hypothesis
that it is absent, there is the possibility that H_1 will be mistakenly accepted when H_0 is actually true, and another possibility
that H_0 will be accepted when H_1 is actually true. The first error
is often referred to as a false alarm (error of the *first* kind)
and the second error as a false dismissal (error of the *second*
kind). Similar types of errors occur in the classification problem.
If there are three different signals to choose amongst, six different misclassification errors are possible.

Let us illustrate a simple signal detection problem in terms
of a three component signal contained in noise. The components are
its amplitudes at three consecutive sampling instants: $s(t)$,
$s(t + 1)$, $s(t + 2)$. The signal is present in background noise, a
combination of background biological activity and instrument noise.
The noise is Gaussian with mean 0 and standard deviation σ. The
signal and noise combine additively to yield the response data,
$x(t) = s(t) + n(t)$. Successive samples of the noise are uncorrelated with one another. On the basis of these properties of the
response data it is desired to construct a test to examine the
hypothesis that in any particular three-sample sequence, there is
a signal of arbitrary structure present in the data. As before,
H_0 is the hypothesis that a signal is absent from the data samples
and H_1 is the hypothesis that it is present. H_0 is known as a

simple hypothesis because it is concerned with only one possible value for the response vector in response space, here 0. H_1, in contrast, is referred to as a composite hypothesis because it is concerned with the signal parameters such as amplitude and latency that have any non-zero value. So long as at least one of these parameters is different from 0 a signal is present. It is possible to have H_1, a simple hypothesis stating, for example, that all sample values of the signal are unity. Usually, however, it is composite hypotheses covering a range of signal parameters that are of greatest interest.

An example of this is the hypothesis that some stimulus-related response of arbitrary waveshape is present in the data vector that we are examining. If Gaussian noise alone is present and its samples at consecutive sample times are independent, the data vector will tend to be found in a spherical region surrounding the origin. We can, from the three-dimensional Gaussian distribution, compute the radius of the sphere that a noise vector falls within some given percent of the time, say 99%. This radius is X_0. Let us then set up the test that we will accept hypothesis H_0 if the observed data vector is within that sphere. That is, we accept H_0 if the observed data, samples of the additive combination of signal

$$x^2(0) + x^2(1) + x^2(2) = X_0 \qquad (1.78)$$

and otherwise we accept H_1, the hypothesis that an arbitrary signal is present. In choosing this and the threshold X_0 we have fixed at 1% the probability of false alarm. The probability of false alarm is called the level of the test. The probability of accepting H_1 when it is true is called the power of the test. It is 1 minus the false dismissal probability and depends upon the strength of the response relative to the noise. Since the test is one involving the squares of the sample amplitudes, the power of the test will be low when the signal energy is small compared to the noise energy, and high when it is large, regardless of how it is apportioned among the three samples.

Fig. 1.8 illustrates these definitions. In it are shown two

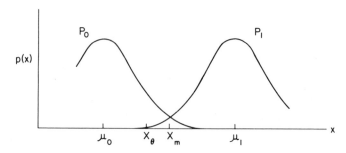

Fig. 1.8. Amplitude probability densities P_0 and P_1 for the data amplitude x, under hypothesis H_0 and H_1. X_θ is a threshold value for choosing H_0 or H_1 on the basis of experimental observation. X_m is the threshold for a maximum likelihood test.

amplitude probability density functions of similar shape but differing means. They correspond to the two hypotheses being tested by a signal measurement of the data x. The left-hand density function is associated with hypothesis H_0 and the other density function with the hypothesis H_1. In this case the strength of the signal is the difference between the two means, $\mu_1 - \mu_0$. Let us somewhat arbitrarily select a decision threshold value along the abscissa such that if a measurement of x yields a value greater than X_θ, hypothesis H_1 will be accepted; if not H_0 will be accepted. Since the two probability densities overlap the threshold, some possibility of error is clearly to be expected. If noise only is present and a measurement exceeds X_θ, an error of the first kind is made. The The probability of this happening is the level of the test and is measured by the area under that part of the H_0 curve to the right of X_θ. If H_1 is true and the measurement exceeds X_θ, H_1 is correctly accepted. The probability of this occurring is given by the area of the H_1 curve to the right of X_0, the power of the test. The area of the H_1 curve to the left of X_θ measures the probability of making an error of the second kind, falsely rejecting H_1.

While we have chosen an arbitrary threshold in this illustration, there is one particular location for it that is usually selected, in a test such as this, that point where the two density curves intersect. Selection of the threshold at this point X_m results in a so-called maximum likelihood test. The value of the likelihood ratio (see below) at X_m is 1. Any measurement to the left of X_m is more likely to have resulted from a situation in which H_0 was correct. But if it fell to the right of X_m, H_1 is more likely to have been correct.

An optimum choice of boundaries in a multidimensional data space to use in accepting one of the hypotheses can be determined by the use of what is called the likelihood ratio. This is a ratio of two conditional probabilities. The one in the numerator, $P_1(X|H_1)$, expresses the probability of having obtained the observed data if H_1 were true (signal present); the one in the denominator is the probability $P_0(X|H_0)$ of having obtained the observed data if only noise were present. Whenever the likelihood ratio equals or exceeds a preset threshold value, hypothesis H_1 is accepted; otherwise H_0 is accepted. The two conditional probabilities are referred to as likelihood functions. The reason is that a conditional probability density is evaluated by inserting into it the observed data values. This yields an expression in which the parameters of the density, its mean and variance, say, are expressed as functions of the data. It is then possible to find values for the density parameters that maximize the conditional probability. The values so obtained are the maximum likelihood estimates, the parameter values which are most likely to have produced the observed data. In the case of the likelihood ratio, the hypotheses being tested are associated with particular values for unknown parameters of the distribution. Then when the observed data values are inserted into each of these likelihood functions, the one which is the more likely will have the larger value. The value of the likelihood ratio can be computed for each observed set of data points only if the form of the conditional probability distributions governing the situation is known. In the particular three-dimensional example of signal detection that we have hosen, one involving the detection of a signal in known Gaussian noise, the likelihood ratio is constant on the surface of a sphere centered on the origin, as is shown in Fig. 1.9. A simpler case is the

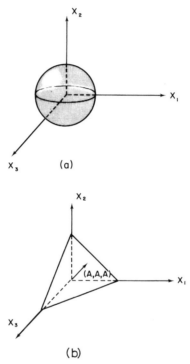

Fig. 1.9. (a) A sphere has constant likelihood ratio for testing for an arbitrary signal in noise. (b) A plane normal to the data vector (A, A, A) has constant likelihood ratio in the test for the presence of that particular signal vector in noise.

situation in which we test the simple hypothesis that a three-sample signal is absent against another simple hypothesis that the signal has a constant value A. In this case the likelihood ratio is constant on a plane as shown in Fig. 1.9. The plane is oriented perpendicularly to the line joining the origin to the point (A, A, A) and its distance from the origin is determined by the choice of the level of the test.

When the decision involves choosing one of several possible
signals in Gaussian noise, the data space is partitioned into
planes, hyperplanes if there are more than three data samples per
data vector, whose orientations and locations are determined by
the statistics of the noise and the parameters of the different
signals. The hyperplanes are the geometric embodiment of the likelihood ratio equations. Signals which vary from one another in
less simple ways can also be separated by data space partitions
which are no longer hyperplanes but more complex surfaces. Nonetheless, the likelihood ratio concept still applies. The acceptance of one hypothesis in preference to the others is dictated by
the location of the data vector in the data space.

Hypothesis testing as described here is performed by the
establishment of decision rules with which to test the observed
data. These rules are established by knowledge of the properties
of the anticipated signals and the interfering noise. The more
comprehensive is this knowledge, the more effective the tests can
be. But as long as there is noise to contend with, the decisions
can never be error-free. Once a decision rule has been adopted for
a particular experiment, the error probabilities are determined by
the properties of the response and noise processes. It is important
to understand that the choice of the decision rule may be crucial to
the success or failure of an experiment, for there are good decision
rules and bad. A bad one will obviously have associated with it
high probabilities of errors. But there are also other aspects to
the choice of decision rules to be concerned with. The first is
that there is generally an optimum decision rule for an experiment,
one which minimizes the error probabilities. No other means of
processing the data can improve upon this decision rule. In some
cases, that optimum decision rule is known or can be calculated
and then relatively simply instrumented; in others, it can be calculated and then instrumented only at great cost. When the latter
is true, it often leads to the search for suboptimum decision rules,
rules which are almost as good theoretically but have the advantage

of being practical to employ. Biological data processing problems are commonly solved by the application of *ad hoc* suboptimum techniques. Great care is advised in considering the use of such techniques for there are often no satisfactory methods for dealing with them analytically. To prove their value in comparison with other techniques it may often be necessary to test them with computer simulated data and trial analyses on pilot data. It often turns out that what seemed on first inspection to be an effective analysis procedure is no better than the method it is meant to replace and sometimes worse. The appealing simplicity of the suboptimum technique must be accompanied by verified adequate performance if it is to be accepted as useful for data processing.

REFERENCES

Cramér, H., "Mathematical Methods of Statistics," Princeton University Press, Princeton, 1946.
Davenport, W. B., Jr. and Root, W. L., "An Introduction to the Theory of Random Signals and Noise," McGraw-Hill, New York, 1958.
Hamming, R. W., "Numerical Methods for Scientists and Engineers," 2nd ed., McGraw-Hill, New York, 1973.
Jenkins, G. M. and Watts, D. G., "Spectral Analysis and its Applications," Holden-Day, San Francisco, 1968.
Mood, A. M., "Introduction to the Theory of Statistics," McGraw-Hill, New York, 1950.

Chapter 2

BASICS OF SIGNAL PROCESSING

2.1. INTRODUCTION

The data arising from an electrophysiological experiment on
the nervous system initially consist of records in continuous analog form of stimulus events and the responses that they give rise
to. If these data are to be analyzed in more than a qualitative
way, digital computation techniques are usually called for. This
means that the analog data have first to be converted to digital,
sampled form. Then the full range of analysis techniques that have
been developed to study dynamic processes can be brought to bear.
These include filtering, averaging, spectral analysis, and covariance analysis. In this chapter we discuss first the properties
of the analog-to-digital conversion processes with particular regard to their effect on the experimental data, and the subsequent
tests the data are subjected to. Then we move to a discussion of
filtering operations, analog and digital, with emphasis on the
latter and how it fits into computer data analysis procedures.
From time to time we consider some of the hardware aspects of
filtering since familiarity with them is quite useful for a fuller
comprehension of filtering procedures.

2.2. ANALOG-TO-DIGITAL CONVERSION

An analog-to-digital converter (ADC) converts a continuous
signal into a sequence of $T-$ and A-discrete measurements. The
two steps of time sampling and amplitude quantizing are usually
performed in a combined procedure. The ADC is first given the
command to sample by the computer and then holds the amplitude of
this sample briefly while quantizing it. We illustrate the
ADC in Fig. 2.1 as performing its operations in the sequence

(a)

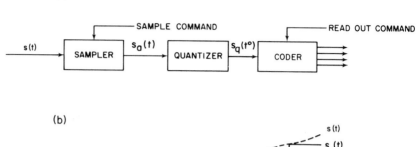

(b)

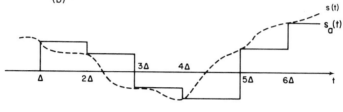

(c)

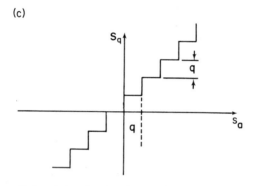

Fig. 2.1. (a) Block diagram structure of an A-D converter. Sampling is initiated periodically. Quantization of the sample is followed by coding it into digital format. When this is complete a read-out command causes delivery of the converted signal to the data processor. (b) The signal s(t) before sampling and its sampled version $s_a(t)$. (c) The input-output relation for the quantizer. The step size is q.

indicated there. The organization of the converter is not intended to describe a particular type of ADC, but to illustrate the function of such a device. In addition, the data analysis problems we are concerned with do not depend upon the detailed circuitry linking the computer to the ADC or upon the structural features of the converter itself. The sampled version of the signal is $x_a(t)$, a sequence of maintained voltage levels lasting the duration between sampling times, Fig. 2.1(b). The amplitude of each level is the signal amplitude at the sampling instant $t^\circ\Delta$. In what follows, we assume Δ to be unity so that $t^\circ\Delta$ can be replaced by the integer valued time variable t°. Sampling devices are often referred to as sample-and-hold circuits because of their ability to hold the sampled value without significant decay until quantization has been completed--a time duration that is often considerably shorter than the interval between samples.

In a number of experimental situations in which a response to a stimulus is being analyzed, the instrumentation is organized so that the stimulator is triggered by the same pulse that initiates A-D conversion of the data. This insures that there will be no jitter (random variation in time) or asynchrony between the onset of the stimulus and the data sampling instants. That is, sampling always occurs at fixed delays from stimulus onset. If, on the other hand, the stimulator is driven independently of the ADC and notifies that device when to initiate sampling, jitter of the sampling instants can occur and tend to result in some temporal smearing of the digitized data. The jitter effect will be small when the cycle time of the computer is small compared with the sampling interval. Here we ignore the effects of jitter in A-D conversion.

The sampled signal $x_a(t)$ is then quantized to yield an output $x_q(t^\circ)$ which can take on only a limited number of, usually, uniformly spaced values. The input-output relationship for the quantizer is shown in Fig. 1(c). The quantization step is q volts in amplitude. The output is 0 as long as the input is greater than 0 and no larger than q; it is q as long as the input is greater than q and no larger than $2q$ and so on. In equation form, the input-output relationship is, at integral values of $t = t^\circ$ (with $\Delta = 1$)

$$x_q(t^\circ) = \begin{cases} Mq, & \text{for } x_a(t^\circ) \geq Mq = Q \\ mq & mq < x_a(t^\circ) \leq (m+1)q, \quad |m| \leq M \quad (2.1) \\ -Mq, & x_a(t^\circ) < -Mq = -Q \end{cases}$$

The maximum and minimum voltage levels that can be handled without saturation are Q and $-Q$ and the total number of levels $2M$ that the output signal can take on is usually some integer power L of 2:

$$2M = 2^L \tag{2.2}$$

The degree of precision of an A-D conversion is referred to in terms of the number of bits in the output word of the converter. A 10-bit converter will quantize voltages between -1 and $+1$ Volt into one of 1024 levels each of whose magnitude is 1.952 mV.

The final step in the conversion is to code $x_q(t°)$ (only the values of x_q at the sampling times are important) into a form acceptable for use by the digital computer. Most often this means that $x_q(t°)$, whether positive or negative, is represented in binary form, L binary digits being adequate for this. Typically, one coded output line is assigned to each binary digit and the value of the voltage on this line at the read-out time indicates whether that binary digit is a 1 or a 0. The time for both sampling and read-out are determined by a clock contained within the computer. "Interrupt" features of the computer assure that the incoming data are accepted after each quantization has been performed.

2.3. QUANTIZATION NOISE

Each conversion has associated with it a discrepancy between the quantized and the true value of the signal. It is useful to consider this error as a form of noise, called quantizing noise, $z_q(t°\Delta)$. We can then write

$$x_q(t°\Delta) = x(t°\Delta) + z_q(t°\Delta) \tag{2.3}$$

z_q is limited in absolute value to 1/2 the size of the quantizing step q. (The properties of quantizing noise in the uppermost and lowermost quantizing levels are different but do not substantially alter this analysis.) We assume the incoming signal to be a random one that is band limited to $F = 1/2$ such that $\Delta = 1$. This means that sampling is done at the Nyquist rate. We also assume that the signal's amplitude is large compared to the size of a quantizing step but small enough not to produce peak value limiting at any time in the converter. Under these reasonable assumptions the following statements hold reasonably well: (1) the quantizing error of a sample is uncorrelated with that of its sequential neighbors; (2) the probability density function for the error z_q of a sample is uniformly distributed over the interval 0 to q. That is, it is equally likely that the magnitude of the error be anywhere in this range. From assumption (2) and the quantization rule of Eq. (2.1), the mean value of the quantizing noise is $q/2$. This is a bias term.

$$\text{var}[z_q] = \int_{-q/2}^{q/2} z_q^2 \, dz = \frac{q^2}{12} \tag{2.4}$$

The lack of correlation between sample errors implies that the autocovariance function for the noise is given by

$$c_{z_q z_q}(\tau^\circ) = \begin{cases} q^2/12, & \text{for } \tau^\circ = 0 \\ 0, & \text{otherwise} \end{cases} \tag{2.5}$$

The power spectrum of the noise, excluding the dc bias term, is flat to $F = 1/2$. To see this, suppose the data consist of N samples of the signal and that we assume the combination of signal and noise to be periodic with period $T = N\Delta = N$. The substitution of Eq. (2.5) into Eq. (1.23) results in spectral terms $C_{z_q z_q}(n)$, which are all equal and independent of n. This is because $c_{z_q z_q}(\tau^\circ)$ is different from 0 only when $\tau^\circ = 0$. Thus the quantizing noise is equally divided among all the $N/2$ frequency components between 0 and $N/2$:

$$C_{z_q z_q}(n) = q^2/12N, \qquad 0 \le n < N/2 \tag{2.6}$$

The ADC converter thus adds noise of its own to the incoming signal, a noise whose covariance and spectral properties are determined solely by the sampling rate and the fineness of quantization. Although quantizing noise has the appearance of being random, it is best to remember that this is not entirely so. To illustrate this point, suppose the incoming signal were a repetitive wave synchronized exactly to some multiple of the sampling period. Samples

taken of the waveform during each period at the same time relative
to the beginning of a period will always produce the same quantizing error and this would not be removable by the process of averaging over successive waveform repetitions. However, as soon as some
background noise is added to the fixed waveform, the situation
changes. The quantizing noise then takes on many of the characteristics of random noise. In a sense, the uncorrelated quantizing
noise is induced into the quantized signal whenever the incoming
signal has a fluctuating random component. Thus, if the input noise
bandwidth were very low relative to 1/2, the quantizing noise would
still exhibit the flat power spectrum indicated by Eq. (2.6). This
induced noise can only be removed by numerical or digital filtering
of the digital data subsequent to the A-D conversion operation, a
topic covered later in this chapter. Since there are many situations in which one is interested in signal peaks which may be small
compared to the largest one present, the existence of quantizing
noise must not be ignored, for it tends to make the small peaks
less detectable. It can, for example, become an important factor
when the biological noise contains a significant amount of low-
frequency components giving rise to what is referred to as baseline
drift in the received data. When this occurs, it is common practice
to reduce the amplification of the signal so as to prevent too
frequent saturation of the signal amplifiers or peak limiting in
the ADC. It is then quite possible that lesser peaks in the signal
will be no larger than a few quantizing intervals, making the quantizing noise a factor of importance.

The fineness of A-D quantization is of importance in still
another way. It affects the ability to reconstruct from the quantized output data, the amplitude probability distribution of the
input data. This issue is somewhat different from that of detecting by response averaging a weak but constant response in a background of noise (Chapter 4). There, one is not interested in determining the nature of the amplitude distribution of the data. Here,
detection of such subtleties in the data is the desideratum, with

response detection being secondary. To find how well this can be
done, it is necessary to know how fine, relative to the peaks in
the amplitude distribution, the quantization steps must be. When
a large number of quantized samples of the input signal are available, the answer, as Tou (1959) has shown, can be arrived at by
considering the signal amplitude distribution as itself a waveform
which is to be represented by a set of uniformly spaced samples
along the amplitude axis. In this approach, the amplitude axis is
analgous to the time axis of conventional waveform sampling. One
can then apply the sampling theorem that states that for perfect
reconstruction of a band limited wave whose highest frequency is
F, sampling should be performed at a rate no lower than $2F$/sec.
In practice, when the experimenter examines the sampled version
of the waveform on an oscilloscope, the Nyquist rate is usually
inadequate to permit satisfactory visual reconstruction of the
waveform. Sampling rates for this purpose should be no lower than
$3F$/sec to $5F$/sec. Although probability distributions of amplitude
are not truly band limited in terms of their Fourier transforms
(called characteristic functions), it is possible to arrive at a
convenient rule-of-thumb in determining what an adequate quantization step or sampling interval should be. Thus, suppose the
narrowest peak in the amplitude probability distribution of the
data is normal in shape, with variance σ^2. The Fourier transform
of this distribution is also Gaussian and has more than 99% of its
area confined to "frequencies" less than $1/3\sigma$. Considering this
to be an adequate approximation to the "bandwidth" of the distribution, simple computations indicate the size of the quantizing step
should then be very nearly σ. Note that though quantizing noise
is present, its variance, $\sigma^2/12$, is small compared to the variance
of the smallest peak in the input distribution. Our rule can now
be stated in terms of the distance D between points three standard
deviations away from the narrowest peak: a sampling width $D/6$ volts
is adequate to represent peaks in the amplitude distribution which
are D volts or more in width. The result holds for overlapping

peaks as long as no component peak is narrower than D. If the peaks are sharper, the rule stated here will produce some distortion of their shapes which will be further contaminated by quantization noise. Sharp peaks therefore require some decrease in the quantization step.

2.4. MULTIPLEXING: MONITORING DATA
SOURCES SIMULTANEOUSLY

Multiplexing is the process whereby several data sources have their information transmitted to the data processor over the same channel. Here the channel is the ADC and the multiplexing is performed by a process of switching the input of the ADC from one signal source to another. The rate at which the switching is performed and the choice of the source to be selected are determined by the data processor which accepts the data from the converter output. Both are constrained, of course, by the data handling capabilities built into the converter. When multiplexing is performed, an additional amount of time is required to perform a data conversion. The additional time arises because the process of switching the data converter from one source to another introduces a brief electrical transient into the signal and it is necessary to wait for this transient to subside before performing a conversion. The multiplexing time can increase the total conversion time by about 10%.

Multiplexing of different data sources is performed most commonly at a uniform rate proceeding from source 1, to source 2, to source 3, etc., and back to source 1 in a recurrent, cyclic fashion. This is the mode of operation when the data from the different sources are signals of comparable bandwidths and whose temporal fluctuations are judged to be of equal interest and importance. When equal sharing of the ADC by the different sources occurs, the minimum period between samples of any one source is increased by a factor equal to the total number of multiplexed channels. As a consequence, the maximum bandwidth which each signal can have without introducing spectral aliasing is $1/2M\Delta$ where M is the number of equally multiplexed sources and $1/M\Delta$ is the effective sampling rate. In addition to being certain that the effective sampling rate is adequate to preserve signal structure, one must also consider the effects of noise in the input data and quantization noise. Ideally, prior to A-D conversion, filtering should be performed to remove from the input data all frequency components higher than $1/2M\Delta$. If this is not done, the higher frequency noise components in the data will, after digitizing, be aliased with the lower frequency ones. Aliasing means that signal components at frequencies greater than 1/2 of the sampling rate will be misinterpreted as components at frequencies less than half the sampling rate. This falsifies the interpretation of signal structure made from the sampled data. Aliasing is discussed more thoroughly in Chapter 3. The net result is a decrease in the signal-to-noise ratio of the digitized data. Suppose, for example, that the sampling rate of the ADC were 1000 samples/sec and that five data channels were being multiplexed. Suppose also that the prefilter had a high frequency cutoff at 500 Hz corresponding to the resolvable bandwidth if only one channel were being digitized. Now, five data sources are being multiplexed. The effective sampling rate of each source is 200/sec and the corresponding resolvable bandwidth is 100 Hz. Even if the response components of the input data have bandwidths less than 100 Hz, all the instrument noise between 100 Hz and the filter cutoff at 500 Hz will be aliased into the spectral region below 100 Hz, producing a degradation of the quantized data from the ADC. This degradation can be eliminated only by reducing the input data bandwidth to 100 Hz. For this reason it is highly desirable when background noise is an important factor to use a prefilter whose cutoff frequency is 1/2 the effective sampling rate.

The total quantizing noise remains unchanged during multiplexing since the quantizing error in each conversion is the same. However, the bandwidth of the digitized output has been reduced so that the spectral intensity of the quantizing noise is increased by the factor M. Filtering prior to A-D conversion cannot reduce this. As basic communications theory shows, this means that when sampling is done at the Nyquist rate, narrow bandwidth data are more affected by quantization noise than are broad bandwidth data.

In some situations, the monitored data sources have widely different bandwidths making it possible to sample the narrow bandwidth signals less frequently than the broad. This often results in a nonuniform rate of sampling of the broader bandwidth signals, there being occasional intervals in which they are not sampled. Usually no serious deterioration in the data analysis results. Infrequent interruptions in sampling can be further minimized by post A-D conversion digital filtering, discussed later in this chapter, which has the effect of interpolating the missed data points in addition to smoothing the data.

If one considers only the spectral properties of the data sources and the sampling rate of the ADC, the problems associated with multiplexing are straightforward. However, another factor, the size of the computer storage area, needs also to be considered when real time data analysis is being performed. As discussed previously, in single channel A-D conversion all real-time data processors have a limited memory capacity in terms of the number of registers available to store data. When multiplexing is employed, these registers are parceled out to the different data sources so that over a given observation epoch, it is never possible to attain the same temporal resolution in each of the several multiplexed channels as it is with just one. The decision to resort to multiplexing must take this into account.

2.5. DATA FILTERING

The operation of data filtering is one in which certain attributes of the data are selected for preservation in preference to others which are "filtered out." To design a satisfactory filtering device or program we must have some knowledge of the structure of both the signal and the noise. In the classical approach to filtering, the spectral components of the signal and noise are of major interest and filters are designed to select or "pass" some spectral components, those containing primarily signal information, and reject or "stop" others, those consisting mostly of noise. While any filtering operation can be described in terms of how it treats the different spectral components of the data, we shall see that this is not the only satisfactory way of dealing with filtration. Prior to the advent of computers, the filtering was concerned primarily with continuous electrical signals and was performed by networks consisting of passive elements (resistors, capacitors, inductors) and active devices (vacuum tubes, transistors). A network of this type is referred to as an analog filter. It operates on continuous data and yields a continuous filtered output. With the advent of the digital computer, it was recognized that analog filters performed computation on their input data which could be carried out equally well and sometimes better by computations on digitized sampled data without the need for constructing specific analog filter devices. In the following sections we discuss some basic attributes of filtering principally from the standpoint of the digital filter but, inasmuch as the continuous analog filter is still of great value in biological data processing, we also consider it to some extent.

2.6. THE DIGITAL FILTER

The history of the digitized version of a signal $x(t)$ over T seconds is represented by N samples of it from $t° = 0$ to $t° = (N-1)\Delta$. They form the set $\{x(t°\Delta)\}$. Once again we assume that the signal is band limited to $F = 1/2$ and that $\Delta = 1$. A filter, digital or otherwise, is a device with input $x(t)$ and output $r(t)$. If the device is digital, it stores a sequence of the past samples of the signal $x(t°)$ in digitized form and operates upon them according to a filtering rule or algorithm to yield the

65

output sequence, $r(t°)$. If the rule does not vary with time, the filter is a time invariant one and if, in addition, the rule involves only the computation of weighted sums of the stored data samples, the filter is linear. The output of a linear, time invariant digital filter can be written as

$$r(t°) = \sum_{\tau°=0}^{N-1} h(\tau°)x(t° - \tau°) \qquad (2.7)$$

In this chapter we are concerned mainly with such filters. Though linearity and time invariance are confining restrictions to put upon a filter's properties, the variety of filtering tasks that can be performed by linear filters is sufficiently rich to satisfy many of our data processing requirements. Linear filtration is easy to understand and perform in both its digital and analog forms. However, it does have deficiencies that limit its ability to deal with time varying processes, and some of them will be made apparent in the discussion.

As Eq. (2.7) indicates, the linear filter consists of a set of N fixed weighting terms $\{h(\tau°)\}$. $h(\tau°)$ multiplies the $\tau°$th most recent sample of the quantized signal and the products when summed yield the filter output. As each new sample of the signal is acquired, the filtered output has to be recomputed, since each of the past samples is now one sampling period older and must be multiplied by the weighting factor corresponding to its age.

An understanding of the nature of the operation of a digital filter can be obtained by a specific example. Let us consider that the sampled $x(t)$, in addition to arising from a band limited signal, is band limited and repetitive with integer valued period T. Its Fourier series representation, valid at the sample times, is then

$$x(t°) = \sum_{n=-N/2}^{N/2-1} X_T(n) \, \exp \frac{j2\pi n t°}{T} \qquad (2.8)$$

We demonstrate how any one of the Fourier components can be filtered from the signal.

A. *FILTERING OF THE CONSTANT COMPONENT*

If the filter output is to be $X_T(0)$, it will have this value regardless of the value of time at which the output is examined. That is, for any integer value of t the output of a filter operating upon M consecutive signal samples is

$$r(t^\circ) = X_T(0) = \sum_{\tau^\circ=0}^{M-1} h(\tau^\circ)x(t^\circ - \tau^\circ) \tag{2.9}$$

Now, since $x(t)$ is periodic and band limited, we need only to have $M = N = T$ equally spaced samples of it since these completely represent the signal. Then Eq. (2.9) becomes

$$r(t^\circ) = X_T(0) = \sum_{\tau^\circ=0}^{N-1} h(\tau^\circ)x(t^\circ - \tau^\circ) \tag{2.10}$$

What we seek is the set of values that the $h(\tau^\circ)$ should have to make this equation an identity. Replacing each sampled value $x(t^\circ)$ by its Fourier series representation, as given in Eq. (2.8), we have

$$r(t^\circ) = X_T(0) = \sum_{\tau^\circ=0}^{N-1} h(\tau^\circ) \sum_{n=-N/2}^{N/2-1} X_T(n) \exp \frac{j2\pi n(t^\circ - \tau^\circ)}{N} \tag{2.11}$$

Interchanging the order of summation gives

$$r(t^\circ) = \sum_{n=-N/2}^{N/2-1} X_T(n) \exp \frac{j2\pi nt^\circ}{N} \sum_{\tau^\circ=0}^{N-1} h(\tau^\circ) \exp \frac{-j2\pi n\tau^\circ}{N} \tag{2.12}$$

If all the $h(\tau^\circ)$ are equal to a constant value h, the inner summation becomes

$$h(0) \sum_{\tau^\circ=0}^{N-1} \exp \frac{-j2\pi n\tau^\circ}{N} = \begin{cases} Nh(0), & n = kN \\ 0, & \text{all other } n \end{cases} \tag{2.13}$$

k is 0 or any other integer. Then, substituting this result into Eq. (2.12) gives

$$r(t^\circ) = X_T(0)Nh(0) \tag{2.14}$$

67

If $h(0) = 1/N$, we obtain the desired identity $r(t^\circ) = X_T(0)$. This means that the digital filter which extracts $X_T(0)$, the average value of a periodic $x(t)$, operates on the N most recent signal samples of $x(t)$, adding them and dividing by N. This particular filter is called a digital integrator since it simply numerically integrates the previous signal sample values. This result holds regardless of the value of Δ.

B. FILTERING THE mTH FREQUENCY COMPONENT

We now wish to filter from the same band limited, periodic signal one of its harmonic components, in particular the component having the frequency $m/T = m/N$. This component is expressed by the sum of two terms, either

$$A_T(m) \cos(2\pi mt/N) + B_T(m) \sin(2\pi mt/N) \tag{2.15}$$

or its identical counterpart

$$X_T(m) \exp(j2\pi mt/N) + X_T(-m) \exp(-j2\pi mt/N) \tag{2.16}$$

We desire to specify a digital filter whose output at each sample time is the same as the amplitude of the mth component of the signal, Eq. (2.16), at that time. Again, because of periodicity only N samples of the signal are necessary:

$$r(t^\circ) = \sum_{\tau^\circ=0}^{N-1} h(\tau^\circ) x(t^\circ - \tau^\circ) = X_T(m) \exp(j2\pi mt/N)$$

$$+ X_T(m) \exp(-j2\pi mt/N) \tag{2.17}$$

The problem is to find if there is a set of values of $h(\tau^\circ)$ which makes this relation an identity. To do this, we proceed as we did previously when determining the average value filter. We obtain the equation (which is identical to Eq. (2.12))

$$r(t^\circ) = \sum_{n=-N/2}^{N/2-1} X_T(n) \exp \frac{j2\pi nt^\circ}{N} \sum_{\tau^\circ=0}^{N-1} h(\tau^\circ) \exp \frac{-j2\pi n\tau^\circ}{N} \tag{2.18}$$

Inspection of this equation reveals that for it to be identical to Eq. (2.16) we need to have

$$\sum_{\tau^\circ=0}^{N-1} h(\tau^\circ) \exp \frac{-j2\pi n\tau^\circ}{N} = \begin{cases} 1, & n = \pm m \\ 0, & \text{otherwise} \end{cases} \qquad (2.19)$$

Let us employ some intuition and guess the form of the solution for $h(\tau^\circ)$:

$$h(\tau^\circ) = \frac{2}{N} \cos \frac{2\pi m\tau^\circ}{N} = \frac{1}{N}\left[\exp \frac{j2\pi m\tau^\circ}{N} + \exp \frac{-j2\pi m\tau^\circ}{N}\right] \qquad (2.20)$$

We substitute this into the left-hand side of Eq. (2.19) and find that

$$\frac{1}{N} \sum_{\tau^\circ=0}^{N-1} \left\{ \exp \frac{j2\pi\tau^\circ(m-n)}{N} + \exp \frac{-j2\pi\tau^\circ(m+n)}{N} \right\}$$

$$= \begin{cases} 1, & n = \pm(m + kn) \\ 0, & \text{otherwise} \end{cases} \qquad (2.21)$$

just as we needed. Since the signal is band limited, only the terms $n = \pm m$ are of interest. Substitution of Eq. (2.20) into Eq. (2.18) gives

$$r(t^\circ) = X_T(m) \exp \frac{j2\pi mt^\circ}{N} + X_T(m) \exp \frac{-j2\pi mt^\circ}{N} , \qquad (2.22)$$

the desired result. The right-hand side may also be expressed in terms of Eq. (2.15). We have thus obtained the digital filter which operates upon the N most recent samples of the signal to yield at its output the sampled sequence representing the mth component of the signal. The values of $A_T(m)$ and $B_T(m)$ can be obtained from the output of the filter, Eq. (2.22), by measuring both the peak value of the output and the time it is 0 and by employing the well-known identity

$$A_T(m) \cos(2\pi mt/N) + B_T(m) \sin(2\pi mt/N)$$

$$= [A_T^2(m) + R_T^2(m)]^{1/2} \cos\{2\pi mt/N + \arctan[A_T(m)/B_T(m)]\}$$

$$(2.23)$$

$X_T(m)$ and $X_T(-m)$ can be obtained if desired by using Eq. (1.12).

Now that we have seen that it is possible to design a digital filter that extracts the mth component of a periodic signal without error, it is possible to demonstrate, though we do not do it here, that any combination of components of such a signal can be filtered by a single compound filter that combines the properties of the individual component filters. Furthermore, this combined filter can weight the contribution of the individual components to the output. Thus, suppose we wish to filter the qth and mth components of the signal $x(t)$ and weight them $V(q)$ and $V(m)$ respectively. The filter output will then be

$$r(t^{\circ}) = V(q) [X_T(q) \exp(-j2\pi q t^{\circ}/N) + X_T(-q) \exp(j2\pi q t^{\circ}/N)]$$

$$+ V(m) [X_T(m) \exp(-j2\pi m t^{\circ}/N) + X_T(-m) \exp(j2 m t^{\circ}/N)] \quad (2.24)$$

Reference to Eq. (2.20) shows that this response can be obtained from a filter whose response is defined by

$$h(\tau^{\circ}) = \frac{V(q)}{N}[\exp(j2\pi q \tau^{\circ}/N) + \exp(-j2\pi q \tau^{\circ}/N)]$$

$$+ \frac{V(m)}{N}[\exp(j2\pi m \tau^{\circ}/N) + \exp(-j2\pi m \tau^{\circ}/N)] \quad (2.25)$$

The output of this filter contains only the qth and mth components of $x(t)$ and in the desired strengths. The result can be generalized to a filter operating upon all the frequency components of the signal.

2.7. IMPULSE RESPONSE OF A DIGITAL FILTER

A convenient way to represent the response of a digital filter is by means of its unit sample response or impulse response $h(t^{\circ})$, its response to a unit amplitude signal sample or discrete time impulse at $t^{\circ} = 0$. All other signal samples, before and after, are 0. As an example, consider the impulse response of a filter which weights equally each of the previous M samples of a signal. This response is

$$h(t^{\circ}) = \begin{cases} K, & 0 \le t^{\circ} \le M - 1 \\ 0, & \text{elsewhere} \end{cases} \quad (2.26)$$

A unit amplitude sample which appeared at the filter input less than M samples ago yields a filter output whose present value is K. If a unit sample at the filter input has occurred more than

M samples in the past, then the present value of the output is 0. Later in the chapter we shall see that the discrete time impulse response described here is closely related to the continuous time impulse response of an analog filter.

When the impulse response of a filter is known, its response to any input signal can be calculated in a straightforward way by taking advantage of the linearity properties of the filter. Thus, to obtain the response at $t° = 0$, $h(1)$ weights the signal amplitude at $t° = -1$, $h(2)$ weights the signal amplitude at $t° = -2$, and so on with all the weighted signal amplitudes then being summed to obtain

$$r(0) = \sum_{\tau°=0}^{\infty} h(\tau°)x(-\tau°) \qquad (2.27)$$

If we are interested in the value of the response at time t, the same procedure follows, each term in the sum being the product of $x(t° - \tau°)$ and $h(\tau°)$. Thus,

$$r(t°) = \sum_{\tau°=0}^{\infty} h(\tau°)x(t° - \tau°) \qquad (2.28)$$

This is the same as Eq. (2.9) if we consider only the first N terms. What we did in the preceding sections, therefore, was to design a digital filter by specifying its impulse response. The computational procedure described in Eq. (2.28) is referred to as convolution of the impulse response with the signal. It is often symbolized mathematically by the notation

$$r(t°) = h(t°) * x(t°) \qquad (2.29)$$

The convolution procedure is illustrated in Fig. 2.2 for a filter which has five terms in its impulse response. To make the procedure more visually comprehensible, we have reversed or folded over the time axis for the plot of $h(t°)$. It tends to bring out the nature of the filter weighting procedure more clearly.

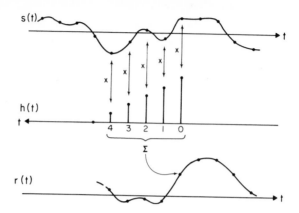

Fig. 2.2. The convolution of a five sample filter with a sampled signal. The filter impulse response is shown in the middle trace with time reversed. The convolution computation is indicated at time t = 8. The continuous lines represent the band limited functions corresponding to the samples.

2.8. SPECTRAL RELATIONS BETWEEN FILTER INPUT AND OUTPUT--THE DISCRETE FOURIER TRANSFORM

The relationship linking a filter's output to its input and its impulse response by the convolution process can also be expressed as a relationship between the corresponding Fourier coefficients. To see this, we again consider a periodic input signal that has period $T = N$ and is bandwidth limited to frequencies less than $1/2$. The signal at sample time $t° - \tau°$ can be represented, as before, by the Fourier series

$$x(t° - \tau°) = \sum_{n=-N/2}^{N/2-1} X_T(n) \exp \frac{j2\pi n(t° - \tau°)}{N} \qquad (2.30)$$

This signal is passed through a digital filter with unit sample response $h(\tau°)$. The output of the filter is given by Eq. (2.28) which has its own Fourier series expansion, also with integer period N.

$$r(t°) = \sum_{n=-N/2}^{N/2-1} R_T(n) \exp \frac{j2\pi n t°}{N} \qquad (2.31)$$

72

Note that the continuous counterpart $r(t)$ of the filter output $r(t^\circ)$ must also be band limited to the same frequency band since the filtering operation only modifies the amplitude and phase of the signal components that are present; *it never introduces new frequencies.* We need consider only filter responses which are less than or equal to the signal period since in the previous sections we have seen that no additional information is gained by making the memory longer than that. If the filter memory is less than the duration of the signal, this can be handled by setting to zero the values of $h(\tau^\circ)$ corresponding to $\tau^\circ \geq N$.

Let us now substitute Eq. (2.30) into Eq. (2.28). We obtain, after changing the upper limit in Eq. (2.28) to $N - 1$,

$$r(t^\circ) = \sum_{\tau^\circ=0}^{N-1} h(\tau^\circ) \sum_{n=-N/2}^{N/2-1} X_T(n) \; \exp \frac{j2\pi n(t^\circ - \tau^\circ)}{N} \qquad (2.32)$$

We now interchange the order of the summations to obtain

$$r(t^\circ) = \sum_{n=-N/2}^{N/2-1} X_T(n) \; \exp \frac{j2\pi nt^\circ}{N} \sum_{\tau^\circ=0}^{N-1} h(\tau^\circ) \; \exp \frac{-j2\pi n\tau^\circ}{N} \qquad (2.33)$$

and then write the inner summation as

$$H_N(n) = \sum_{\tau^\circ=0}^{N-1} h(\tau^\circ) \; \exp \frac{-j2\pi n\tau^\circ}{N} \qquad (2.34)$$

The right hand side of Eq. (2.34) is referred to as the discrete Fourier transform of the impulse response, $h(\tau^\circ)$. $H_N(n)$ and $h(\tau^\circ)$ are further related by the inverse discrete Fourier transform:

$$h(\tau^\circ) = \frac{1}{N} \sum_{n=-N/2}^{N/2-1} H_N(n) \; \exp \frac{j2\pi n\tau^\circ}{N} \qquad (2.35)$$

We call $H_N(n)$ the transfer function or system function of the filter. When Eq. (2.35) is substituted into Eq. (2.33) and the result compared to Eq. (2.31), the Fourier coefficients of the filter's output are seen to be given by

$$R_T(n) = H_N(n) X_T(n) \qquad (2.36)$$

Clearly, the output never has frequency components where the signal has none so that if the input is band limited, so is the output,

and to the same bandwidth or less. The properties of the direct
and inverse Fourier transform will be discussed more thoroughly
in Chapter 3.

2.9. FILTERING APERIODIC SIGNALS

A. *SHORT DURATION SIGNALS*

Digital filtering has been discussed in terms of periodic
signals that persist indefinitely. Under these circumstances a
filter whose memory can store the waveform samples of a single
period of a band limited signal will have an output which is also
periodic and whose Fourier components are related, as shown in the
previous sections, to those of the input signal by the weighting
factors built into the filter. Often, however, we are confronted
with signals that are transitory in nature, having a definite
beginning and end. More often than not, in neurobiology, such
signals occur in a background of noise and are of great interest.
We would like therefore to build a filter which, essentially,
passes the transitory signal but suppresses the noisy background.
An example of such a situation arises when we wish to devote attention to alpha bursts in an ongoing EEG. The bursts occur infrequently and persist for relatively short periods of time while the
EEG process is itself aperiodic. It persists indefinitely and may
in this situation be considered noise. It also differs substantially from the alpha burst in its frequency content, and so a
filtering operation on a sampled representation of the data can
help to suppress the noise with respect to the alpha burst. Another example of a transitory potential is the action potential
of an individual neuron. This is also often observed in a background of noise arising both from unrelated electrical activity
of the nervous system and from the microelectrode and its associated amplifier. Here again, because the noise differs substantially in its frequency content from the signal, filtering can
serve to enhance the size of the signal relative to the noise.
In either example the goal is to preserve the structure of the

74

signal and eliminate, as much as possible, the noise. However, a necessary consequence of filtering short duration signals is that there always occurs a certain amount of alteration in the structure of the signal, even when sampling is performed without distortion and at the Nyquist rate. The alteration is ascribable to the memory of the filter. Because of it, the filter's response to a brief signal has a longer onset than the signal and, likewise, a longer decay. The filter may be said to smear the signal out in time. This temporal smearing increases with the length of the filter's memory. Let us illustrate this with a digital filter designed to extract a brief burst of a 10 Hz sine wave from background noise, an idealization of an alpha burst in the EEG. The filter memory consists of 20 samples taken at a rate of 100/sec. The filter's unit sample response illustrated in Fig. 3(a) is two cycles of a

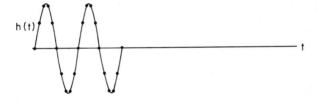

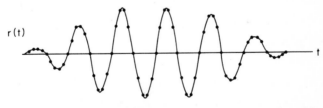

Fig. 2.3. (a) The impulse response (dots) of a 10 Hz digital filter with a 20 sample memory two cycles in duration. (b) The response of this filter to a burst of four cycles of a 10 Hz sine wave. Note the response onset and decay. In both (a) and (b) a continuous line is drawn through the dots to aid visualization.

sampled sine wave. If the filter were operating upon a periodic signal whose period corresponded to the memory duration of the filter, 0.2 sec, 10 Hz would correspond to the second harmonic, $n = 2$, of the 0.2 sec interval. The filter passes this component of a periodic signal and rejects all the other *harmonically related* ones. The filter's output when the actual signal is a burst of four cycles of a 10 Hz sine wave is shown in Fig. 3(b). It can be seen that the filter output exhibits transient behavior over the first two cycles of the response and then is transient-free for the next two cycles. This is followed by a transient decay to zero output for the time lasting from the end of the burst until 0.2 sec later, the duration of the filter's memory. Note that the original four-cycle burst has been stretched by the filter into one of six cycles duration with slower onsets and offsets than were exhibited by the original signal.

B. MAINTAINED SIGNALS

Let us move from the transient, short duration signals to signals which last indefinitely. Periodic signals, as previously pointed out, are of this class and we showed how we could analyze them completely with a restricted number of samples. For a band limited signal of T seconds and bandwidth $1/2$, $N = T$ samples are necessary for this. Suppose we now consider the filter memory to be limited to these N samples and let the period of the signal gradually increase beyond T seconds to T' seconds while still maintaining its bandwidth limitation. It is clear, first of all, that one result of lengthening the period is that the signal acquires an increased number of signal components equally spaced between 0 and $1/2$ Hz, $T'/2$ to be exact, and that these are not harmonically related to the original fundamental frequency $1/T$ (except when the extended period is a multiple of T). In the limit as T' becomes indefinitely large, the signal becomes aperiodic and has its frequency components spread throughout the continuum of frequencies between 0 and $1/2$. If we examine how the N sample filter operates upon an arbitrary frequency $f = 1/T'$ in this frequency region, we find that it passes frequencies other than those which are integral multiples of the fundamental frequency $1/T$. To see this, let us consider a filter designed to pass only the mth harmonic of a periodic signal with period $N = T$. We know from

Eq. (2.20) that its impulse response is given by

$$h(\tau^\circ) = (2/N) \cos(2\pi m\tau^\circ/N) \tag{2.37}$$

Let the input to this filter be the single frequency signal $x(t) = \cos 2\pi ft$. Then the output of the filter is, by Eq. (2.7)

$$r(t^\circ) = \frac{2}{N} \sum_{\tau^\circ=0}^{N-1} \cos \frac{2\pi m\tau^\circ}{N} \cos[2\pi f(t^\circ - \tau^\circ)] \tag{2.38}$$

This equation is easiest to deal with when complex notation is used for the cosine terms. We can then simplify the right hand side in a straightforward manner that is, however, somewhat tedious. The simplification makes use of the identity arising from the summation of a geometric series,

$$\sum_{\tau^\circ=0}^{N-1} \exp j2\pi g\tau = \exp[j\pi(N-1)g] \frac{\sin \pi Ng}{\sin \pi g} \tag{2.39}$$

The result is that the output of the filter is found to be

$$r(t^\circ) = \frac{\sin \pi N(f - m/N)}{N \sin \pi(f - m/N)} \cos 2\pi\left[ft + \frac{N-1}{2} f - \frac{m}{N}\right]$$
$$+ \frac{\sin \pi N(f + m/N)}{N \sin \pi(f + m/N)} \cos 2\pi\left[ft + \frac{N-1}{2} f + \frac{m}{N}\right] \tag{2.40}$$

In this formidable looking equation it is the first term that is of major importance since it makes the principal contribution to the filter output in most circumstances. This can be seen by referring to our previously discussed 10 Hz filter. That filter has a 20-sample impulse response (Δ = .01 sec) that covers two cycles of a 10 Hz wave. Thus $m = 2$ and $N = 20$. To evaluate the filter's performance let us plot the expressions

$$\frac{\sin \pi N(f - m/N)}{N \sin \pi(f - m/N)} \quad \text{and} \quad \frac{\sin \pi N(f + m/N)}{N \sin \pi(f + m/N)} \tag{2.41}$$

as a function of frequency f for the chosen values of m and N. This is done in Fig. 2.4. (The phase shift terms in Eq. (2.40) are of minor importance.) There are several important properties to note:

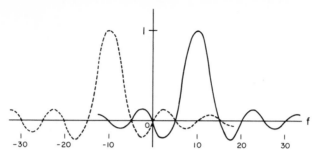

Fig. 2.4. The two expressions of Eq. (2.41) plotted as a function of frequency. They show how the amplitudes of the two response components of Eq. (2.40) vary with signal frequency.

1. The filter has unity transmission at the single frequency $f = m/N = 1/10$. (This corresponds to a data frequency of $m/N\Delta$ = 10 Hz.)

2. The filter has no transmission (infinite attenuation) at other frequency multiples of $1/N = 1/20$.

3. There is significant transmission of other signal frequencies that are located in the frequency band between $(m - 1)/N$ and $(m + 1)/N$, here 1/20 and 3/20. (This corresponds to data frequencies of 5 and 15 Hz.)

4. There exist other frequency bands on either side of this central band or main lobe where signal components can also be passed though with significant attenuation. These bands are often referred to as the side lobes of the filter. Their size is an important consideration in the design of filters that are used in spectral analysis.

The second term defining the filter response in Eq. (2.40) represents a contribution to the output effect that arises from the fact that a cosine wave is the sum of two complex frequency terms: $\exp j2\pi ft$ and $\exp(-j2\pi ft)$ that are equal in magnitude. The filter's cosine unit sample response has the same representation. Note that when the signal frequency is in the filter's main lobe, $(m/N) - f$ is small while $(m/N) + f$ tends to be large. This

means, as already noted, that the contribution of the second term
to the filter output is usually negligible except in filters that
are designed to pass frequencies near 0.

Suppose now that the memory of the filter of Fig. 3 were
increased in duration by a factor of 5. Its unit sample response
would then be 10 cycles of a 10 Hz sine wave. We then have $M = 100$
and $m = 10$ (since we are interested in that harmonic of the fundamental period). If we examine expression (2.41) we find that it
still has unit amplitude at $f = m/N$ but that now the zero transmission frequencies defining the main lobe are at $f = 9/100$ and
$11/100$ (corresponding to data frequencies of 9 and 11 Hz). We
have thus narrowed the pass band of the filter by a factor of 5.
From this it can be surmised that there is an inverse relationship
between the length of a filter's unit sample response (at a given
sample rate) and its bandwidth. This general relationship between
temporal and frequency properties always needs to be kept in mind
when data filtering is employed..

2.10. DATA SMOOTHING BY DIGITAL FILTERING

Let us now consider a slightly different filtering situation.
Here the incoming data to the sampler is bandwidth limited to
1/2 Hz by a preamplifier and sampling is performed at a 1/sec rate.
We know, however, that the bandwidth of the response we are interested in is somewhat less than 1/2 Hz. Without adjustment of
either the preamplifier or the sampling rate, we would like to
design a digital filter that passes only the lower frequencies
present in the response and rejects the higher frequencies as
much as possible. We would like to do this using as little memory
as possible and without introducing phase distortion which alters
the response waveform. A filter which does this is called a
smoothing filter and it has broadly useful properties. Its
smoothing action results from its weighted averaging of a usually
short sequence of consecutive signal samples.

A simple smoothing filter that computes the average of three consecutive samples of the signal has its response given by

$$r(t^\circ) = \sum_{\tau^\circ=0}^{2} h(\tau^\circ)x(t^\circ + 1 - \tau^\circ) \qquad (2.42)$$

This way of representing the signal samples simplifies the analysis. $t^\circ + 1$ is the most recent sample time and $r(t^\circ)$ is the smoothed version of the signal one second ago. For simplicity let $x(t)$ have period $T >> 1$. We then substitute its complex Fourier series representation for it and interchange the order of summation to obtain

$$r(t^\circ) = \sum_{n=-N/2}^{N/2-1} X_T(n) \exp \frac{j2\pi nt^\circ}{N} \sum_{\tau^\circ=0}^{2} h(\tau^\circ) \exp \frac{-j2\pi n(\tau^\circ - 1)}{N} \qquad (2.43)$$

When the inner sum is expanded into its three terms, we have

$$h(0) \exp(-j2\pi n/N) + h(1) + h(2) \exp j2\pi n/N = H_N(n) \qquad (2.44)$$

See Eqs. (2.34) - (2.36) and the accompanying text. $H_N(n)$ is a spectral component weighting factor, possibly complex, for each term in the Fourier series representation for $r(t^\circ)$:

$$r(t^\circ) = \sum_{n=-N/2}^{N/2-1} X_T(n)H_N(n) \exp \frac{j2\pi nt}{N} \qquad (2.45)$$

Now let us choose the values of the $h(\tau^\circ)$ so that (a) there is unity gain at 0 frequency and (b), the frequency component in $x(t)$ at $f = 1/2$ is completely removed from $r(t^\circ)$. A simple filter which meets these constraints has $h(1) = 1/2$, $h(0) = h(2) = 1/4$, and, from Eq. (2.44)

$$H_N(n) = \frac{1}{2} [1 + \cos(2\pi n/N)] \qquad (2.46)$$

This weighting filter $H_N(n)$ is plotted in Fig. 2.5 as a function of $f = n/N$. The nth frequency component in $r(t^\circ)$ is $H_N(n)$ times the nth component in $x(t)$. Note that the weighting factor is always real and positive so that none of the frequency components in $r(t^\circ)$ is different in phase from those of the original signal. Also, the low frequency components near 0 are passed almost without attenuation and the higher frequency components, those above 1/4, are highly attenuated, meaning that if there is noise present and

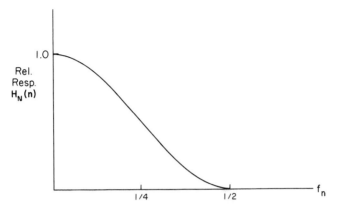

Fig. 2.5. The frequency response $H_N(n)$ of the three component filter with weights 1/4, 1/2, 1/4. The frequency axis is $f_n = n/N$.

it is uniformly distributed in the spectrum, a large fraction of it has been removed without adversely affecting the low frequencies in the signal waveform. The noise reducing effects can be exemplified by referring to the statistics of the original noise. If its bandwidth were 1/2 and its variance unity, the variance of the noise at the filter output would be

$$\text{var}[r(t^\circ)] = (1/4)^2 + (1/2)^2 + (1/4)^2 = 3/8 \tag{2.47}$$

This reduction in noise has been obtained without changing the bandwidth of the preamplifier preceding the digital filter. It is also important to remember that if the sampling rate had been reduced to be commensurate with the bandwidth of the response component of the data, there would have been no change in the variance of the noise per output sample. Instead, the noise at the output would have had its bandwidth compressed (by aliasing of the higher frequency components) to produce increased contamination in the spectral region occupied by the signal. Thus, when signal bandwidth is considerably less than noise bandwidth, digital filtering can yield significant reductions in noise, including that introduced by quantization, that would not be obtainable by alterations in sampling rate.

Although the preceding discussion was based upon $x(t)$ being periodic, the results obtained also apply to stochastic band limited signals in general. The response properties of the filter are such as to inherently pass low frequencies and attenuate high frequencies regardless of the signal structure.

The digital filter described here is one example of a type encountered often in problems dealing with signal smoothing (Hamming, 1973). A certain amount of improvement in removing the higher frequencies can be obtained by increasing the filter memory to 5, 7, 9, etc., samples. Such filters can be designed to have a variety of transfer functions with different filtering characteristics, to have no phase shift, to pass the 0 frequency component without loss, and to attenuate the 1/2 Hz component completely. Such filters can be quite useful, but an adequate discussion of them is beyond the scope of this book. The interested reader is referred to Oppenheim and Schafer (1975). We note, however, that as the memory and complexity of the filter increases, the amount of time required to perform the computations also increases. When the data are being processed in real time, the amount of time available to compute each filtered data value can be no greater than the length of the sampling interval minus the time required to sample and perform A-D conversion. The computation time required for any given filter will depend upon the speed and structure of the computer employed. For these reasons, there can be no hard and fast formula relating sampling rate to allowable filter characteristics.

In addition to being used for spectral filtering of a response from the background noise contained in the data, digital filters may at times be useful for interpolating purposes. This use arises in situations in which the data occasionally contain brief spikelike transients that are perhaps artifactual in origin and unrelated to the response of interest. In this case an inter-

polating filter can act to minimize the effect of the transients
by discarding the data sample amplitude at the time of the transient. An example of a three-sample interpolating filter is one
whose weighting coefficients are 1/2, 0, 1/2. Postexperimental
use of this filter upon those data points where the transients
are suspected can be of value. But it is not a filter to be used
with abandon. The reason is that its transfer function, evaluated
according to the methods employed above, is

$$H_N(n) = \cos(2\pi n/N) \qquad (2.48)$$

Note that there is complete attenuation of frequencies near 1/4 Hz
and that all frequency components above that are phase shifted by
180° at the filter output. This can produce severe distortion in
the filtered version of the data. A five-sample interpolating
filter with weighting coefficients 1/4, 1/4, 0, 1/4, 1/4 can reduce this distortion somewhat but it also produces 180° phase
shifts over half the frequency band and weights negatively the
frequency components near $f = 1/2$.

Digital filters have been applied with good success to spectral analysis of random processes such as the EEG. In this type
of application which is discussed in more detail in Chapter 3, the
spectral characteristics of the filter are of equal importance to
its temporal response properties. The filter is spoken of as providing a spectral window through which to view the random process.
The spectral shape of this window is one of the factors that determine how well one can estimate the spectrum of the random process
from a sequence of its sampled values. There are a number of window filters which have been proposed and used for this type of
analysis. In general they have not been applied to spectral analysis of neurological processes in real time because even with fast
Fourier transform techniques the speed of computation required is
beyond the capabilities of present day computers. Their predominant use is off-line with recorded data. This means that the filters are not constrained to operate upon a small temporal segment
of the data and can have substantially large memories in order to

of the data and can have substantially large memories in order to compute the estimates necessary to a spectral analysis.

2.11. DIGITAL FILTERS WITH FEEDBACK--
RECURSIVE FILTERS

The filters discussed above have used the N most recent samples of the signal. Their finite impulse response means that they possess no memory of data that occurred more than N samples ago. This situation can be modified without increasing the physical size of memory of the filter by the use of data feedback from the filter's output. A filter employing feedback is often called a recursive filter. It turns out to have an infinitely long response to a unit sample. An example is given in Fig. 2.6.

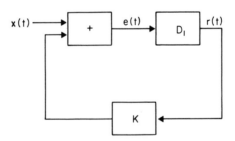

Fig. 2.6. A digital recursive filter with a single storage element D_1. The output of the storage element is equal to its input one time interval earlier.

Here the filter has a single storage element or shift register, D_1. The output, $r(t^\circ)$, of the register is the value its input, $e(t^\circ)$, had at the previous sampling time. The input to the register is the weighted sum of the signal and the register output:

$$e(t^\circ) = x(t^\circ) + Kr(t^\circ) \qquad (2.49)$$

where K is the weighting factor applied to the output of the storage element. The output of the filter is just

$$r(t^\circ) = e(t^\circ - 1) \qquad (2.50)$$

If we substitute for $e(t^\circ - 1)$ in the above expression:

$$r(t^\circ) = x(t^\circ - 1) + Kr(t^\circ - 1) \qquad (2.51)$$

We then substitute $e(t° - 2)$ for $r(t° - 1)$ using Eq. (2.50) and substitute for $e(t° - 2)$ using Eq. (2.49). We find that

$$r(t°) = x(t° - 1) + Kx(t° - 2) + K^2 r(t° - 2) \qquad (2.52)$$

Continuing on in this manner for earlier and earlier values of r, we see that

$$r(t°) = \sum_{\tau°=0}^{\infty} K^{\tau°} x(t° - 1 - \tau°) \qquad (2.53)$$

The impulse response of the filter yielding this response is

$$h(\tau°) = K^{\tau°} \qquad (2.54)$$

The single shift register filter is thus theoretically equivalent to a filter storing all the past signal samples each of which it weights according to the power of K that corresponds to the age of the sample. Great flexibility can be obtained in feedback filters by using several shift registers in various feedback configurations. The theoretical response of such configurations can be obtained without undue difficulty, although we shall not do so here. For more details, see Oppenheim and Schafer (1975). In practice there are distinct limitations to the amount of memory realizable with such a filter. Suppose, for example, we let $K = 1/2$. As the age of the sample increases, the value of the corresponding power of K decreases until it becomes so small that the weighted sample is not representable in a computer by a fixed point number. The smaller the size of the computer word, the smaller is the number of past samples that can be usefully represented. There are also problems encountered in the round-off errors of the products resulting from the multiplication by K called for in Eq. (2.49) and in the time requirements to perform them. These increase if floating point multiplication is employed to circumvent the limitations imposed by fixed point arithmetic. It can be seen that such problems require careful consideration when one is designing a feedback digital filter to meet a given response specification.

2.12. THE LINEAR ANALOG FILTER

The continuous analog filter preceded the digital in its application to signal analysis and its use remains widespread, the growth in the use of the digital filtration notwithstanding. The reason is that solid state technology has made analog filters easy to design and apply, usually at a modest cost, to specific filtering problems. The concepts of the spectrum and impulse response of a filter and the relationship between them were first understood in terms of the linear, time-invariant analog filter. These were later adapted and extended to the linear, time-invariant digital filter.

The most common biological instrumentation application of the analog filter is in preamplifiers and amplifiers which link the biological preparation to the data analyzing system. As such, it produces the requisite signal amplification and some preliminary filtering, though at the unavoidable cost of adding instrument noise to the biological signal. Amplification is produced by the active power-producing elements. Filtering is produced by electrical circuits composed of passive resistors, capacitors, and, occasionally, inductors acting in conjunction with active amplifying elements. The configuration of these circuits and the relative sizes of the elements in them determine the characteristics of the filter. When the elements involved are linear, i.e., when their parameters are independent of the voltage across them or the current passing through them, the filters are referred to as linear. The relationship between the output and input of a linear filter is described by a linear ordinary differential equation with constant coefficients. An example of a linear filter is the low-pass filter illustrated in Fig. 2.7. The triangular symbol is commonly employed to indicate an active circuit element, usually an operational amplifier, which amplifies the incoming signal by a factor of K and inverts its phase. If we employ (a) Kirchhoff's rule that the sum of the currents entering a circuit junction is equal to the currents leaving, (b) Ohm's law, and (c) the current-voltage

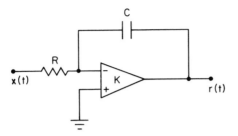

Fig. 2.7. A linear low-pass filter constructed from an operational amplifier, a resistor R, and a capacitor C.

relation for a capacitor, $i = C\ dv/dt$, and if we assume that there is no current entering the input terminals of the amplifier, it is a simple matter to show that the differential equation for this configuration is given by

$$[K/(K + 1)]\ RC(d/dt)r(t) + (1/K)r(t) = x(t) \qquad (2.55)$$

The characteristics of this filter are obtained by solving the differential equation. As will be shown, this filter is a low-pass filter because it tends to pass the low frequency components of the data with little attenuation while, at the same time, it attenuates the high frequency components.

2.13. THE LAPLACE TRANSFORM, THE FILTER TRANSFER FUNCTION, AND IMPULSE RESPONSE

In order to obtain the solution of the linear differential equation and, thereby, the explicit response of the filter to any arbitrary input signal, the most useful mathematical technique to employ is that of the Laplace transform.

The Laplace transform when applied to a suitable function of time $f(t)$ yields a new function $F(s)$ defined by the transform equation

$$F(s) = \int_0^\infty f(t)\ \exp(-\ st)\ dt \qquad (2.56)$$

There are many valuable properties of this transform that show up in the transformed function $F(s)$. Among them is the fact that the

nth time derivative of $f(t)$ turns out to be $s^n F(s)$. [We ignore here consideration of the initial condition of $f(t)$ and its derivatives at $t = 0$.] This means that the Laplace transform of a linear ordinary differential equation for $f(t)$ yields an algebraic equation in s and $F(s)$. Thus the Laplace transform of Eq. (2.55) is

$$[K/(K + 1)]RCsR(s) + (1/K)R(s) = X(s) \qquad (2.57)$$

where $R(s)$ and $X(s)$ are Laplace transforms of $r(t)$ and $x(t)$ respectively. The solution for $R(s)$ in terms of $X(s)$ is

$$R(s) = \frac{X(s)}{[K/(K + 1)]RCs + (1/K)} \qquad (2.58)$$

This equation can then be inverse transformed to yield the temporal response $r(t)$ as given by the inverse Laplace transform

$$r(t) = \int_{-\infty}^{\infty} R(s) \exp st \, ds \qquad (2.59)$$

Tables of the Laplace transform and its inverse have been compiled for the more common functions of t and s and they can often be used to advantage. See Abramowitz and Stegun (1965) for example. In practice, the application of Laplace transforms can be involved and direct solution of the differential equation may be preferable. One way to do this is by computer simulation methods, digital or analog. We shall not consider this further.

The Laplace variable s is a complex one with real and imaginary parts: $s = \sigma + j\omega = \sigma + j2\pi f$. Among other things this means that the integration in Eq. (2.59) is in the complex plane. It should also be noticed that if $\sigma = 0$, the Laplace transform resembles the Fourier transform closely. The resemblance is more than coincidental. The two are actually intimately related and this is important in deriving the properties of filters. A more complete discussion of the Laplace transform is beyond the scope of this book but can be found in many standard texts, Spiegel (1965) and Milsum (1966) for example. Simon (1972) provides an introduction to the Laplace transform at a more basic level.

If we know nothing about the properties of a filter except that it is linear, an examination of the relationship between its input signal and its output can reveal the filter's exact mathematical structure. In this regard, a particularly important input to the filter is the unit impulse, $\delta(t - \tau)$. This is an infinitesimally short pulse occurring at time τ whose amplitude is inversely proportional to its duration so that its area is 1:

$$\int_{-\infty}^{\infty} \delta(t - \tau) \, dt = 1 \qquad (2.60)$$

This impulse, or delta function, is also called the Dirac delta function. One of its important properties is that the time integral of its product with another time function $f(t)$ yields the value of that other function at time τ:

$$\int_{-\infty}^{\infty} \delta(t - \tau) \, f(t) \, dt = f(\tau) \qquad (2.61)$$

The Laplace transform of $\delta(t - \tau)$ is easily shown by Eq. (2.56) to be $\exp(-s\tau)$. Note that when $\tau = 0$, this becomes unity.

If an impulse is applied at $t = 0$ to the input of a filter, the filter output at time t is, appropriately enough, its impulse response, $h(t)$. If the impulse is applied at time τ, the response of the filter at time t to this delayed impulse is $h(t - \tau)$. Suppose we are interested in the output of the filter at time t to some arbitrary input $x(t)$. We may determine this response by the following line of reasoning. Any signal can be considered to be composed of a steady stream of short pulses $\Delta\tau$ sec in duration, each of whose strength (area) at time $t - \tau$, τ sec earlier than t, is $x(t - \tau)\Delta\tau$. The response of the filter τ sec after such a pulse has been delivered is approximately $x(t - \tau)$ $h(\tau)\Delta\tau$. Now, the linearity property of the filter assures us that at any time t the response of the filter to the entire past signal is the sum of its responses to the individual impulses of which that signal is composed. If we pass to the limiting situation by letting $\Delta\tau$, the pulse duration, become very small, we have

$$r(t) = \int_0^\infty x(t - \tau) \, h(\tau) \, d\tau \tag{2.62}$$

Note that the integration is over the past history of the signal. The response of the filter $h(\tau)$ is thus 0 when τ is negative. This means that the filter cannot anticipate what its input will be in the future and this is a property of all real filters. It is not to be confused with the fact that, under suitable circumstances, a properly designed filter may predict future values of the signal on the basis of the signal's past behavior. That is another matter. Equation (2.62) shows that the output of the filter is the convolution of the input with the impulse response of the filter. This is the analog version of Eq. (2.28) obtained for the digital filter. Using the convolution notation of Eq. (2.29) we have

$$r(t) = h(t) * x(t) \tag{2.63}$$

If we take the Laplace or Fourier transform of both sides of Eq. (2.62) we find that

$$R(f) = H(f) \, X(f) \tag{2.64}$$

(It is not necessary here to distinguish between the two, beyond noting that the Laplace transform is evaluated for $s = j2\pi f$.) This is an analog counterpart of Eq. (2.36). An important facet of of these analog filter relationships is that there are no bandwidth restrictions on the incoming signal and as a result no aliasing problems to be concerned with. The relations are independent of both signal bandwidth and filter impulse response.

Let us now return to the filter described by the differential equation, Eq. (2.55). The solution of this equation indicates that the impulse response of the filter is given by

$$h(t) = \begin{cases} \exp(-t/RC), & t \geq 0 \\ 0 & , \quad t < 0 \end{cases} \tag{2.65}$$

The quantity RC whose dimension in sec is the time constant of the filter. This filter is the analog of the digital feedback filter whose impulse response was given in Eq. (2.54). That this is so can be seen by considering $h(1)$ as obtained from Eq. (2.65).

$$h(1) = \exp(-1/RC) = K \qquad (2.66)$$

Then, for integer values t

$$h(t) = \exp(-t/RC) = K^t \qquad (2.67)$$

which is the same as Eq. (2.54). Thus while the digital filter weights the past of the signal exponentially at the sample times t, the continuous analog filter does the same type of weighting for all values of time into the infinite past. In this sense the digital filter is a sampled version of the continuous one. At the sample times, it performs indistinguishably from the continuous filter provided the bandwidth of its input signal is properly limited.

The Fourier or Laplace transform (with $s = j2\pi f$) of Eq. (2.65) is the transfer function of the filter and is given by

$$H(f) = \frac{RC}{1 + j2\pi fRC} = |H(f)| \exp(j\theta) \qquad (2.68)$$

Note that if the incoming signal is a unit amplitude sine wave of frequency f, the output of the filter will be another sine wave of the same frequency:

$$r(t) = |H(f)| \sin(2\pi ft + \theta) = \left[\frac{RC}{1 + (2\pi fRC)^2}\right]^{1/2} \sin(2\pi ft + \theta) \qquad (2.69)$$

The amplitude of the sine wave is the amplitude of $H(f)$ at the signal frequency f, and there is a shift θ in phase of the output relative to the input. In this case, the phase shift is given by

$$\theta = -\arctan 2\pi fRC \qquad (2.70)$$

The filter $H(f)$ has a pass band and a stop band. The pass band is defined as that band of frequencies in which a sine wave signal is attenuated by less than $2^{-1/2}$. This amount of attenuation in decibels is $20 \log_{10} 2^{-1/2} = -3$dB. The band of frequencies where attenuation is greater than 3 dB is defined as the stop band. The frequency marking the boundary between pass and stop bands is the cutoff frequency, here the 3 dB cutoff frequency. (Other attenuation levels are sometimes used to define the limits of a pass band.) At the 3 dB cutoff frequency, the phase shift produced by the filter is 45° or $\pi/4$ radians. In the simple low-pass

RC filter, the maximum phase shift occurs at very high frequencies and is -90°. The characteristics of filter performance can be summarized in the pair of curves called Bode plots (see Fig. 2.8),

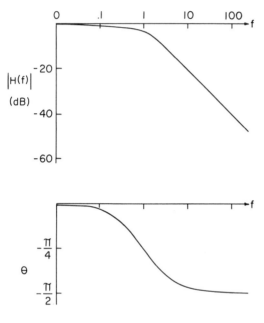

Fig. 2.8. Bode plots for the low pass filter of Eq. (2.69). RC = 1. The frequency axis is logarithmic. The upper diagram plots the gain in dB; the lower diagram, the phase shift in radians. The 3 dB cutoff frequency is at f = 1 Hz.

which relate its amplitude and phase properties to frequency. The upper curve plots $20 \log_{10} |H(f)|$, the decibel value of $H(f)$, as a function of frequency while the lower plots the phase angle θ. *RC* is taken to be 1/2π. The decibel gain measure is preferred because when filters are cascaded, both their logarithmic gains and their phase shifts add. [This is true as long as the individual filter stages are properly isolated from one another (buffered) so that they do not interact.] As can be seen, the slope of the log gain curve in the region somewhat above $f = 1/2\pi$ is nearly linear. Thus, a simple low-pass, single time constant *RC* filter has a gain slope of -20 dB/decade of frequency. That is, each time the frequency increases tenfold, the gain is reduced one-tenth. Equivalently, each time the frequency doubles, the gain halves, a 6 dB change in gain per octave frequency change. This is characteristic of a filter described by a linear first order differential equation.

It is possible to increase the rate of attenuation of a filter in the stop band to -40 dB/decade by designing a filter represented by a second order differential equation, to -60 dB/decade
by a third order filter, etc. As mentioned above, one simple way
of achieving the higher cutoff rates is to cascade filter units or
stages. However, there are now far more elegant techniques for
designing inexpensive filters that have sharp cutoff properties.
The more prominent types of filters are of the Butterworth and
Chebychev types. The principles behind their designs can be found
in standard texts on filter design. See Brown *et al.* (1973) and
the Federal Telephone and Radio Handbook (1963), for example.

Besides the low-pass filter, there are two other general
types of filters which find wide application in studying dynamic
processes. These are the high-pass and the bandpass filter. The
former is characterized by being able to pass high frequencies with
little or no attenuation while substantially attenuating low frequencies. It has a low frequency cutoff and a log gain-versus-
frequency curve which is essentially a mirror image of the high-
pass filter. So is its phase-versus-frequency characteristic.
High-pass filters are typically used to remove slow-wave activity
from single unit records. They are also used to remove from the
data spurious very low frequency components as might arise from
electrode instabilities or from the amplifier components themselves. The bandpass filter, on the other hand, is characterized
by being able to pass only a limited band of frequencies located
between low and high cutoff frequencies. The attenuated frequencies are in the stop bands located beyond these cutoff frequencies. Filters of this type are employed when there is a more
or less narrow range of frequencies of primary interest in the
signal data as is the case, for example, in studying the alpha frequency component of the EEG.

The inverse of a bandpass filter is a stop band filter. One
common application of it is to remove power line interference from
recordings of EEG data. Although these filters have a very narrow

stop band, their phase characteristics inherently introduce phase distortion of frequency components of the signal which may be relatively remote from the stop band. An inevitable consequence is that there is some waveform distortion of the filtered signal. Thus, one should use such remedial filters with caution and only when other techniques for interference suppression at the source have failed.

2.14. THE OPERATIONAL AMPLIFIER

Our brief discussion of the linear analog filter has presented only its essential properties in outline. Since the linear analog filter is so widespread in the prefiltering operations that precede A-D conversion, it is useful also to consider the analog filter from a more instrumentational point of view. Here we consider some of the properties of the active amplifying element that forms the heart of the analog filter, the operational amplifier. This device has simplified linear filter design in many instances to little more than cookbook complexity. Consequently an understanding of its basic properties will help the neurobiologist in applying these recipes to his own requirements.

The operational amplifier's name derives from its original use in analog computers where it was developed to help perform the mathematical operations of summation, integration, and differentiation. These are accomplished by incorporating the amplifier into feedback networks which take advantage of the amplifier's most important property, extremely high gain or amplification. The applications of the operational amplifier have by now been greatly diversified so that it finds extensive use wherever analog filtering applications occur. At present, the most common configuration of the operational amplifier is the differential configuration shown in Fig. 2.7. The output of the amplifier is $-K$ times the voltage difference between the inverting (-) and the noninverting (+) inputs. Practical values for K range from 10,000 to considerably higher. Another basic property of the operational

amplifier is that its input terminals draw negligible current from
the electrical networks connected to them. In Fig. 2.9 the opera-

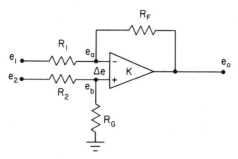

*Fig. 2.9. An operational amplifier configured to function
as a differential amplifier. The voltages at the inverting and
non-inverting inputs are e_a and e_b, respectively. R_F is the
feedback resistor.*

tional amplifier is shown in a four resistor network which makes
it function as a differential amplifier with respect to the two
signal sources e_1 and e_2. Some simple network relations show how
this comes about. First,

$$e_0 = K(\Delta e) = -K(e_a - e_b) \qquad (2.71)$$

The voltages e_a and e_b are derivable from the signals e_1 and e_2
and the output e_0, assuming that the resistances of these sources
are very small compared to the network resistors. Thus,

$$e_a = e_0 \frac{R_1}{R_1 + R_F} + e_1 \frac{R_F}{R_1 + R_F} \qquad (2.72)$$

$$e_b = e_2 \frac{R_G}{R_2 + R_G} \qquad (2.73)$$

Substituting Eqs. (2.72) and (2.73) into Eq. (2.71) and simplifying somewhat, gives

$$e_0\left(1 + \frac{K}{R_1 + R_F}\right) = -K\left(e_1 \frac{R_F}{R_1 + R_F} - e_2 \frac{R_G}{R_2 + R_G}\right) \qquad (2.74)$$

We now divide both sides by the coefficient of e_0 and simplify it
a little further

$$e_0 = \frac{-(R_1 + R_F)}{[(1 + K)/K]R_1 + (R_F/K)}\left(e_1 \frac{R_F}{R_1 + R_F} - e_2 \frac{R_G}{R_2 + R_G}\right) \quad (2.75)$$

Since K is very large, Eq. (2.75) can be accurately approximated by

$$e_0 = \frac{-(R_1 + R_F)}{R_1}\left(e_1 \frac{R_F}{R_1 + R_F} - e_2 \frac{R_G}{R_2 + R_G}\right) \quad (2.76)$$

The differential relationship can now be obtained by setting $R_G = R_F$ and $R_2 = R_1$. Then

$$e_0 = (-R_F/R_1)(e_1 - e_2) \quad (2.77)$$

This is the defining relation for the differential amplifier. As long as K is large, the amplification is determined by the sizes of the resistors in the network and not by the gain of the operational amplifier. Changes in the sizes of R_2 and R_G from those selected here weight the contribution of e_2 differently from that of e_1. Note, however that the output is always in phase with e_2 and in phase opposition to e_1. Moderate variations in K, as inspection of Eq. (2.75) will indicate, do not materially alter the differential operation. This arises from the negative feedback from the output to the inverting input via R_F.

When a number of inputs are to be added in phase with one another and amplified, they may all be brought to the inverting input terminal of the amplifier of Fig. 2.9 through their own input resistors. The inverting input is thus also referred to as the *summing junction*. The contribution of each input to the amplifier output is in proportion to the Ohmic value of the resistor connecting it to the summing junction. Thus if e_1, e_3 and e_4 are connected to the summing junction by resistors R_1, R_3 and R_4, the amplifier output will be proportional to $R_1 e_1 + R_3 e_3 + R_4 e_4$. It should also be noted that if the noninverting input is connected directly to ground, the summing junction is at "virtual ground" potential in that its potential is the output voltage divided by the gain of the amplifier. Under normal circumstances the summing junction is never more than one or two millivolts from ground.

Another important use of the operational amplifier is as a buffer between signal and load. In this type of use, the amplifier is used to furnish more power to a load than the signal source can. The amplifier isolates the load from the signal and thereby prevents the load from distorting the signal waveform properties and from interfering with the properties of a biological preparation. Because of its low output impedance the buffer amplifier tends to suppress transient artifactual potentials which may be generated in the load. This can be the case where the load is an ADC. The switching transients which occur in these devices may, unless properly guarded against, corrupt the signal being digitized. A more complete discussion of the characteristics of operational amplifiers may be found in Brown *et al.* (1973).

2.15. THE AMPLITUDE COMPARATOR

It is common in the examination of single and multiple unit activities to have to assign an occurrence time or epoch to each individual waveform, be it a spike from a neuron or some particular feature of an EEG wave. The major difficulty in occurrence time measurement arises when the events are waveforms occurring amidst other activity such as background noise. Error-free estimation of the epoch is impossible; but the epochs of events whose waveforms are larger in amplitude than those of the background noise can be measured quite accurately with an amplitude comparator, a device which operates upon the instantaneous amplitude of the observed signal.

The output of the comparator changes rapidly from one voltage level to another when the amplitude of its input signal increases through some reference threshold level. The reverse transition in output occurs when the signal amplitude decreases through this threshold. Thus, both these time instants can be marked by the comparator. Many of the common amplitude comparators are based on the bistable Schmitt trigger circuit and are further specialized so that they generate a brief pulse only at the time of the upward threshold crossing. Bistable means that the circuit has two stable states, one when the input is below threshold, the other when the input exceeds the threshold. The transition time is very rapid. In Fig. 2.10 is shown the action of such an amplitude comparator

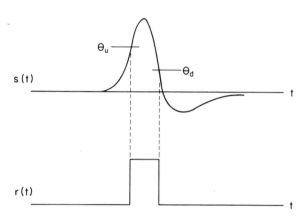

Fig. 2.10. Above, the input to a Schmitt trigger circuit. θ_u is the upward going threshold; θ_d, the downward. The difference between the two, here exaggerated, is the hysteresis. Below, the output of the circuit. The pulse exists as long as the input exceeds θ_u and has not gone below θ_d.

on a brief, pulselike signal. The downward threshold crossing time is disregarded when only onset times are of interest. Also, comparators of the bistable Schmitt trigger type exhibit a hysteresis phenomenon: the threshold for a downward crossing is at a different lower level from the upward threshold. The hysteresis may be minimized by careful design and adjustment, but it can never be eliminated. Any measurement which requires accurate determination of upward and downward crossings of the same threshold must therefore employ amplitude comparators which effectively remove hysteresis.

The epoch time estimated by an amplitude comparator is subject to errors introduced by the presence of noise in the data and by inherent fluctuations in the observed spike waveform itself.

As the noise and waveform fluctuations increase, errors increase. The temporal distribution of the epoch estimate of a spike is dependent upon the properties of the noise and upon the spike shape and how it fluctuates from spike to spike.

Amplitude comparators can also be used to separate pulselike waveforms of different amplitudes that are mixed together in the electrode signal. This often occurs in extracellular microelectrode records. The activity of different neurons observed by the electrode will differ most obviously in the amplitudes of the action potentials from the different units. If the action potential peaks from each of these units occupy nonoverlapping ranges in amplitude, the spikes from each unit can be filtered from the others by the use of paired amplitude comparators, often referred to as an amplitude window circuit. One comparator is set at a low level A_1, and the other at a higher level A_2. The amplitude interval between them is the window and covers the range of amplitude variation exhibited by one unit. If the peak of a spike falls in the A_1 to A_2 window, its waveform will ascend and descend through A_1 without passing through A_2 in the intervening interval. Spikes which are larger than A_2 in amplitude will pass through both the A_1 and A_2 levels, and those which are too low will pass through neither. The decision on whether a peak falls within the selected window must await the recrossing of the lower level. An output pulse is generated by the discriminator only if there has been no crossing of A_2 between the upward and downward crossings of A_1. The delay is generally not significant.

A pair of amplitude comparators can be used to filter out each spike amplitude range of interest. The window width of each pair is set experimentally to pass only those spikes thought to be associated with a particular single unit. Each pair operates independently of the others and their ranges must not overlap. In many experimental situations, however, overlap does exist in the amplitude ranges of the spikes generated by the different units. This is due to the intrinsic variability of the spike

99

amplitudes themselves, as observed by the electrode, and to the presence of background noise. The overlap greatly reduces the utility of the filtering scheme since spikes arising from one neuron can be improperly attributed to another. A noise spike can also be mistakenly classified as arising from a unit and occasionally, the combination of noise and spike activity can cause a unit spike to be missed entirely. These standard misclassification errors can degrade the analysis of unit and interunit activity with a severity that depends upon the frequency of their occurrence. Except in exceptional circumstances, three units with nonoverlapping amplitude ranges seem to be the practical limit that can be satisfactorily filtered by amplitude comparators. More powerful techniques are available for filtering spikes from one another on the basis of their waveform shapes. These techniques are discussed in Chapter 7.

2.16. TIME-VARYING AND NONLINEAR FILTERS

With the exception of the amplitude comparator, the filters that have been discussed are linear. That is, the output is a weighted sum of the input signal, its time derivatives and integrals. The properties of a particular linear filter are determined by the assignment of weight to each of these terms. Once assigned, these weights are not changed during a filtering procedure. The filter is thus both linear and time invariant. These filters are usually referred to simply as linear filters in contrast to time-varying linear filters. We do the same here. The mathematics describing the properties of the filter are those of linear difference equations, where computer operations on sampled signals are concerned, or upon linear differential equations, where operations on the original continuous signals are concerned. One of the key facts to keep in mind with respect to linear filters is that their best application is to situations in which the signal and the background noise are stationary. In certain instances of this type, mainly where the noise is Gaussian, it has been shown that a linear

100

filter is the best filter that can be employed to extract response information. However, few of the neurological signals of interest can be said to fit completely the description of stationarity; nor is biological noise purely Gaussian. Linear filters perform data processing that is less than optimum in these situations. More satisfactory solutions to the problems encountered in dealing with nonstationarity and non-Gaussian processes require the application of a variety of filtering operations which may be either time-varying, nonlinear, or both.

A time-varying linear filter is one whose weights (or coefficients in the defining filter differential equation) may be systematically altered as a function of time according to some prescribed recipe. This is done in the case of adaptive or learning filters. These can be used to achieve better response estimates in the situation in which either the response or the noise properties vary with time. A nonlinear filter is one that performs operations which cannot be described by linear differential or difference equations. The amplitude comparator is an example of such a filter. Products, quotients, and powers of derivatives and integrals are among those that may be encountered in nonlinear filtration; so are logical operations. A moment's consideration will indicate that the class of nonlinear filters is vastly greater than that of linear filters. Nonlinear filtering operations are implicitly involved in a number of statistical data processing techniques that have been applied to response estimation. The consideration of these tests from the filtering point of view can have conceptual advantages for it helps provide a concise description of how signal data are processed.

REFERENCES

Abramowitz, M. and Stegun, I. A., "Handbook of Mathematical Functions," Dover, New York, 1965.
Brown, P. B., Maxfield, B. W. and Moraff, H., "Electronics for Neurobiologists," MIT Press, Cambridge, 1973.
Federal Telephone and Radio Corp., "Reference Data for Radio Engineers," American Book-Stratford Press, New York, 1963.

Hamming, R. W., "Numerical Methods for Scientists and Engineers,"
    2nd ed., McGraw-Hill, New York, 1973.
Milsum, J. H., "Biological Control Systems Analysis," McGraw-Hill,
    New York, 1966.
Oppenheim, A. V. and Schafer, R. W., "Digital Signal Processing,"
    Prentice-Hall, Englewood Cliffs, 1975.
Simon, W., "Mathematical Techniques for Physiology and Medicine,"
    Academic Press, New York, 1972.
Spiegel, M. R., "Laplace Transforms," Schaum, New York, 1965.
Tou, J. T., "Digital and Sampled Data Control Systems," McGraw-
    Hill, New York, 1959.

Chapter 3

POWER SPECTRA
AND COVARIANCE FUNCTIONS

3.1. INTRODUCTION

In the introductory chapter we pointed out the usefulness of
covariance functions and spectral representations as ways of describing continuous data that are mixtures of signal and noise.
These two ways of representing continuous dynamic processes lead
to powerful methods of signal analysis. However, we indicated
that the analysis procedures are generally performed not upon specimen functions of the original continuous processes, processes that
are essentially infinite in duration, but upon finite segments of
their sampled versions. The results and conclusions drawn from
these analyses are then used to draw inferences about the original
processes: the waveform of a response, its spectrum, its correlation with another response, its dependence upon a stimulus parameter, etc. The question is, how good are these inferences?
Although we made some effort to point out the legitimacy of the
procedures under many circumstances of practical interest, it is
important that we establish their validity somewhat more securely.
Once this is done we can examine specific applications of covariance functions and spectral analysis in more depth and detail.
This will permit us in addition to move to related methods of
signal analysis, such as coherence functions, which also have found
applicability in studying the relationships between pairs of processes. Finally, these methods are applicable not only to the
study of continuous processes such as the EEG but also form the
basis for the analysis of certain aspects of single and multiple
unit activity. Thus an understanding of how continuous processes
are analyzed forms a basis for studying unit activity.

3.2. DISCRETE FOURIER REPRESENTATIONS
OF CONTINUOUS PROCESSES

At the outset it is important to state a basic attribute of band-limited signals that is of fundamental importance: Whether periodic or not, such signals must be infinite in duration. This fact follows directly from the properties of the Fourier transform for continuous signals. On the other hand, the properties of the Fourier transform also guarantee that the spectrum of a finite duration signal, such as a segment of an infinite duration signal, cannot be band-limited even when the infinite duration signal is. This means that there is an inherent contradiction built into our procedures for analyzing infinite duration signals from their finite segments. The contradiction is only resolved when the infinite duration signal is truly periodic. In all other cases we are forced to settle for errors of estimation. The sampling procedure does not alleviate these errors but introduces problems of its own, the kinds of problems we deal with here.

Although it may be a fiction, we have assumed that the processes we are studying are stationary mixtures of signals and noise with at least the noise being a random process. The analysis procedures are by necessity performed upon their finite duration segments. And here we invoke the next assumption, a true fiction. This is that the finite duration segment is a single period of a periodic specimen function. As objectionable as this might seem at first, it does no real harm since we have no knowledge of the specimen function's behavior outside this observed interval. Because of stationarity, the statistical behavior of the specimen function outside this observed interval is not likely to be much different. Thus we are not disregarding any information that we have concerning the specimen's behavior. In the first chapter we assumed that the repetition period was equal to the time of observation T. Other periodicity assumptions are also possible. If we want, we can consider the repetition period to be longer than T, T' say, by padding out the observed segment with a zero amplitude data segment lasting $T' - T$ sec. In a sense this is falsifying the data, but we know exactly how we have falsified it and we can take this into consideration in the subsequent analyses in order to avoid arriving at erroneous conclusions. Padding out the data with zero amplitude segments is a routine procedure when dealing with the estimation of the covariance functions. In this case, as we shall see, it is convenient to make $T' = 2T$. For the moment, however, let the repetition period be T. Let us keep in mind, then, the fact that we have forced periodicity upon the process and that for practical purposes we can make this periodicity length T or longer. Later on we shall use a $2T$ repetition period to deal with autocovariance function estimation.

In Chapter 1 we introduced the Fourier series representation for a T-continuous periodic signal and showed that if the signal were band-limited, its waveform could be completely represented by a finite number of parameters. Specifically, if the period of the signal is T and its bandwidth is F, then $N = 2FT$ terms are involved in either the real or complex Fourier series representation. It was also demonstrated that the signal could be completely represented by N consecutive sample amplitudes spaced Δ sec apart where $\Delta = 1/2F$ sec. The Fourier and time sample representations are closely related, the relationship between the two involving what is called the discrete Fourier transform. We introduce it here and show that in the bandwidth-limited situation, it leads to the same Fourier coefficients as would be obtained from a Fourier series representation of the original T-continuous signal.

We start with a single T sec segment of a band-limited signal which we consider to have period T. We obtain N samples of this signal at times Δ sec apart starting at the beginning of the segment, $t = 0$. Using these samples we can partially reconstruct the original signal by means of weighted sinc functions. The partial representation is

$$x(t) \simeq \sum_{t°=0}^{N-1} x(t°\Delta) \frac{\sin[\pi(t - t°\Delta)/\Delta]}{\pi(t - t°\Delta)/\Delta} \tag{3.1}$$

The reason for the reconstruction being partial is that we have ignored the tails of the weighted sinc functions outside the T sec segments. We can, however, insert them because of the assumed periodicity of $x(t)$. The complete reconstruction takes in all the weighted sinc functions throughout time:

$$x(t) = \sum_{t°=-\infty}^{\infty} x(t°\Delta)\ \frac{\sin[\pi(t - t°\Delta)/\Delta]}{\pi(t - t°\Delta)/\Delta} \tag{3.2}$$

This now holds for all t. Now let us take the complex Fourier series representation of a single period from 0 to $T = N\Delta$:

$$X_T(n) = \frac{1}{T} \int_0^T \sum_{t°=-\infty}^{\infty} x(t°\Delta)\ \frac{\sin[\pi(t - t°\Delta)/\Delta]}{\pi(t - t°\Delta)/\Delta}\ \exp(-j2\pi nt/T)\ dt$$

$$= \frac{1}{T} \sum_{t°=-\infty}^{\infty} x(t°\Delta) \int_0^T \frac{\sin[\pi(t - t°\Delta)/\Delta]}{\pi(t - t°\Delta)/\Delta}\ \exp(-j2\pi nt/T)\ dt$$

$$\tag{3.3}$$

This is actually a simple equation to deal with, given the periodicity of $x(t)$. Because of periodicity we have $x[(N + t°)\Delta] = x(t°\Delta)$. When this fact is taken into account for values of $t°$ outside the range 0 to $N - 1$, Eq. (3.3) simplifies, after some elementary substitutions, to

$$X_T(n) = \frac{\Delta}{T} \sum_{t°=0}^{N-1} x(t°\Delta)\ \exp(-j2\pi nt°\Delta) \int_{-\infty}^{\infty} \frac{\sin \pi x}{\pi x} \cos \frac{2\pi nx}{N}\ dx \tag{3.4}$$

As long as $n/N < 1$, which is true for the band-limited signal, this further reduces to

$$X_T(n) = \frac{1}{N} \sum_{t°=0}^{N-1} x(t°\Delta)\ \exp(-j2\pi nt°/N) \tag{3.5}$$

The original integration operation upon $x(t)$ has thus been modified into a summation operation upon $x(t°\Delta)$.

This is an opportune time to reconsider the steps that led us to Eq. (3.5). Our data specimen was a T sec segment of an ongoing process band-limited to real frequencies between 0 and $1/2\Delta$. We assumed, solely for the purpose of analysis, that this segment was one period of a periodic process. We then sampled the segment at intervals Δ sec apart to obtain an N sample representation of it. Because of the bandwidth limitation and the periodicity assumption, we need only N Fourier components at complex frequencies spaced equally from $-1/2\Delta$ to $1/2\Delta$ to represent the data completely. Now, in the majority of situations, the data do not arise from a periodic process but are specimens of an aperiodic process with power distributed at all frequencies up to $1/2\Delta$ (or at all the complex frequencies between $-1/2\Delta$ and $1/2\Delta$). Hence, our periodicity assumption has in a sense falsified the data. It has produced a representation of the signal requiring only N Fourier components. This is not a serious falsification, however. What it amounts to is saying that all the frequency components in the narrow frequency band between $(n - 1/2)/N\Delta$ and $(n + 1/2)/N\Delta$, a band $1/N\Delta$ wide, are considered to be concentrated at the single frequency $n/N\Delta$, and represented by $X_T(n)$. $X_T(n)$ is therefore essentially the product of the frequency density of the Fourier representation times the incremental bandwidth $1/N\Delta$. The density in that frequency region can then be obtained by dividing $X_T(n)$ by $1/N\Delta$. This gives

$$N\Delta X_T(n) = \Delta \sum_{t°=0}^{N-1} x(t°\Delta) \exp(-j2\pi n t°/N) \tag{3.6}$$

Δ is a constant independent of the duration of the specimen and plays only a minor role in the reconstruction of $x(t)$ from the Fourier representation. For this reason we define the discrete Fourier transform (DFT) of $x(t)$ as $X_N(n)$:

$$X_N(n) = NX_T(n) = \sum_{t°=0}^{N-1} x(t°\Delta) \exp(-j2\pi n t°/N) \tag{3.7}$$

The elimination of the factor N that appeared in Eq. (3.5) means that in order to recover $x(t°\Delta)$ from $X_N(n)$, we must define the inverse DFT as

$$x(t^\circ\Delta) = \frac{1}{N} \sum_{n=-N/2}^{N/2-1} X_N(n) \, \exp(j2\pi nt^\circ/N) \tag{3.8}$$

To see this, we multiply both sides of Eq. (3.7) by $\exp(j2\pi nu^\circ/N)$ and sum over all the values of n between $-N/2$ and $(N/2) - 1$, the range of the complex Fourier expansion. We obtain

$$\sum_{n=-N/2}^{N/2-1} X_N(n) \, \exp(j2\pi nu^\circ/N)$$

$$= \sum_{n=-N/2}^{N/2-1} \left[\sum_{t^\circ=1}^{N-1} x(t^\circ\Delta) \, \exp(-j2\pi nt^\circ/N) \right] \exp(j2\pi nu^\circ/N) \tag{3.9}$$

We then interchange the order of the two summations on the right-hand side and consider the summation with respect to n. This is

$$\sum_{n=-N/2}^{N/2-1} \exp[j2\pi n(u^\circ - t^\circ)/N]$$

For any value of t° different from u°, this summation is zero (as can be seen by using the summation formula for a geometric series). But when $t^\circ = u^\circ$, the summation is N. Thus, Eq. (3.9) reduces to Eq. (3.8) which is what we wished to show.

Equations (3.7) and (3.8) are a discrete Fourier transform pair and have been justified on a heuristic basis. Later in the chapter we shall establish the validity of the relation somewhat more carefully, paying closer attention to the properties of continuous processes. It is also worth noting that the definition of the DFT varies from author to author according to the handling of the factor N. The definition adopted here seems to be the most common one.

The cosine and sine versions of the DFT are given by

$$A_N(n) = 2\sum_{t^\circ=0}^{N-1} x(t^\circ\Delta) \, \cos(2\pi nt^\circ/N) \tag{3.9a}$$

$$B_N(n) = 2\sum_{t°=0}^{N-1} x(t°\Delta)\ \sin(2\pi n t°/N) \qquad (3.9b)$$

These are associated with the complex relations $A_N(n) = X_N(n) +$ $X_N(-n)$ and $B_N(n) = j[X_N(n) - X_N(-n)]$. It is worthwhile pointing again that $X_N(n)$, the direct DFT, is a periodic function of n, period N, and its inverse $x(t°\Delta)$ is a periodic function of time. That is, $X_N(-N + n) = X_N(N + n)$, etc. and $x[(-N + t°)\Delta] =$ $x[(N + t°)\Delta]$, etc. In the previous chapters we considered the index for the direct DFT to run from $-N/2$ to $(N/2) - 1$. It is clear now that because of the periodicity it is equally satisfactory to consider n to range from 0 to $N - 1$.

The periodicity of the direct and inverse DFT emphasizes the fact that when the DFT is applied to an N sample sequence of data points, it is done under the assumption that the data arise from a periodic process, period N. Sometimes the period can be considered to be greater than N by appending or "padding" a sequence of zero amplitude samples, $N' - N$ of them so that the overall length of the resulting sequence is N'. This padding with zeros is a technique commonly employed in digital filtering and in the estimation of the acvf and spectrum of a specimen function, as we shall see later. The resulting sequence of sample values can be considered to arise from a periodic band-limited signal $\tilde{x}(t)$, period N', which is zero at $L = N' - N$ consecutive sample times. The DFT of this signal is

$$\tilde{X}_{N'}(m) = \sum_{t°=0}^{N'-1} \tilde{x}(t°\Delta)\ \exp(-j2\pi m t°/N') \qquad (3.10)$$

Because of the fact that $\tilde{x}(t) = x(t)$ for values of $t°$ ranging from 0 to $N - 1$ and is zero for values of $t°$ ranging from N to $N' - 1$, we have

$$\tilde{X}_{N'}(m) = \sum_{t°=0}^{N-1} x(t°\Delta)\ \exp(-j2\pi m t°/N') \qquad (3.11)$$

109

An especially important case is $N' = 2N$. Here we have

$$\tilde{X}_{2N}(m) = \sum_{t°=0}^{N-1} x(t°\Delta) \exp(-j2\pi mt°/2N) \tag{3.12}$$

Because of the $2N$ periodicity of $\tilde{x}(t)$, the values of n range from $-N$ to $N - 1$ instead of from $-N/2$ to $(N/2) - 1$. If we examine Eqs. (3.7) and (3.10), we see that when $m = 2n$, i.e., it is an even number or zero,

$$\tilde{X}_{2N}(2n) = \sum_{t°=0}^{N-1} x(t°\Delta) \exp(-j2\pi nt°/N) = X_N(n) \tag{3.13}$$

This shows that the even index terms for $\tilde{X}_{2N}(n)$ are completely determined by the values of the $X_N(n)$. But what about the odd index terms? Some reflection on this reveals that these terms arise solely because of the padding procedure. They are necessary to force $\tilde{x}(t)$ to be zero at the sample times between N and $N' - 1$. They provide no additional information about $x(t)$, but, interestingly enough, are an essential ingredient for obtaining an estimate of the acvf from the estimated spectrum. This point will be discussed later. Finally, it is easy to see that similar results would be obtained if N' were any other multiple value of N.

3.3. ALIASING

As we discussed in Chapter 1, the necessity for sampling a signal at a rate compatible with its bandwidth, the Nyquist rate, is vital to a meaningful interpretation of a spectral analysis. Here we wish to establish this point somewhat more securely and show in what way improper sampling, sampling at too low a rate for a given bandwidth, obscures and falsifies spectral analysis.

Let us begin by considering the continuous signal $x(t)$ to be periodic T, and to have an unlimited bandwidth. The Fourier series representation for such a signal is given by

$$x(t) = \sum_{n=-\infty}^{\infty} X_T(n) \, \exp(j2\pi nt/T) \tag{3.14}$$

where

$$X_T(n) = \frac{1}{T} \int_0^T x(t) \, \exp(-j2\pi nt/T) \, dt \tag{3.15}$$

We wish to deal with the sampled representation $x(t°\Delta)$ and so we sample $x(t)$ every Δ sec, obtaining N samples such that $T = N\Delta$. We then blindly take the DFT,

$$x^{\dagger}(n) = \sum_{t°=0}^{N-1} x(t°\Delta) \, \exp(-j2\pi nt°/N) \tag{3.16}$$

We have used the dagger symbol to indicate our suspicion that something may be amiss in this representation, i.e., that $X_T^{\dagger}(n)$ may not be the same as $X_T(n)$. That such is the case may be seen by substituting for each sample value its Fourier series expansion as given by Eq. (3.14):

$$x^{\dagger}(n) = \sum_{t°=0}^{N-1} \left[\sum_{m=-\infty}^{\infty} X_T(m) \, \exp(j2\pi mt°\Delta/T) \, \exp(-j2\pi nt°/N) \right]$$

$$= \sum_{t°=0}^{N-1} \sum_{m=-\infty}^{\infty} X_T(m) \, \exp[j2\pi(m-n)t°/N] \tag{3.17}$$

The exponential term here has the important property that when $m - n = 0$ or some integer multiple of N, the summation over $t°$ is equal to N; otherwise it is identically 0. That is, for fixed m,

$$\sum_{t°=0}^{N-1} \exp[j2\pi(m-n)t°/N] = \begin{cases} N, & m = kN + n \\ 0, & m \neq kN + n \end{cases} \tag{3.18}$$

where k is an integer. Using this fact in Eq. (3.17), it can be seen that

$$x^{\dagger}(n) = N \sum_{k=-\infty}^{\infty} X_T(kN + n) \tag{3.19}$$

111

This means that each term in the DFT of $x(t)$ is the sum of a possibly infinite set of Fourier coefficients associated with the higher frequency components in $x(t)$. The higher frequency components are those corresponding to frequencies that are greater than N by an amount kN. If $x(t)$ has no Fourier series components for values of n equal to or greater than $N/2$ (corresponding to frequencies $1/2\Delta$ or greater), $X_N^{\dagger}(n) = NX_T(n) = X_N(n)$; otherwise, $X_N^{\dagger}(n) \neq NX_T(n)$. This means that the DFT for $x(t)$ yields correct results only if $x(t)$ is band-limited to frequencies below $1/2\Delta$. When $x(t)$ has a greater bandwidth, the high frequency components add to the low frequency ones, an effect that is called aliasing because the high frequency components are misrepresented or misinterpreted as low frequency ones. Once aliasing occurs, there is no way to properly sort out the $X_T(n)$ components from the $X_N^{\dagger}(n)$. This is why the cutoff frequency F of the analog prefilter must be matched to the sampling rate such that $F \leq 1/2\Delta$. It is essential to the proper analysis of continuous data by sampling techniques. The numerical value of n corresponding to the highest frequency representable by the sampling procedure is $N/2$. As shown previously, it is determined by the relation $n/T = 1/2\Delta$. To see the effect of aliasing more clearly, consider Fig. 3.1 which shows a

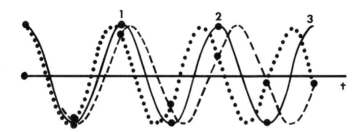

Fig. 3.1. A cosine wave of frequency F (solid line) sampled at its Nyquist rate. A higher frequency (dotted) wave, frequency F + a, is shown sampled at the same rate. At the sample times it is indistinguishable from a lower frequency (dashed) wave, frequency F - a.

cosine wave of frequency $F = 1/2\Delta$ being sampled at the negative and positive peaks. If the frequency of the wave increases a little above F to $F + a$ (dotted line), sine waves of frequency $F + a$ and $F - a$ can be drawn through the sampling points equally well. This gives us reason to suspect that a wave of real frequency $F + a$ will, after sampling, be confused with a wave of real frequency $F - a$. With this in mind, let us examine Eq. (3.19) when n has a value of $(N/2) - i$. Then all the $X_T(kN + n)$ such that

$$kN + n = kN + (N/2) - i = (k + 1/2)N - i$$

will contribute to the terms $X_N^{\dagger}[(N/2) - i]$. A real frequency term at $(N/2) - i$ corresponds to complex frequency terms $X_T[(N/2) - i]$ and $X_T[(-N/2) + i]$. The aliases of $X_T[(N/2) - i]$ are at frequencies ... , $(-3N/2) - i$, $(-N/2) - i$, $(3N/2) - i$, ... while the aliases of $X_T[(-N/2) + i]$ are at frequencies ... , $(-3N/2) + i$, $(N/2) + i$, $(3N/2) + i$, ... If we group these aliasing terms in pairs, one term from each sequence, we find that $X_T[(-N/2) - i]$ pairs with $X_T[(N/2) + i]$ to give a real frequency term at $(N/2) + i$. Similarly, there are real frequency terms at $(3N/2) + i$, $(3N/2) - i$, $(5N/2) + i$, $(5N/2) - i$, etc. Thus a real frequency data component at $(N/2) - i$ will have alias contributions from whichever of these higher frequency terms that are present in the data input to the ADC. In effect the original Fourier representation of $x(t)$ has been folded in accordion fashion about frequencies that are multiples of $1/2\Delta$ and collapsed into the frequency region extending from 0 to $1/2\Delta$ which is also called the folding frequency. (Fig. 3.2)

It is of some interest that aliasing effects can also enter into sampled representations of data that are band-limited to the Nyquist frequency. We have seen previously how the discrete Fourier transform is a completely adequate representation of a continuous periodic band-limited signal as long as the signal samples are taken frequently enough to eliminate the possibility of aliasing. But in actuality, few of the data one analyzes are

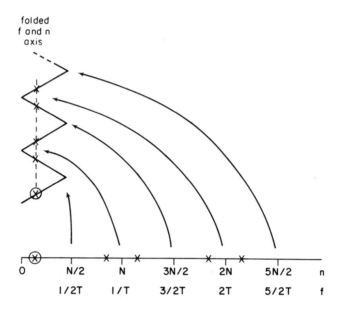

Fig. 3.2. The accordionlike folding of the frequency (or n)
axis due to sampling of a continuous signal. Frequency components
of the original signal marked with x's on the f axis are interpreted
in the sampled version as belonging to the lowest frequency, an
encircled x.

periodic or band-limited, although the latter condition can be
approached as closely as desired by analog prefiltering prior to
sampling. Periodicity is another matter. Even when periodic
stimulation is employed and the response or signal component of
the data is periodic, the remainder, the noise, is not. Periodicity is then lacking in the data. What the data analysis procedure does in this situation is to effectively create periodic data
from the T sec data segment we have available to study. That is,
we analyze the T sec segment as though it originated from a process with period T or greater. This introduces some complications
which we need to consider. The "periodicized" process created
from a T sec segment of data (1) is generally not band-limited
even if the original data are, (2) can contain frequency components, apart from aliases, that are not present in the original

data. Let us deal with these complications in order, using as an illustration a signal that is both band-limited and periodic, a cosine wave whose period is $3T/8$, T being the period of its observation. The periodicized version of this signal is shown in Fig. 3.3. It is clear that there are discontinuities in the

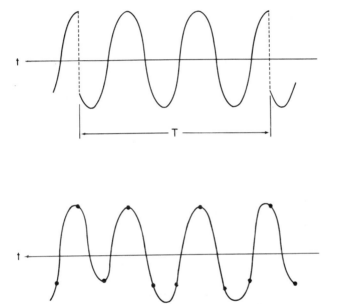

Fig. 3.3. Top, a periodicized segment of a cosine wave. T is the observation time and $3T/8$ the period of the wave. Note the discontinuities at 0 and T. Bottom, a continuous and periodic band-limited wave drawn through the sample points $\Delta = T/16$ sec apart.

periodicized signal which guarantee that it will not be band-limited. In fact, it may be stated that unless the original signal has rather special properties, i.e., that its amplitude and time derivatives at $t = 0$ are the same as those at $t = T$, there will be discontinuities in the periodic waveform and its derivatives that guarantee that the periodicized signal will not be band-limited. We know that if we sample this process, every Δ sec such that $T = N\Delta$, we are sure to encounter aliasing, its severity depending upon the sampling rate. If we apply the DFT to the samples and treat the resulting Fourier coefficients as though there were no aliasing involved, we effectively consider the data as having arisen from a periodic band-limited process, i.e., one that has no discontinuities of any kind at the ends of the interval. This recreated signal is also shown in Fig. 3.3 for $N = 16$, $\Delta = T/16$. This means that the sampling has distorted the original data, primarily at the ends of the interval. The high frequency components associated with the discontinuities at 0 and T have been aliased into the spectral representation. The numeric results obtained from the DFT show the results of this aliasing. Both covariance and spectral analysis of the data can be affected. Fortunately, the larger N is, the smaller the end effects tend to become. They also diminish as the severity of the discontinuities diminishes.

3.4. LEAKAGE

A. FOURIER SERIES

Besides the aliasing that is introduced into the DFT representation of a time-limited segment of a nonperiodic signal, we must deal with another form of signal misrepresentation, referred to as spectral leakage. It occurs with all aperiodic data and even with periodic band-limited data whose period is not integrally related to the time of observation. In the Fourier analysis procedures, the frequency composition of the data is computed to be a set of frequency constituents harmonically related to $1/T$, the fundamental of the time of observation. The frequency components that are closest to the original frequencies in the data contribute most to the analysis, but more remote frequencies may also be interpreted as being present when in fact they are not. To see a specific example of this, consider the signal to be the cosine wave whose period is $3T/8$ (Fig. 3.3). We compute the Fourier series representation of this signal first because it avoids all aliasing effects. The Fourier series coefficients are given by

$$X_T(n) = \frac{1}{T} \int_0^T \cos\left(2\pi\frac{8}{3T} t\right) \exp\left(-j2\pi\frac{n}{T} t\right) dt$$

for $-(N-1)/2 \leq n \leq (N-1)/2$.

$$A_T(n) = \frac{2}{T} \int_0^T \cos\left(2\pi\frac{8}{3T} t\right)\cos\left(2\pi\frac{n}{T} t\right) dt \qquad (3.20)$$

$$B_T(n) = \frac{2}{T} \int_0^T \cos\left(2\pi\frac{8}{3T} t\right)\sin\left(2\pi\frac{n}{T} t\right) dt$$

for $0 \leq n \leq (N-1)/2$. The values for $A_T(n)$ and $B_T(n)$ are obtained by standard integration formulas and are tabulated in Table 3.1 for $n = 1, 2, \ldots 8$.

TABLE 3.1

FOURIER SERIES AND DFT
COEFFICIENTS FOR $\cos(2\pi 8t/3T)$

	$A_T(n)$	$A_N(n)$		$B_T(n)$	$B_N(n)$		$\lvert X_T(n)\rvert$	$\lvert X_N(n)\rvert$	
N		16	256		16	256		16	256
n									
1	-.120	-.017	-.114	-.078	-.085	-.078	.143	.086	.139
2	-.236	-.133	-.230	-.307	-.320	-.307	.387	.347	.384
3	.389	.493	.395	.758	.738	.758	.852	.888	.855
4	.083	.188	.089	.215	.187	.215	.230	.265	.232
5	.041	.147	.047	.134	.098	.133	.140	.177	.141
6	.026	.133	.031	.099	.055	.099	.102	.144	.104
7	.018	.127	.024	.080	.025	.080	.082	.129	.083
8	.013	.125	.019	.067	.000	.067	.068	.125	.070

Inspection of the Fourier components as determined by
Eq. (3.20) reveals that the analysis has decomposed the original
cosine wave into frequency components at all values of n. None
of these corresponds to the frequency of the original signal which
lies slightly below $n = 3$, but the coefficients are largest at
$n = 3$ and next largest at $n = 2$. There is a gradual diminution of
component amplitudes as n departs from these values. What has
happened is that the power of the original signal has been dispersed or "leaked" out from the original signal frequency into the
neighboring frequencies of the Fourier analysis. No spurious
power is added by the analysis, for if all the $A_T(n)$ and $B_T(n)$
were squared and summed, their total contribution would equal that
of the original signal in the T sec interval. The net effect,
however, is a rather serious misrepresentation of the original
signal whose spectrum is a single real frequency component at
$8/3T$. The cause of the misrepresentation is that only a finite
length of the signal segment has been used for the analysis. It
is possible to show that the Fourier representation of a T sec
segment of data results from a convolution of the spectrum of the
original, infinite duration signal with the sinc function
$\sin(\pi nt/T)/(\pi nt/T)$. To see how this comes about, we refer back
to the expression for $X_T(n)$ in Eq. (3.20) where we replace the
illustrative frequency $8/3T$ by the general frequency f so that
$x(t) = \cos 2\pi ft$. We can calculate the $A_T(n)$ and $B_T(n)$ for this
signal and find them to be

$$A_T(n) = \frac{1}{T}\left[\frac{\sin 2\pi T\{f - (n/T)\}}{2\pi\{f - (n/T)\}} + \frac{\sin 2\pi T\{f + (n/T)\}}{2\pi\{f + (n/T)\}}\right]$$

$$B_T(n) = -\frac{1}{T}\left[\frac{\cos 2\pi T\{f - (n/T)\} - 1}{2\pi\{f - (n/T)\}} - \frac{\cos 2\pi T\{f + (n/T)\} - 1}{2\pi\{f + (n/T)\}}\right]$$

$$(3.21)$$

The terms containing $f - n/T$ and $f + n/T$ are a manifestation of
the fact that cosine and sine waves consist of positive and negative complex frequency terms. We are considering real (positive)

frequency data and so both f and n are greater than 0. In most cases f will be sufficiently greater than 0 to make the second term of Eq. (3.21) negligible compared to the first. This results in the approximation

$$A_T(n) \simeq \frac{1}{T} \; \frac{\sin 2\pi T\{f - (n/T)\}}{2\pi\{f - (n/T)\}}$$

$$B_T(n) \simeq -\frac{1}{T}\left[\frac{\cos 2\pi T\{f - (n/T)\} - 1}{2\pi\{f - (n/T)\}}\right]$$

(3.22)

From this we obtain the spectral power at real frequency n/T:

$$\left|X_T(n)\right|^2 + \left|X_T(-n)\right|^2 = \frac{1}{2}\left[\left|A_T(n)\right|^2 + \left|B_T(n)\right|^2\right]$$

$$\simeq \frac{1}{2}\left[\frac{\sin \pi T\{f - (n/T)\}}{\pi T\{f - (n/T)\}}\right]^2 \qquad (3.23)$$

The total power of $x(t) = \cos 2\pi f t$ is 1/2 and is concentrated solely at frequency f. The Fourier analysis has in effect dispersed or leaked this power out into neighboring frequencies that are harmonically related to $1/T$. This also means that if one is interested in estimating the spectral component of the data at a particular frequency, there will be included in the estimate a contribution from nearby spectral components that have had their power leaked into the frequency where the estimate is being made. The weighting factor for these extraneous contributions is that given by the bracketed term in Eq. (3.23). It shows that the larger T becomes, the smaller is the frequency range over which leakage is a significant factor.

Leakage may also magnify the undesirable effects of 60 Hz or other single frequency artifacts in the data. These may arise from a variety of causes: ineffective electrical shielding, stray coupling of stimulus frequencies into the responses, and so on. An important attribute of a signal with a line spectrum, one expressed by delta functions in the spectrum, is that a rather substantial amount of power is confined to an infinitesimally narrow

frequency band rather than being spread out over a broader range
of frequencies. It is this concentration of power that can be so
potent in producing leakage into the estimates of power density
in the neighboring regions of the spectrum. The leakage occurs,
as Eq. (3.23) indicates, if the line component is not exactly located at a harmonic of the fundamental analysis interval. To see
this, suppose a spurious line component is located midway between
adjacent harmonic frequencies of the analysis interval and that
the rms strength of the line is σ_a. The leakage of this component
into the neighboring frequency terms is well approximated by
Eq. (3.23) as long as the line is reasonably far from 0 frequency.
It can be seen that the larger N is, the narrower will be the frequency range over which significant amounts of leakage occur. Because of the side lobes of the sinc function, leakage effects can
occur between rather widely spaced frequencies when σ_a is large.
It is also true that the closer the frequency of a line component
is to a harmonic of the analysis interval, the smaller is the leakage effect. The most generally useful way of minimizing leakage
is by means of spectral "windowing" techniques of which more will
be said later. These techniques, which are another form of linear
filtering, have the effect of estimating the spectrum in a way
that greatly minimizes the side lobe contributions to the spectral
estimate.

B. DISCRETE FOURIER TRANSFORMS

Leakage is not alleviated by resort to the DFT. Rather,
the situation persists and is also overlayed with aliasing effects
so that the resulting data representation contains both, inextric-
ably combined. To see this we refer again to the signal
$x(t) = \cos 2\pi 8t/3T$ and represent it by its DFT as given by
Eqs. (3.7) and (3.9), rewritten here for $N = 16$:

$$X_N(n) = \sum_{t°=0}^{15} \cos(2\pi t°/6) \exp(-j2\pi n t°/16) \qquad (3.24a)$$

$$A_N(n) = \sum_{t°=0}^{15} \cos(2\pi t°/6) \cos(2\pi n t°/16) \qquad (3.24b)$$

$$B_N(n) = \sum_{t°=0}^{15} \cos(2\pi t°/6) \sin(2\pi n t°/16) \qquad (3.24c)$$

In Table 3.1 we show the DFT coefficients for n ranging from 1 to 8 when there are two different sample intervals, the first being $T/16$ with $N = 16$, and the second $T/256$ with $N = 256$. The discrepancy between the tabulated values for either situation and those obtained from the continuous Fourier series expansion arises from the aliasing introduced by sampling. As the sampling interval becomes shorter, the discrepancy diminishes and what remains is the pure leakage effect. Again, what causes it is the finite length of the signal segment, N samples in duration. If we let $x(t) = \cos 2\pi ft$ and perform a calculation similar to that just done for the Fourier series, we find that power has leaked from frequency f into frequency n/N. The amount that has leaked is given by

$$\left|X_N(n)\right|^2 + \left|X_N(-n)\right|^2 = \frac{1}{2}\left[\left|A_N(n)\right|^2 + \left|B_N(n)\right|^2\right]$$

$$\approx \frac{1}{2}\left[\frac{\sin \pi N(f\Delta - n/N)}{N \sin \pi(f\Delta - n/N)}\right]^2 \qquad (3.25)$$

The approximation arises as before because of the fact that we have ignored the usually small terms involving $f + (n/N)$. From Eq. (3.25) we see that the leakage from frequency f into the nth component of the DFT has very nearly the same behavior as it had for the Fourier series representation. Thus leakage in the two cases is comparable although the leakage in the DFT tends to be the larger of the two because the denominator of Eq. (3.25) is smaller than that of Eq. (3.22).

Another aspect of leakage is associated with the presence of a constant dc component in the data. If only the spectrum of the data is of interest, leakage is not a factor because the steady component shows up only in the $n = 0$ term of the Fourier representation. But when one uses the spectrum as an intermediary step for obtaining an estimate of the acvf (or ccvf) of the data, then leakage does become a factor. Such a procedure is quite common when one employs the fast Fourier transform to first obtain the spectral estimate and then the acvf from it. The reason that leakage becomes a factor is that in this procedure it is necessary to pad out the original sequence of N data points with a sequence of zero amplitude samples, L of them if one wishes to estimate the acvf for lags up to $L\Delta$. This means that the DFT that one works with is

$$X_{N'}(n) = \sum_{t°=0}^{N-1} x(t°\Delta) \exp(-j2\pi nt°/N') \qquad (3.26)$$

The upper limit is $N - 1$ rather than $N' - 1$, $(N' = L + N)$, because the last L values of $x(t°\Delta)$ are taken to be 0. When $x(t)$ has an average value a, the contribution of this to $X_N(n)$ is

$$[X_{N'}(n)]_{dc} = a\sum_{t°=0}^{N-1} \exp(-j2\pi nt°/N') = \frac{a[1 - \exp(-j2\pi nN/N')]}{1 - \exp(-j2\pi n/N')} \qquad (3.27)$$

The contribution to the raw spectral estimate $[C_{xx}(n)]_{dc} = |[X_N(n)]_{dc}|^2$ follows directly. It is

$$\left| [X_{N'}(n)]_{dc} \right|^2 = a^2 \left[\frac{\sin(\pi nN/N')}{\sin(\pi n/N')} \right]^2 \qquad (3.28)$$

For $n = 0$, the result is $(aN)^2$ as is to be expected. If a data record of length $N = 1000$ were padded with 10 zeros to permit estimation of the acvf out to 10Δ, the dc leakage at $n = 1$ would be $100a^2$. If the record were padded with 100 zeros, the dc leakage at $n = 1$ would be $1.053 \times 10^4 a^2$. The effect obviously depends upon the strength of the dc term. In the second case, if

a is 5 times the amplitude of the real component at $n = 1$, one could expect an error in the spectral estimate amounting to about 24%, a rather serious matter. To eliminate leakage, a good procedure is to first remove the average value from the data before padding it with zeros.

3.5. TREND

Another effect that we need to be aware of is one that is brought about by the presence of very low frequency components in the data, frequencies that are less than that of the fundamental frequency of the analysis interval. Such components are referred to as producing trends in the data. These are progressive changes in the short term mean of the data, a mean that is calculated over a relatively small segment of the data. Trends may also be found in other properties of the data such as the variance and covariance functions, but here we are concerned only with trends in the mean and, more specifically, linear trends, i.e., those trends that can be described by data having the form $x(t) = bt + v(t)$, bt being the trend component and $v(t)$ the component one normally considers in a trend-free situation. It is also possible to take into account trends which are not linear (Otnes and Enochson, 1974) but here we are only interested in seeing how linear trends affect a spectrum analysis. When a linear trend is present in an N sample sequence of data, it will contribute to the DFT according to

$$[X_N(n)]_{trend} = \sum_{t°=0}^{N-1} bt° \exp(-j2\pi nt°/N) \tag{3.29}$$

The expression can be summed without difficulty. When n is small compared to N, we find that

$$\left[C_{xx}(n)\right]_{trend} = \left|\left[X_N(n)\right]_{trend}\right|^2 \approx (bN/2\pi n)^2 \tag{3.30}$$

In effect the trend leaks into the nearby low frequency components in a manner that is inversely proportional to n^2. Note that bN is the total trend in the data from the beginning to the end of the sequence. To eliminate contamination of the spectral estimates by trends, the trends should be estimated and removed before a spectrum analysis. Procedures for doing this are given in Otnes and Enochson (1974) and Blackman and Tukey (1958).

3.6. THE POWER SPECTRUM, GENERAL CONSIDERATIONS

When investigating the properties of samples of random variables, it is useful to characterize them by population statistics. In the case of a simple, univariate random variable, the mean is a measure of its location (from zero), and the variance is a measure of its dispersion about the mean. These two statistics are also of use when investigating random signals. The mean specifies a baseline about which the signal fluctuates. If the physical signal is an electrical one, then the mean corresponds to the dc level of the signal. The variance provides a measure of the magnitude of the signal's fluctuation about its mean. For electrical signals, the variance corresponds to the power of the ac component of the signal. While the mean and variance are useful and readily computed statistics, they provide no information concerning the temporal character of the fluctuation of a random signal. We cannot infer from them whether the signal's fluctuations are slow or rapid or whether they possess some rhythmicity or a high degree of irregularity. However, as we noted in Chapter 1, if the signal is wide sense stationary, such information can be provided by the power spectrum of the signal.

The power spectrum provides a statement of the average distribution of power of a signal with respect to frequency. If the signal varies slowly, then its power will be concentrated at low frequencies; if the signal tends to be rhythmic, then its power will be concentrated at the fundamental frequency of the rhythm, perhaps at its harmonic frequencies; if the signal lacks rhythmicity, then its power will be distributed over a broad range of frequencies.

A way of obtaining an estimate of the power spectrum of a signal at a given frequency is to pass the signal through a narrow band linear filter centered at the frequency of interest, and then to compute the variance (power) of the filter output. This operation can be performed at any frequency of interest. The variance of the output of the filter will be proportional to the amount of power in the signal at frequencies close to the filter center frequency. The variance can then be plotted as a function of the filter's center frequency and the resulting graph will be an approximate indication of the frequency distribution of the signal's power. This filtering approach was the traditional way of analyzing spectra before the advent of high speed digital computers. It is still useful conceptually although the mechanization of the filtering techniques has been changed drastically by the computer.

The concept of a power spectrum applies to both T-continuous and T-discrete signals. Because we are usually interested in continuous signals, we will begin with a discussion of the power spectra of wide sense stationary continuous signals. Then we move to consider more fully the computation and interpretation of power spectra from wide sense stationary sampled data. This is the representation of continuous signals that digital computers usually operate upon.

Illustrations of how a power spectrum characterizes the temporal behavior of a signal are provided in the following examples. First, consider an EEG recording from a subject in deep sleep (Fig. 3.4a). In such a case the EEG consists primarily of slowly fluctuating, high amplitude delta wave activity. Consequently, most of the power is concentrated at low frequencies and so the spectrum will be relatively large at those frequencies, and small elsewhere (Fig. 3.4b). As a second example, consider the EEG of an awake but resting subject. In this case the EEG may consist of primarily rhythmic, quasisinusoidal alpha wave activity in the 9 to 12 Hz frequency range (Fig. 3.5a). The associated power spectrum will have a peak in the 9 to 12 Hz range and be

125

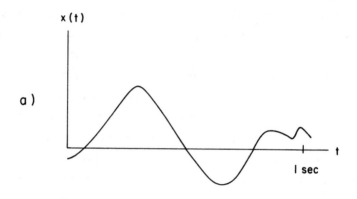

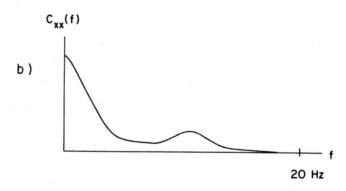

Fig. 3.4. (a) A hypothetical example of a low frequency EEG waveform recorded from an individual in deep sleep. (b) Power spectrum corresponding to the low frequency EEG process.

relatively small elsewhere (Fig. 3.5b). In the third example, consider the EEG of an alert subject. Here the EEG tends to consist of low amplitude waves with rapid, irregular fluctuations (Fig. 3.6a). No predominant rhythms or slow fluctuations are apparent. The corresponding power spectrum will tend to be broadly distributed over the frequency range of the EEG (Fig. 3.6b), a range which extends to an upper frequency of about 30 to 50 Hz.

x(t)

a)

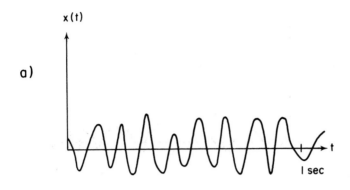

I sec

$C_{xx}(f)$

b)

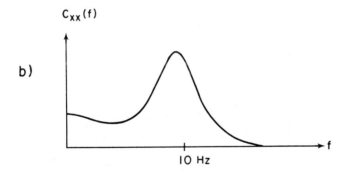

IO Hz

*Fig. 3.5. (a) A hypothetical example of EEG alpha activity.
(b) Power spectrum corresponding to an EEG process with pronounced
alpha activity.*

The three foregoing examples illustrate how the power spectrum provides a characterization of the "average" temporal behavior
of a random signal. But it does not uniquely specify the signal it
is derived from. One cannot reconstruct the signal given only its
power spectrum because the power spectrum does not preserve the
phase information in the signal. In effect, the spectrum specifies

127

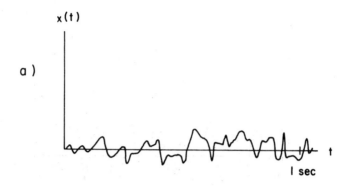

a)

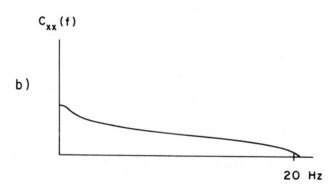

b)

Fig. 3.6. (a) A hypothetical example of rapid, irregularly fluctuating EEG recorded from an alert individual. (b) Power spectrum corresponding to the rapid, irregularly fluctuating EEG.

the average strength of a signal at each frequency. The average strength at a given frequency reflects both the amount of time during which there is activity at that frequency and the strength of that activity. For example, consider Fig. 3.7 which illustrates both a persistent, relatively low amplitude rhythmic random signal (a), and a signal in which relatively high amplitude bursts of rhythmic activity occur irregularly (b). The magnitudes of the

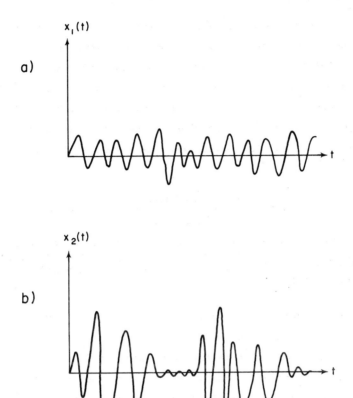

Fig. 3.7. Hypothetical example of (a) a low amplitude
random process with persistent rhythmic activity, and (b) a
random process with irregularly occurring bursts of high
amplitude rhythmic activity.

power spectra corresponding to the two signals may be the same
near the frequency of the rhythm. Although the signal in Fig.
3.7b has higher amplitudes during the bursts of rhythmic activity,
the average power near the frequency of the rhythm is no greater
than that of the signal in Fig. 3.7a because the duration of the
rhythmic activity in (b) is less than in (a).

3.7. POWER SPECTRUM OF CONTINUOUS RANDOM SIGNALS

In the above discussion we presented the concept of the power spectrum from an empirical point of view. We held that the variance of the output signal of a narrow band linear filter provides a measure of the power of the components of the input signal whose frequencies are in the pass band of the filter. We now examine this statement more closely, taking a mathematical point of view. Consider Fig. 3.8. $x(t)$ is a wide sense stationary ran-

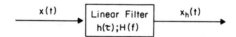

$$x(t) \longrightarrow \boxed{\begin{array}{c} \text{Linear Filter} \\ h(\tau); H(f) \end{array}} \xrightarrow{x_h(t)}$$

Fig. 3.8. Block diagram of a linear filtering operation. The input signal is x(t) and the output is $x_h(t)$. The filter transfer function is H(f) and the corresponding weighting function is h(τ).

dom signal whose power spectrum is of interest to us. For simplicity, we assume that the mean value of $x(t)$ is zero. $H(f)$ is the transfer function and $h(\tau)$ the corresponding impulse response (weighting function) of the linear filter used to obtain a spectral estimate of $x(t)$. We shall compute the variance of the filter's output $x_h(t)$ and relate it to $x(t)$ as well as to $h(\tau)$ and $H(f)$ and to the power spectrum of $x(t)$, $C_{xx}(f)$.

We first state the output signal in terms of the convolution relation between output and input, established in Chapter 2:

$$x_h(t) = \int_{-\infty}^{\infty} h(\tau)x(t - \tau) \, d\tau \qquad (3.31)$$

The variance of the output can be expressed in terms of the variance of the input signal and the filter impulse response function, as given above. Since the output, like the input, has zero mean,

$$\text{var}\left[x_h(t)\right] = \text{E}\left[x_h^2(t)\right] = \text{E}\left\{\left[\int_{-\infty}^{\infty} h(\tau)x(t - \tau) \, d\tau\right]^2\right\}$$

$$(3.32)$$

Now the square of an integral can be expressed as the product of two identical integrals, differing only in the symbols used to denote the variable over which the integration is performed. Then we have

$$\text{var}\Big[x_h(t)\Big] = \text{E}\left[\int_{-\infty}^{\infty} h(\tau)x(t - \tau)\ d\tau \int_{-\infty}^{\infty} h(u)x(t - u)\ du\right] \tag{3.33}$$

Since the averaging operation is with respect to the random variable $x(t)$, Eq. (3.33) can be rearranged so that the averaging operation is performed prior to integration over τ and u.

$$\text{var}\Big[x_h(t)\Big] = \int_{-\infty}^{\infty} h(\tau)\ d\tau \int_{-\infty}^{\infty} h(u)\ \text{E}[x(t - \tau)x(t - u)]\ du \tag{3.34}$$

$\text{E}[x(t - \tau)x(t - u)]$ is the autocovariance function (acvf) of $x(t)$. Since $x(t)$ is wide sense stationary, the acvf is a function only of the difference between τ and u. Denote the acvf by $c_{xx}(t)$ and substitute $c_{xx}(\tau - u)$ into Eq. (3.34). This gives

$$\text{var}\Big[x_h(t)\Big] = \int_{-\infty}^{\infty} h(\tau)\ d\tau \int_{-\infty}^{\infty} h(u)c_{xx}(\tau - u)\ du \tag{3.35}$$

Equation (3.35) indicates that the variance of $x_h(t)$, the filter output, is determined solely by the filter characteristics and the second-order statistics (acvf) of the input signal. However, Eq. (3.35) does not show clearly just how the filter's action upon the input signal determines the variance of $x_h(t)$. This can be brought out if Eq. (3.35) is expressed in terms of the frequency response of the filter and the spectrum of the signal as we shall do in the next step. But some comments upon this step are first in order. Up to this point we have used a deductive argument to arrive at Eq. (3.35). We have assumed nothing about the nature or even the existence of the power spectrum. We have only assumed that the input process is stationary and that it has the acvf $c_{xx}(t)$. We now make use of the fact, first mentioned in Chapter 1, that the power spectrum and the acvf of a wide sense stationary process constitute a Fourier transform pair. The power spectrum is the direct Fourier transform of the acvf, and the acvf is the inverse Fourier transform of the power spectrum. The latter is indicated below, with the power spectrum of $x(t)$ denoted by $C_{xx}(f)$.

$$c_{xx}(t) = \int_{-\infty}^{\infty} C_{xx}(f) \exp(j2\pi ft) \, df \tag{3.36}$$

Substitution of Eq. (3.36) into Eq. (3.35) yields an expression which relates the variance of the filter output to the power spectrum of the input signal:

$$\text{var } x_h(t) = \int_{-\infty}^{\infty} h(\tau) \, d\tau \int_{-\infty}^{\infty} h(u) \, du$$

$$\int_{-\infty}^{\infty} C_{xx}(f) \exp[j2\pi f(\tau - u)] \, df \tag{3.37}$$

Equation (3.37) can be further simplified by changing the order of integration, as follows:

$$\text{var}\left[x_h(t)\right] = \int_{-\infty}^{\infty} C_{xx}(f) \, df \int_{-\infty}^{\infty} h(\tau) \exp(j2\pi f\tau) \, d\tau$$

$$\int_{-\infty}^{\infty} h(u) \exp(-j2\pi fu) \, du \tag{3.38}$$

The two right-most integrals in Eq. (3.38) are Fourier transforms of the filter impulse response, and hence may be stated in terms of the filter's transfer function:

$$\int_{-\infty}^{\infty} h(u) \exp(-j2\pi fu) \, du = H(f) \tag{3.39a}$$

$$\int_{-\infty}^{\infty} h(\tau) \exp(j2\pi f\tau) \, d\tau = H(-f) = H^*(f) \tag{3.39b}$$

Note that $H*(f)$ is the complex conjugate of $H(f)$. Since the product of a complex quantity and its conjugate equals the squared magnitude of the quantity, substitution of Eqs. (3.39a and b) into Eq. (3.38) yields

$$\text{var}[x_h(t)] = \int_{-\infty}^{\infty} C_{xx}(f) |H(f)|^2 df \tag{3.40}$$

This can be seen to specify the variance of the filter's output in terms of both the power spectrum of the input signal and the squared magnitude of the filter's transfer function.

Equation (3.40) indicates that the power spectrum of a random signal is the density of average power at a given frequency. The units are power per Herz. To see this, suppose that the filter transfer function is unity over a narrow band b of frequencies centered at frequency f_c and zero elsewhere. Then,

$$|H(f)| = \begin{cases} 1, & f_c + \dfrac{b}{2} \le f \le f_c + \dfrac{b}{2} \\ 0, & \text{elsewhere} \end{cases} \tag{3.41}$$

Substitution of Eq. (3.41) into Eq. (3.40) yields

$$\text{var}[x_h(t)] = \int_{f_c - b/2}^{f_c + b/2} C_{xx}(f) \, df \tag{3.42}$$

Since b is small, the integral in Eq. (3.42) can be approximated by

$$\text{var}[x_h(t)] \simeq bC_{xx}(f_c) \tag{3.43}$$

Rearranging Eq. (3.43), and taking the limit as b becomes infinitesimally small, yields

$$C_{xx}(f_c) = \lim_{b \to 0} \frac{\text{var}[x_h(t)]}{b} \tag{3.44}$$

Note that $\text{var}[x_h(t)]$ represents the total average power of the random process in the narrow pass band of the filter: $f_c - (b/2)$ to $f_c + (b/2)$. Thus, from Eq. (3.44) it can be seen that the power spectrum is a density function.

The integral of $C_{xx}(f)$ over all frequencies equals the total power of the random process. This can be inferred from Eq. (3.40) by setting $|H(f)|^2 = 1$ for all f. Passing a signal through a filter with a transfer function of unity magnitude in no way alters the amount or the frequency distribution of the average power of a signal. Hence, for this case Eq. (3.40) reduces to

$$\text{var}[x(t)] = \int_{-\infty}^{\infty} C_{xx}(f) \ df \tag{3.45}$$

It is useful here to reconsider two important properties of the power spectrum previously discussed in Chapter 1.

(1) As Eqs. (3.40) and (3.42) indicate, $C_{xx}(f)$ is non-negative at all frequencies.

(2) It is an even function of frequency.

With regard to the first property, if negative values could occur, then by suitable filtering one could obtain an output signal with negative power. However, this is impossible since the power of a signal is the signal's variance, and variance, being the average of a squared quantity, can never be negative. The second property can be inferred from the Fourier transform relationship between the power spectrum and acvf, as follows.

$$C_{xx}(f) = \int_{-\infty}^{\infty} c_{xx}(t) \ \exp(-j2\pi ft) \ dt \tag{3.46}$$

Replacing the exponential in Eq. (3.46) with its Euler identity yields

$$C_{xx}(f) = \int_{-\infty}^{\infty} c_{xx}(t)(\cos 2\pi ft - j\sin 2\pi ft) \ dt \tag{3.47}$$

Since $c_{xx}(t)$ is an even function of t and $\sin 2\pi ft$ is an odd function of t, the integral of the product of the acvf with the sinusoid will be zero. Hence

$$C_{xx}(f) = \int_{-\infty}^{\infty} c_{xx}(t) \ \cos 2\pi ft \ dt \tag{3.48}$$

Changing f to $-f$ in Eq. (3.48) does not alter the cosine and therefore does not alter the integral. Consequently, $C_{xx}(f)$ must be a real, even function of f.

3.8. THE POWER SPECTRUM OF T-DISCRETE RANDOM SIGNALS

Use of a digital computer for power spectrum computations requires that the continuous signal be sampled. It is important that aliasing errors be avoided if an accurate estimate of the power spectrum is to be obtained. When the signal is band-limited, sampling at the Nyquist rate or faster will insure that aliasing will not occur. If the signal is not band-limited or cannot be sampled at twice its upper band-limit, then it should be low-pass filtered prior to sampling, so that activity at frequencies above one-half the sampling frequency will be effectively eliminated. A power spectrum estimate that is free of aliasing errors can then be obtained for frequencies below one-half the sampling frequency. However, information concerning activity at higher frequencies will necessarily be lost. Although the power spectrum properties of T-discrete signals are closely related to those of the original continuous signals, there are important differences which it is most useful to discuss.

The two approaches commonly used to estimate power spectra via digital computation are:

(1) The estimation first of the acvf and from it the power spectrum by the use of the discrete Fourier transform (DFT).

(2) The computation of the periodogram, the "raw" spectrum estimate, by applying the DFT to a finite N sample segment of the signal.

With the advent of the fast Fourier transform algorithm (Oppenheim and Schafer, 1975), the periodogram approach is usually the more rapid one. Once the periodogram has been obtained, further steps are necessary to improve the goodness of the spectral estimate. We will discuss these after paying initial attention to the properties of the periodogram.

3.9. THE FOURIER TRANSFORM
FOR T-DISCRETE SIGNALS

The Fourier transform relationship between the power spectrum and the acvf for T-continuous signals has been developed and discussed in Chapter 1. The Fourier transform pair is restated here.

$$C_{xx}(f) = \int_{-\infty}^{\infty} c_{xx}(t) \, \exp(-j2\pi ft) \, dt \tag{3.49}$$

$$c_{xx}(t) = \int_{-\infty}^{\infty} C_{xx}(f) \, \exp(j2\pi ft) \, df \tag{3.50}$$

An analogous relationship can be shown to hold for T-discrete signals. If the period between samples is Δ sec and the upper bandlimit of the signal is less than or equal to $1/2\Delta$, then Eq. (3.50) becomes

$$c_{xx}(t°\Delta) = \int_{-1/2\Delta}^{1/2\Delta} C_{xx}(f) \, \exp(j2\pi ft°\Delta) \, df \tag{3.51}$$

The acvf is defined only at the discrete times of $t°\Delta$, where $t°$ is an integer that can range from minus to plus infinity. However, $C_{xx}(f)$ is a continuous function of frequency. Note that Eq. (3.51) is obtained from Eq. (3.50) by direct substitution of $t°\Delta$ for t and setting the limits of integration to correspond to one-half the Nyquist frequency.

The discrete analog of Eq. (3.49) is a summation over the discrete set of acvf values:

$$C_{xx}(f) = \Delta \sum_{t°=-\infty}^{\infty} c_{xx}(t°\Delta) \, \exp(-j2\pi ft°\Delta) \tag{3.52}$$

When Eq. (3.52) is compared with Eq. (3.49), we see that $t°\Delta$ replaces t, a summation replaces the integral, and the finite time

increment Δ replaces the infinitesimal dt. The correspondence
between Eq. (3.52) and (3.49) has been given here by making some
intuitively reasonable changes in the original T-continuous transform pair. We will now demonstrate that the relationship is a
mathematically valid one. This is done by substituting for $C_{xx}(f)$
in Eq. (3.51) the right side of Eq. (3.52).

$$c_{xx}(t°\Delta) = \int_{-1/2\Delta}^{1/2\Delta} \Delta \sum_{\tau=-\infty}^{\infty} c_{xx}(\tau°\Delta) \, \exp(-j2\pi f\tau°\Delta) \, \exp(j2\pi ft°\Delta) \, df$$

(3.53)

Interchange of the order of integration and summation yields

$$c_{xx}(t°\Delta) = \Delta \sum_{\tau=-\infty}^{\infty} c_{xx}(\tau°\Delta) \int_{-1/2\Delta}^{1/2\Delta} \exp[j2\pi f(t° - \tau°)\Delta] \, df$$

(3.54)

The integral on the right side is easily shown to be

$$\frac{1}{\Delta} \frac{\sin \pi(t° - \tau°)}{\pi(t° - \tau°)} = \int_{-1/2\Delta}^{1/2\Delta} \exp[j2\pi f(t° - \tau°)\Delta] \, df \qquad (3.55)$$

When both $t°$ and $\tau°$ are integers, the above integral is zero
except for $t° = \tau°$, for which case the integral equals $1/\Delta$.
Hence, substitution of Eq. (3.55) into Eq. (3.54) results in the
elimination of all terms in the summation over $\tau°$, except the
$\tau° = t°$ term. The Δ and $1/\Delta$ factors cancel. What is left is
an identity proving the equality of Eq. (3.54) and demonstrating
the validity of the Fourier transform pair for T-discrete signals,
Eqs. (3.51) and (3.52).

We noted above that $C_{xx}(f)$ is a continuous function. Examination of Eq. (3.52) also indicates that $C_{xx}(f)$ is a periodic
function of frequency, since all the complex exponentials in the
summation are periodic with the fundamental frequency being $1/\Delta$.
This property was to be expected in view of the discussion of
aliasing in Section 3.3. Note that only the frequency components
between $-1/2\Delta$ and $1/2\Delta$ are needed to describe the signal.

3.10. THE PERIODOGRAM

The intention of this section is to show that the power spectrum of a stationary random process can be estimated through use of
the periodogram without having first to estimate the acvf. We will
show that the periodogram is equivalent to a Fourier transform of
the acvf. To do this we first discuss (1) the properties of an
estimated acvf which is based upon a finite segment of a T-discrete
waveform; and (2) the properties of an estimated power spectrum
which is based upon the Fourier transform of such a specimen acvf.

An estimate of the acvf of a stationary random process can
be computed from a T sec segment of the process. A set of N consecutive samples spaced Δ sec apart is used as follows:

$$\hat{c}_{xx}(\tau°\Delta) = \frac{1}{N} \sum_{t°=0}^{N-|\tau°|-1} x(t°\Delta)x[(t° + \tau°)\Delta], \quad |\tau°| \leq N - 1 \qquad (3.56)$$

Note that the upper limit of the summation is a function of $\tau°$.
This is because there are only a finite number of sample products
available. For example, in the $\tau° = 0$ case, all N points can be
used to compute the cross products $x(t°\Delta)x(t°\Delta)$. In the $\tau° = 1$
case, only $N - 1$ points can be used to compute the cross products
since, when $t° = N - 1$, the cross product becomes $x[(N - 1)\Delta]x(N\Delta)$.
The only data samples available are for the time points at 0
through $(N - 1)\Delta$. There is no $N\Delta$ time sample available unless, as
noted in Section 3.2, the data are periodicized. This will be
discussed further in Section 3.18. Thus the summation over the
cross products must be limited to the range of $t° = 0$ to $t° = N - 2$
when $\tau° = 1$. Similar reasoning is applicable to larger magnitudes
of $\tau°$, in which case still fewer sample cross products are available. The expected value of $\hat{c}_{xx}(\tau°\Delta)$ is

$$E[\hat{c}_{xx}(\tau^\circ\Delta)] = \frac{1}{N} \sum_{t^\circ=0}^{N-|\tau^\circ|-1} E\{x(t^\circ\Delta)x[(t^\circ + \tau^\circ)\Delta]\}$$

$$= \frac{1}{N} \sum_{t^\circ=0}^{N-|\tau^\circ|-1} c_{xx}(\tau^\circ\Delta)$$

$$= \frac{c_{xx}(\tau^\circ\Delta)}{N} \sum_{t^\circ=0}^{N-|\tau^\circ|-1} 1 \tag{3.57}$$

Since the summation consists of $N - |\tau^\circ|$ terms, all equal to unity, the sum equals $N - |\tau^\circ|$ and so Eq. (3.57) becomes

$$E[\hat{c}_{xx}(\tau^\circ\Delta)] = \left(1 - \frac{|\tau^\circ|}{N}\right) c_{xx}(\tau^\circ\Delta) \tag{3.58}$$

Equation (3.58) indicates that Eq. (3.56) is a biased estimator of the acvf, and that as the number of sample times N becomes large with respect to $|\tau^\circ|$, the bias becomes small.

An estimate of the power spectrum can then be obtained by using Eq. (3.52) to compute the Fourier transform of the acvf estimate, Eq. (3.56). The summation index τ° is confined to the range $- (N - 1)$ to $(N - 1)$ since only N time points are available in the original sampled data segment and positive and negative values of τ° are permitted up to $N - 1$. We then have for the estimate of the power spectrum,

$$\hat{C}_{xx}(f) = \frac{\Delta}{N} \sum_{\tau^\circ=-(N-1)}^{N-1} \sum_{t^\circ=0}^{N-|\tau^\circ|-1} x(t^\circ\Delta)x[(t^\circ + \tau^\circ)\Delta] \exp(-j2\pi f\tau^\circ\Delta) \tag{3.59}$$

This equation forms a basis for estimating the power spectrum although, as will be shown, some modifications are needed so as to obtain statistically acceptable results.

From a practical point of view, evaluation of Eq. (3.59) can entail relatively large amounts of computer time when N is large. For this reason it may be advantageous to estimate the power spectrum directly by means of the periodogram of the waveform specimen, as expressed by the following equation:

139

$$P_{xx}(n) = \frac{\Delta}{N} \left| \sum_{t°=0}^{N-1} x(t°\Delta) \, \exp(-j2\pi n t°/N) \right|^2 \qquad (3.60)$$

$P_{xx}(f)$ is the symbol for the periodogram. It arises from the Fourier transform of the unsampled T sec data segment of $x(t)$,

$$P_{xx}(f) = \frac{1}{T} \left| X(f) \right|^2 \qquad (3.61)$$

When $x(t)$ is band-limited, we can resort to the sampled representation and the Fourier transform,

$$P_{xx}(f) = \frac{\Delta}{N} \left| \sum_{t°=0}^{N-1} x(t°\Delta) \, \exp(-j2\pi f t°\Delta) \right|^2 \qquad (3.62)$$

Usually only the harmonic frequencies $f_n = n/T = n/N\Delta$ are of interest to us (by periodicizing the original data), and we can obtain the periodogram from the DFT:

$$P_{xx}(f_n) = \frac{\Delta}{N} \left| X_N(n) \right|^2$$

$$= \frac{\Delta}{N} \left| \sum_{t°=0}^{N-1} x(t°\Delta) \, \exp(-j2\pi n t°/N) \right|^2 \qquad (3.63)$$

On occasion we shall write $P_{xx}(f_n)$ as $P_{xx}(n)$ so that the two notations are equivalent.

We will now show that $P_{xx}(f)$ is equal to the $\hat{C}_{xx}(f)$ defined in Eq. (3.59). As a first step, we note that the square of the magnitude of a complex quantity is equal to the product of that quantity and its complex conjugate. Hence,

$$P_{xx}(f_n) = \frac{\Delta}{N} \sum_{t°=0}^{N-1} x(t°\Delta) \, \exp(-j2\pi f_n t°\Delta) \sum_{u°=0}^{N-1} x(u°\Delta) \, \exp(j2\pi f_n u°\Delta)$$

$$= \frac{\Delta}{N} \sum_{t°=0}^{N-1} \sum_{u°=0}^{N-1} x(t°\Delta) x(u°\Delta) \, \exp[-j2\pi f_n(t° - u°)\Delta] \qquad (3.64)$$

We now make a change of variables, substituting $\tau°$ for $t° - u°$. Since both $t°$ and $u°$ range from 0 to $N - 1$, the range will be

- $(N - 1)$ to $(N - 1)$. Hence, Eq. (3.64) becomes

$$P_{xx}(f_n) = \frac{\Delta}{N} \sum_{\tau°=-(N-1)}^{N-1} \sum_{u°=0}^{N-|\tau°|-1} x(u°\Delta)x[(u° + \tau°)\Delta] \exp(-j2\pi f_n \tau°\Delta)$$

(3.65)

Note that the upper limit of the summation over $u°$ has been reduced by $|\tau°|$. The reasons are the same as for the summation in Eq. (3.56). Comparison of Eq. (3.59) with Eq. (3.65) indicates that the periodogram $P_{xx}(f_n)$ is identical with the spectral estimate $\hat{C}_{xx}(f)$ obtained by means of the Fourier transform of the sample acvf. The reason for preferring the periodogram as the vehicle for spectral estimation is that it can be computed more rapidly, provided that a fast Fourier transform algorithm is used.

3.11. STATISTICAL ERRORS
OF THE PERIODOGRAM--BIAS

We previously indicated that the specimen or sample acvf, which is used explicitly in Eq. (3.59) and implicitly in Eq. (3.60), provides a biased estimate of the acvf. Consequently, the periodogram will provide a biased estimate of the power spectrum. The expected value of the periodogram can be obtained by substituting Eq. (3.58), the expected value of the sample acvf, into Eq. (3.65).

$$E[P_{xx}(f_n)] = \Delta \sum_{\tau°=-(N-1)}^{N-1} \left(1 - \frac{|\tau°|}{N}\right) c_{xx}(\tau°\Delta) \exp(-j2\pi f_n \tau°\Delta) \quad (3.66)$$

Comparison of this equation with Eq. (3.52), which defines $C_{xx}(f)$ as the Fourier transform of $c_{xx}(\tau°\Delta)$, yields

$$E[P_{xx}(f_n)] = C_{xx}(f_n) - \sum_{\tau°=-\infty}^{-N} c_{xx}(\tau°\Delta) \exp(-j2\pi f_n \tau°\Delta)$$

$$- \sum_{\tau°=N}^{\infty} c_{xx}(\tau°\Delta) \exp(-j2\pi f_n \tau°\Delta)$$

$$- \frac{\Delta}{N} \sum_{\tau°=-(N-1)}^{N-1} |\tau°| c_{xx}(\tau°\Delta) \exp(-j2\pi f_n \tau°\Delta)$$

(3.67)

The three right-most terms in Eq. (3.67) constitute the bias. Assuming that $x(t)$ is a zero mean random process, the bias will tend toward zero as N becomes large.

To examine the nature of the bias in the frequency domain, we can rewrite Eq. (3.66) in a somewhat more general form, as follows:

$$E[P_{xx}(f_n)] = \Delta \sum_{\tau\degree=-\infty}^{\infty} w_B(\tau\degree\Delta) c_{xx}(\tau\degree\Delta) \exp(-j2\pi f_n \tau\degree\Delta) \qquad (3.68)$$

where

$$w_B(\tau\degree\Delta) = \begin{cases} 1 - \dfrac{|\tau\degree|}{N}, & |\tau\degree| < N \\ 0 & , \quad |\tau\degree| \geq N \end{cases} \qquad (3.69)$$

The function $w_B(\tau\degree\Delta)$ can be thought of as a "lag window" function which multiplies or weights the set of acvf terms, and, since it is different from unity, "causes" the periodogram to be a biased estimate of the power spectrum. Since we showed in Chapter 1 that multiplication in the time domain is the equivalent of convolution in the frequency domain, Eq. (3.68) can be stated in the frequency domain as

$$E[P_{xx}(f_n)] = \Delta \int_{-1/2\Delta}^{1/2\Delta} C_{xx}(f) W_B(f_n - f) \, df \qquad (3.70)$$

where $W_B(f)$ is the Fourier transform of $w(t)$. It can be shown that

$$W_B(f) = \sum_{\tau\degree=-(N-1)}^{N-1} \left(1 - \frac{|\tau\degree|}{N}\right) \exp(-j2\pi f\tau\degree\Delta)$$

$$= \frac{1}{N} \left(\frac{\sin \pi N\Delta f}{\sin \pi\Delta f}\right)^2 \qquad (3.71)$$

$W_B(f)$ can be thought of as a "frequency window" function. Substituting Eq. (3.71) into Eq. (3.70) gives

$$E[P_{xx}(f_c)] = \Delta \int_{-1/2\Delta}^{1/2\Delta} \frac{1}{N} \left(\frac{\sin \pi N\Delta(f_c - f)}{\sin \pi\Delta(f_c - f)}\right)^2 C_{xx}(f) \, df \qquad (3.72)$$

A plot of $W_B(f)$ is provided in Fig. 3.9a. Note that within

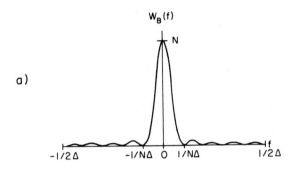

a)

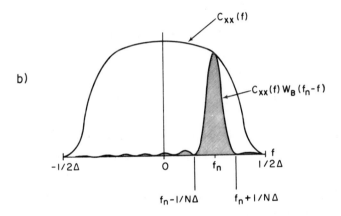

b)

Fig. 3.9. (a) Plot of the window function, $W_B(f) =$ $(\sin \pi N \Delta f)^2 / N(\sin \pi \Delta f)^2$, for $N = 10$. (b) An illustration of how the product of $C_{xx}(f)$ and $W_B(f_n - f)$ determines the expected value of the estimate of the power spectrum.

the frequency band of interest, $-1/2\Delta$ to $1/2\Delta$, $W_B(f_n - f)$ is near zero except at $f = f_n$. Hence, only that portion of $C_{xx}(f)$ which is near frequency f_n will contribute much to the periodogram esti-mate of the power spectrum. This is illustrated in Fig. 3.9b. Note that $E[P_{xx}(f_c)]$ is equal to an area determined by the product of $C_{xx}(f)$ and $W_B(f_n - f)$. As N becomes large, the area becomes more closely confined to frequencies that are near to f_n. This means that by increasing N we can obtain a high resolution, small bias estimate whose expected value is close to $C_{xx}(f_n)$. If N is small, the expected value of the estimate will contain spectral components covering a broad range of frequencies. In this circumstance only a low resolution, large bias estimate can be obtained, and nuances such as sharp peaks in the spectrum may not be detected.

A rough guide to the size of N necessary for the bias to become negligible can be obtained from consideration of Eq. (3.72), Fig. 3.9b, and the fact that

$$\Delta \int_{-1/2\Delta}^{1/2\Delta} W_B(f_n - f) \, df = \int_{-1/2\Delta}^{1/2\Delta} \frac{\Delta}{N} \left[\frac{\sin N\Delta(f_n - f)}{\sin \pi\Delta(f_n - f)} \right]^2 df = 1.0$$

This means that if $C_{xx}(f)$ is relatively constant over the band of frequencies where the frequency window function is markedly greater than zero, then the right side of Eq. 3.72 is approximately equal to $C_{xx}(f_n)$. Inspection of Fig. 3.9b suggests that N should be such that $C_{xx}(f)$ does not vary significantly over a frequency bandwidth of about $4/N\Delta$ Hz.

The concept of leakage that was discussed in Section 3.4 is simply another way of describing bias or resolution. Examination of Fig. 3.9b indicates that the low resolution, large bias situation is one in which activity at frequencies other than the one of interest contributes to (i.e., leaks into) the estimate of $C_{xx}(f_n)$.

3.12. STATISTICAL ERRORS
OF THE PERIODOGRAM--VARIANCE

Since $P_{xx}(f_n)$ is a function of the set of N random variables, the $x(t°\Delta)$, $P_{xx}(f_n)$ is also a random variable. We already know that as N becomes large, the mean of $P_{xx}(f)$ approaches $C_{xx}(f)$, the power spectrum of $x(t)$. We now arrive at a troublesome property of the periodogram, namely, that its variance does not become small as N increases. Instead, the estimation errors contained in $P_{xx}(f)$ will be of the same order of magnitude as the $P_{xx}(f)$

itself, regardless of N. Consequently, the raw periodogram is not
a consistent estimate of the power spectrum $C_{xx}(f)$. For $P_{xx}(f)$ to
be a consistent estimate in the statistical sense, its mean must
approach the true spectrum and its variance must become small as N
becomes large. The periodogram meets the former but not the latter
criterion. However, by application of suitable averaging procedures the latter criterion can also be satisfied. We will now discuss the basis of such averaging procedures.

First, to gain insight into the nature of the variance of the
periodogram, let us consider the case of a zero mean, white
Gaussian process. In this case, the samples $x(t°\Delta)$ are independent
of one another and the power of the process is uniformly distributed
over the frequency band from $-1/2\Delta$ to $1/2\Delta$. The acvf, $c_{xx}(\tau°\Delta)$,
is zero for all $\tau°$ except $\tau° = 0$, at which point it has the value
σ_x^2. The spectrum $C_{xx}(f)$ of such a process is easily seen to be
equal to $\sigma_x^2 \Delta$ for all f.

We find the mean and variance of the periodogram at zero
frequency by setting $f = 0$ in Eq. (3.60). This yields

$$P_{xx}(0) = \frac{\Delta}{N} \left[\sum_{t°=0}^{N-1} x(t°\Delta) \right]^2 \tag{3.73}$$

In Section 1.13 it was pointed out that the distribution of the
sum of N identically distributed normal (μ, σ) random variables is
normal ($N\mu$, $\sqrt{N}\sigma$). Hence, the distribution of $\sum_{n=0}^{N-1} x(t°\Delta)$ is
Gaussian with a mean of zero and variance equal to $N\sigma_x^2$. It was
further shown in Section 1.13 that the square of a zero mean, unit-
standard-deviation Gaussian random variable has a chi-squared distribution with one degree of freedom. Thus inspection of Eq. (3.73)
indicates that it can be expressed as the product of a constant
times a chi-squared random variate, as follows:

$$P_{xx}(0) = \Delta\sigma_x^2 \left[\frac{1}{\sqrt{N}\sigma_x} \sum_{t°=0}^{N-1} x(t°\Delta) \right]^2 \tag{3.74}$$

The square of the quantity within the brackets has a chi-squared distribution with one degree of freedom. Two other results from Section 1.13 are useful here. The first is that the mean of a chi-squared variable with m degrees of freedom equals m and its variance equals $2m$. The second is that the product of a constant α times a chi-squared random variate with m degrees of freedom has a mean equal to αm and a variance equal to $2\alpha_m^2$. Applying these to Eq. (3.74), we have

$$E[P_{xx}(0)] = \Delta\sigma_x^2 \qquad (3.75)$$

$$\text{var}[P_{xx}(0)] = 2\Delta^2\sigma_x^4 \qquad (3.76)$$

Hence, the standard deviation of $P_{xx}(0)$ is $\sqrt{2}\Delta\sigma_x^2$. Since $C_{xx}(0)$ equals $\Delta\sigma_x^2$, the standard deviation of $P_{xx}(0)$ equals $\sqrt{2}C_{xx}(0)$. This shows that although the expected value of $P_{xx}(0)$ equals $C_{xx}(0)$, the variance of $P_{xx}(0)$ is independent of N, the number of time samples. The coefficient of variation of $P_{xx}(0)$ is $\sqrt{2}$.

The above result applies only to the estimate at zero frequency. A basically similar but computationally more tedious development can be made for the value of a periodogram of a white, Gaussian process at any arbitrary frequency. The mean and variance of the periodogram are (Oppenheim and Schafer, 1975)

$$E[P_{xx}(f)] = \Delta\sigma_x^2 \qquad (3.77)$$

$$\text{var}[P_{xx}(f)] = \Delta^2\sigma_x^4\left[1 + \left(\frac{\sin 2\pi f\Delta N}{N \sin 2\pi f\Delta}\right)^2\right] \qquad (3.78)$$

Equation (3.78) reduces to Eq. (3.76) when f equals zero or $1/2\Delta$. Since $[\sin 2\pi f\Delta N/N \sin(2\pi f\Delta)]^2$ ranges between zero and one, we find that $\text{var}[P_{xx}(f)]$ does not become small, viz.,

$$\Delta^2\sigma_x^4 \leq \text{var}[P_{xx}(f)] \leq 2\Delta^2\sigma_x^4$$

In practice it is only necessary to compute the periodogram at the discrete set of frequencies $f = n/N\Delta$, where n is an integer. This makes it possible to use a fast Fourier transform algorithm. At these frequencies, var$[P_{xx}(n/N\Delta)]$ equals $\Delta^2 \sigma_x^4$. Hence for a zero mean, white Gaussian process the expected value of the periodogram equals $C_{xx}(f)$ while its standard deviation is also approximately equal to $C_{xx}(f)$. Increasing N will not reduce the standard deviation.

For a nonwhite random process the results are quite similar. The periodogram again provides a biased estimate of $C_{xx}(f)$, as indicated by Eqs. (3.67), (3.68) and (3.72). An approximate expression for the variance of the periodogram is (Oppenheim and Schafer, 1975)

$$\text{var}[P_{xx}(f)] \simeq C_{xx}^2(f) \left[1 + \left(\frac{\sin 2\pi f \Delta N}{N \sin 2\pi f \Delta} \right)^2 \right] \tag{3.79}$$

Thus, as in the case of a white Gaussian process, the standard deviation of the periodogram is equal to $C_{xx}(f)$ at frequencies $n/N\Delta$ and is slightly larger at other frequencies. While increasing N will decrease the bias, as indicated by Eq. (3.72), it will not effectively decrease the standard deviation of the periodogram estimate.

3.13. AVERAGING THE PERIODOGRAM-- THE BARTLETT ESTIMATOR

It is apparent from the preceding discussion that since the periodogram is not a consistent estimator of the power spectrum, a procedure is required that will attenuate the random fluctuations associated with the periodogram and produce a useful spectrum estimate. One such procedure is to divide the signal specimen into a series of subsegments, compute a periodogram for each of them and then average the periodograms. This approach, first suggested by Bartlett (Oppenheim and Schafer, 1975), also gives one the opportunity of testing for stationarity. It is implemented as follows. Let the signal segment be divided into M subsegments, each $N\Delta$ sec long. Denote the signal in the mth subsegment by

$$x^{(m)}(t°\Delta) = x\left([t° + N(m - 1)]\Delta\right), \quad 0 \leq t° \leq N - 1$$
$$1 \leq m \leq M \qquad (3.80)$$

The corresponding periodogram for the mth subsegment is

$$P_{xx}^{(m)}(f) = \frac{\Delta}{N}\left|\sum_{t°=0}^{N-1} x^{(m)}(t°\Delta)\exp(-j2\pi ft°\Delta)\right|^2 \qquad (3.81)$$

Thus, using Bartlett's method, the estimate of the power spectrum of $x(t)$ is

$$B_{xx}(f) = \frac{1}{M}\sum_{m=1}^{M} P_{xx}^{(m)}(f) \qquad (3.82)$$

The expected value of the Bartlett estimator at frequency f_n is

$$E[B_{xx}(f_n)] = \frac{1}{M}\sum_{m=1}^{M} E[P_{xx}^{(m)}(f_n)] \qquad (3.83)$$

The expected value of the periodogram, $P_{xx}^{(m)}(f_n)$, is the same for all m and is given by Eq. (3.72). Hence, the expected value of the Bartlett estimator is the same as the expected value of the individual periodograms and is given by

$$E[B_{xx}(f_n)] = \Delta\int_{-1/2\Delta}^{1/2\Delta} \frac{1}{N}\left[\frac{\sin \pi N\Delta(f_n - f)}{\sin \pi\Delta(f_n - f)}\right]^2 C_{xx}(f)\ df$$
$$(3.84)$$

The bias leakage properties of the Bartlett estimator are also the same as that of the individual periodograms so that the remarks following Eq. (3.72) concerning bias and leakage of raw periodograms apply here as well. What is most important is that the variance of the Bartlett estimator is less than that of the periodogram, as we shall show in the next section. The argument is based upon the assumption that there is a total of $N_m M$ data points available, N_m being the number of data points in each of the M subsegments.

3.14. VARIANCE OF THE BARTLETT ESTIMATOR

If N_m, the number of time points in a subsegment, is suffi-
ciently large so that $c_{xx}(\tau^\circ \Delta)$ is small for $\tau^\circ > N_m$, then the various subsegment periodograms, $P_{xx}^{(m)}(f)$, will tend to be statistically
independent of one another. This means that the variance of the
average of the M periodograms will be approximately equal to the
variance of the individual periodograms divided by M. (See Sections 1.13 and 4.1.) Using this and Eq. (3.79), it follows that
the variance of the Bartlett estimator is approximately

$$\text{var}\,[B_{xx}(f)] = \text{var}\,[P_{xx}^{(m)}(f)]/M = \frac{c_{xx}^2(f)}{M}\left[1 + \left(\frac{\sin 2\pi f \Delta N_m}{N_m \sin 2\pi f \Delta}\right)^2\right] \qquad (3.85)$$

Thus, for $f_n = n/N_m \Delta$ and unequal to zero or $1/2\Delta$,

$$\text{var}\,[B_{xx}(f_n)] \simeq c_{xx}^2(f_n)/M \qquad\qquad (3.86a)$$

and when $f_n = 0$ or $1/2\Delta$,

$$\text{var}\,[B_{xx}(0)] = 2c_{xx}^2(0)/M \qquad\qquad (3.86b)$$

$$\text{var}\,[B_{xx}(1/2\Delta)] = 2c_{xx}^2(1/2\Delta)/M \qquad\qquad (3.86c)$$

This means that Bartlett's method is a consistent estimator of the
power spectrum since, as the total number of data points $N = N_m M$
increases, both the bias and variance of the estimate become small.
The bias, as given by Eq. (3.84), is determined solely by the
length of the subsegments N_m, and diminishes as N_m increases.
The variance is determined by the number of subsegments M to which
it is inversely proportional.

Since only a fixed number of time samples $N_m M$ is available
for estimation of the power spectrum, however it is done, there
is a trade-off between the size of the variance and the resolution
of the Bartlett estimator. Variance is reduced by dividing the
data segment into as many subsegments as possible, thereby increasing M. But by so doing, one shortens the length of the sub-

segments N_m, and hence increases the bias and decreases the resolution. Thus, the size of variance and bias are inversely related to one another: as one increases, the other decreases. Variance itself is related closely to spectral resolution, the ability to detect fine structure in the spectrum. Decreasing the variance of an estimate is brought about by decreasing the length N_m of a data subsegment. This means that the periodograms have fewer frequency components in them (smaller N_m) so that the frequency resolution decreases. Reduced resolution is therefore concomitant with reduced variance. Later we shall show this is another way by speaking of frequency resolution in terms of bandwidth.

3.15. THE FAST FOURIER TRANSFORM AND POWER SPECTRUM ESTIMATION

We mentioned in Section 3.8 that the main reason for using the periodogram approach to power spectrum estimation is that it can be carried out more rapidly than by computing the acvf and then taking its Fourier transform. The savings in time come about by use of the fast Fourier transform algorithm (Bergland, 1969; Oppenheim and Schafer, 1975) to compute the Fourier transforms of the original data, as specified by Eqs. (3.60) and (3.81). In order to take advantage of the fast Fourier transform or FFT, we must confine the frequencies for which the spectral estimate is computed to the discrete set of $f_n = n/N\Delta$, $n = 0, \ldots, N - 1$, where $N\Delta$ is the duration of the segment. This is no restriction since the periodogram of a band-limited process is completely represented by its sample values at frequencies $n/N\Delta$. We must emphasize the fact that the value of the spectral estimate at each frequency does not depend upon whether the FFT or some other algorithm is used. Neither are the bias and variance of the estimate affected by the choice of the algorithm. The only difference may be in computational round-off error, which may be smaller with the FFT, since the FFT entails fewer steps.

3.16. SMOOTHING OF SPECTRAL ESTIMATES BY WINDOWING

We have shown above that although the periodogram itself is not a consistent estimator of the power spectrum, a way of obtaining one is to average across a set of sequentially obtained periodograms. Here we shall develop a different approach to a smoothing of the periodogram which also yields a consistent spectral estimate. Our argument will apply mainly to estimates obtained at the discrete set of frequencies $f_n = n/N\Delta$.

Rather than dividing the data into numerous time sequential subsegments and averaging across time, the periodogram can be smoothed by averaging over narrow bands of frequency. One important property of periodogram estimates that we make use of here is that $P_{xx}(f_n)$ for a white Gaussian process is the sum of the square of two identical and independent Gaussian random variables (Jenkins and Watts, 1968), except when $f_n = 0$, $1/2\Delta$. This property is also approximately valid when the Gaussian restriction is eliminated and any peak in the spectrum is broad compared to $1/N\Delta$. This means that in most situations of interest, $P_{xx}(f_n)$ is proportional to a chi-squared random variable with two degrees of freedom. Since

$$E[P_{xx}(f_n)] = C_{xx}(f_n)$$

and

$$\text{var}[P_{xx}(f_n)] = C_{xx}^2(f_n)$$

$2P_{xx}(f_n)/C_{xx}(f_n)$ is a χ_2^2 random variable. A second important property of periodogram estimates is that for a white Gaussian process $\text{cov}[P_{xx}(f_n), P_{xx}(f_m)] = 0$ when $n \neq m$. This property is also approximately valid for nonwhite and some non-Gaussian processes. Thus one can treat values of the periodogram at integer multiples of $1/N\Delta$ as uncorrelated random variables. For more details, see Jenkins and Watts (1968).

Let us now consider a spectral estimate made up of a weighted sum of periodogram values:

$$\hat{C}_{xx}(f_n) = \sum_{k=n-K}^{n+K} P_{xx}(f_k)W(f_n - f_k) \qquad (3.87)$$

The $W(f_k)$ are the weights of a spectral smoothing filter which weights and sums the periodogram estimates from f_{n-K} to f_{n+K}. $\hat{C}_{xx}(f_n)$ is a new random variable, and when the process is Gaussian, its mean and variance are given by

$$E[\hat{C}_{xx}(f_n)] = \sum_{k=n-K}^{n+K} E[P_{xx}(f_k)]W(f_n - f_k) \qquad (3.88a)$$

$$\text{var}[\hat{C}_{xx}(f_n)] = \sum_{k=n-K}^{n+K} \text{var}[P_{xx}(f_k)]W^2(f_n - f_k) \qquad (3.88b)$$

Since frequency averaging is usually applied to periodograms obtained from long data segments, the results of Section 3.12 indicate that Eqs. (3.88a and b) can be approximated by

$$E[\hat{C}_{xx}(f_n)] = \sum_{k=n-K}^{n+K} C_{xx}(f_k)W(f_n - f_k) \qquad (3.89a)$$

$$\text{var}[\hat{C}_{xx}(f_n)] = \sum_{k=n-K}^{n+K} C_{xx}^2(f_k)W^2(f_n - f_k) \qquad (3.89b)$$

These equations can be further simplified when the process is a white one (even if only in the range of frequencies covered by the summation), in which case its mean and variance are given by

$$E[\hat{C}_{xx}(f_n)] = C_{xx}(f_n) \sum_{k=-K}^{K} W(f_k) \qquad (3.90a)$$

$$\text{var}[\hat{C}_{xx}(f_n)] = C_{xx}^2(f_n) \sum_{k=-K}^{K} W^2(f_k) \qquad (3.90b)$$

It is convenient to use only positive weights and to set $\sum_k W(f_k) = 1$. This results in no loss of generality. Since each weight must be no larger than unity, the variance of $\hat{C}_{xx}(f_n)$ must be less than the variance of $P_{xx}(f_n)$. A rectangular filter, one which weights equally all the periodogram values from f_{n-K} to f_{n+K} has weights $W(f_k) = 1/(2K + 1)$. For a white noise process, the variance of $C_{xx}(f_n)$ with such a filter is $1/(2K + 1)$ that of $P_{xx}(f_n)$.

Because $\hat{C}_{xx}(f_n)$ is the weighted sum of a set of $P_{xx}(f_k)$ and each $P_{xx}(f_k)$ is closely proportional to a χ_2^2 random variable, $\hat{C}_{xx}(f_n)$ is itself closely proportional to a $\chi_{d.f.}^2$ random variable and can be dealt with in this way. This was discussed earlier in Section 1.13. The degrees of freedom d.f., and the constant proportionality α for the random variable are given by

$$\text{d.f.} = \frac{2\{E[\hat{C}_{xx}(f_n)]\}^2}{\text{var}[\hat{C}_{xx}(f_n)]} \simeq \frac{2}{\sum\limits_{k=-K}^{K} W^2(f_k)} \qquad (3.91a)$$

$$\alpha = \frac{E[\hat{C}_{xx}(f_n)]}{\text{d.f.}} \simeq \frac{C_{xx}(f_n)}{\text{d.f.}} \qquad (3.91b)$$

This means that we can consider d.f. $[\hat{C}_{xx}(f_n)/C_{xx}(f_n)]$ to be a $\chi_{d.f.}^2$ random variable. Applying this result to a rectangular smoothing filter, one which weights equally the periodogram values from f_{n-K} to f_{n+K}, we find d.f. $= 2(2K + 1)$. This was to be expected since $2K + 1$ periodogram values, each with 2 degrees of freedom, were used to construct the estimate. Computations of this sort can be carried out for any smoothing window of interest. For example, a Bartlett estimator which is obtained by sectioning an N sample record into M segments, each of length N/M, can be shown to have $3M$ degrees of freedom.

Equation (3.91a) shows that the degrees of freedom and the variance of the estimator are inversely related. The equation also bears a close relationship to the number of frequency components being summed over: the greater the number, the greater the degrees of freedom and the smaller the variance. We may assign to the smoothing filter a generalized bandwidth parameter. This is the bandwidth (or the number of frequency components averaged over) that a uniformly weighted filter would have in order to yield an estimator with the same variance as the actual smoothing filter. This assumes the data have a flat spectrum over the range of the smoothing filter. The bandwidth and variance are inversely related so that their product is a constant. This can be readily seen for a white noise process being smoothed by a uniformly weighted filter. The bandwidth = $2K + 1$ and the variance = $\text{var}[P_{xx}(f_n)]/(2K + 1)$. This means that there is always a trade-off between variance and bandwidth. Small variance is obtained at the cost of large bandwidth (or low resolution) and vice versa.

The trade-offs between variance and resolution are much the same whether a Bartlett estimator, Eq. (3.82), or a more general windowing approach, Eq. (3.87), is used. However, there are differences in details. Inspection of Eq. (3.84) indicates that the Bartlett estimator is the equivalent of using a frequency smoothing filter of the form $(\sin \pi N \Delta f/N \sin \pi \Delta f)^2$, referred to as the Bartlett window. While the Bartlett window has been widely used and provides a reasonable balance between variance and resolution, in some instances other window shapes may be more desirable. An advantage of the averaging over the frequency approach is that a wide variety of window functions can be devised according to the particular spectral smoothing problem at hand. Details such as the precise width of the window function can be controlled by direct specification of the $W(f_k)$ terms.

Although there is some latitude in selecting a spectral window function $W(f_k)$ for a given application, there are practical constraints that should be evaluated. Thus, while a window that extends over a broad frequency range will yield a low variance estimate, it is associated with leakage from frequencies that are far from the one at which the spectrum is being estimated. If these distant spectral components are large, the window width should be narrowed to reduce the leakage. Another consideration has to do with the values of the $W(f_k)$. There are relatively common window functions that have negative values for some of the $W(f_k)$. Such windows must be used with caution since they can lead to negative spectrum estimates.

From Eqs. (3.90b) and (3.91a) it can be seen that the magnitude of $\sum_{k=-K}^{K} w^2(f_k)$ is crucial in determining the variance of the spectrum estimate. The smaller the sum of the squares, the smaller the variance. Given the constraint that $\sum_{k=-K}^{K} W(f_k) = 1.0$, it can be shown that the sum of the $w^2(f_k)$ terms will be smallest when all $W(f_k) = 1/(2M + 1)$, in which case the sum of the squares equals $1/(2M + 1)$.

Spectral windowing can also be implemented in the time domain by dealing with the acvf. Since convolution in the frequency domain is equivalent to multiplication in the time domain, the time domain equivalent of Eq. (3.87) is

$$C_{xx}(f) = \Delta \sum_{t°=-(N-1)}^{N-1} w(t°\Delta)\hat{c}_{xx}(t°\Delta) \exp(-j2\pi ft°\Delta) \qquad (3.92)$$

where $\hat{c}_{xx}(t°\Delta)$ is given by Eq. (3.56), and $w(t°\Delta)$, commonly referred to as a "lag window," is in effect the Fourier transform of $W(f)$. Prior to the late 1960s, when the FFT became widely known, windowing was usually implemented in the time domain, via Eq. (3.92). It is the Fourier transform of these lag windows that sometimes yields negative $W(f_k)$. A detailed discussion of the properties of spectral and lag window functions and their implementation can be found in Jenkins and Watts (1968), Otnes and Enochson (1972), and Welch (1967).

3.17. THE CROSS SPECTRUM

In Chapter 1 we discussed the concept of the cross covariance function (ccvf). The Fourier transform of the ccvf is referred to as the cross spectrum. The cross spectrum provides a statement of how common activity between two processes is distributed across frequency. The cross spectrum is the Fourier transform of the ccvf, as indicated by Eq. (1.69). As an example, consider two processes each of which consists of a quasiperiodic signal embedded in wide band noise processes. Suppose the quasiperiodic signals are due to a common phenomenon so that they are closely related. The wide band noise processes, on the other hand, are due to random fluctuations that are unique to each process and so are unrelated. The cross spectrum of the two processes would be relatively large in the frequency band of the shared, quasiperiodic signal and small at other frequencies, since the wide band noise processes are independent and not shared activity.

To some extent the cross spectrum can provide insight into the relationships between a pair of random processes. Further insight can be obtained from the coherence function, which is derived from the power spectra and cross spectrum of the pair of random processes. The coherence function will be discussed in Section 3.19.

The procedures and problems in estimating cross spectra are similar to those described in the preceding discussion of the power spectra. It can be computed by Fourier transform of the sample ccvf. However, with the availability of the FFT algorithm, a periodogram approach in some instances may be preferable. The bias-resolution and variance properties of the cross spectrum are the same for both approaches and are similar to those of the power spectrum.

For example, consider the ccvf and cross spectrum for two wide sense stationary random signals, $x(t)$ and $y(t)$. The sample ccvf may be computed in the same manner as an acvf [see Eq. (3.56)], as follows,

$$\hat{c}_{xy}(\tau^\circ\Delta) = \frac{1}{N} \sum_{t^\circ=0}^{N-|\tau^\circ|-1} x(t^\circ\Delta)y[(t^\circ + \tau^\circ)\Delta], \quad |\tau^\circ| \leq N - 1 \qquad (3.93)$$

The sample cross spectrum can be obtained in the same manner as the sample power spectrum [see Eq. (3.59)], as follows,

$$\hat{C}_{xy}(f) = \Delta \sum_{\tau°=-(N-1)}^{N-1} \hat{c}_{xy}(\tau°\Delta) \, \exp(-j2\pi f\tau°\Delta) \qquad (3.94)$$

The expected value of the above cross-spectrum estimate can be found by the same steps used to arrive at Eq. (3.72), the expected value of the periodogram estimate. The result is

$$E[\hat{C}_{xy}(f_n)] = \Delta \int_{-1/2\Delta}^{1/2\Delta} \frac{1}{N} \left(\frac{\sin \pi NT(f_n - f)}{\sin \pi T(f_n - f)} \right)^2 C_{xy}(f) \, df$$

$$(3.95)$$

Eq. (3.95) is directly comparable to Eq. (3.72), the expression for the expected value of the periodogram estimate of the power spectrum. As in the case of the periodogram, increasing the length of the epoch segment N will decrease the bias of the cross-spectral estimate but its variance will not be effectively decreased. Consequently, averaging and/or windowing techniques, as described earlier for estimation of the power spectrum, must also be employed when estimating the cross power spectrum. Further details about cross-spectral estimates may be found in Chapters 8 and 9 of Jenkins and Watts (1968).

3.18. COVARIANCE FUNCTIONS

The auto- and cross covariance functions were introduced in Chapter 1 and shown to be a way of representing the temporal relationships within an individual dynamic process and also between different dynamic processes. The Fourier relationship between the cvfs and power spectra was also established for continuous stationary processes and for T sec realizations of them. To do this for the power spectra we resorted to the artifice of considering a T sec segment of data to be one period of a periodic process. This provided us with an estimator for the cvf and the spectrum of the continuous aperiodic process. The properties of the spectral estimators have been discussed in the preceding section. Now we move to a more detailed consideration of the covariance function, pointing out some essential features of its estimation and how

this estimation is related to power spectrum estimation. We begin
with the autocovariance function.

A. *SOME STATISTICAL PROPERTIES*
   OF THE ACVF ESTIMATOR

The representation of a T sec segment of data as one period
of a periodicized specimen function $x(t)$ means that the estimated
acvf is given by

$$\tilde{c}_{xx,N}(\tau^\circ) = \frac{1}{N} \sum_{t=0}^{N-1} \tilde{x}(t^\circ)\tilde{x}*(t^\circ + \tau^\circ) \qquad (3.96)$$

and is itself periodic, N. We use the tilde to denote that the
acvf has arisen from periodicized data $\tilde{x}(t)$. The subscript N
indicates the periodicity. (Throughout this discussion we will
assume the original specimen function to be band limited, $F = 1/2$,
and sampled at the Nyquist rate so that $\Delta = 1$.) Whenever $t^\circ + \tau^\circ$
exceeds $N - 1$, $t^\circ + \tau^\circ$ is to be considered as having its value
taken "modulo N." That means, in this instance, that if $t^\circ + \tau^\circ$
$= 117$ and $N = 100$, the value taken for $t^\circ + \tau^\circ$ is 17 and $\tilde{x}(117)$
$= x(17)$. This follows from the periodicity of $\tilde{x}(t^\circ)$. The estimated acvf that results from the use of Eq. (3.96) is sometimes
referred to as a circular covariance function because of this
method of computation--the data are in effect considered to be
wrapped around a cylinder whose circumference is $T = N\Delta$. The
circular covariance function estimator has a serious deficiency
that limits its usefulness. The nature of this deficiency can be
seen by representing it as two summations:

$$\tilde{c}_{xx}(\tau) = \frac{1}{N}\left[\sum_{t^\circ=0}^{N-1-|\tau^\circ|} \tilde{x}(t^\circ)\tilde{x}*(t^\circ + \tau^\circ) \right.$$

$$\left. + \sum_{t^\circ=N-|\tau|}^{N-1} \tilde{x}(t^\circ)\tilde{x}*(t^\circ + \tau^\circ - N) \right] \qquad (3.97)$$

The absolute value sign serves to make the equation applicable to
both positive and negative delays, though from the symmetry of

the acvf about $\tau = 0$, only positive values need be considered. Using this fact, it can be seen that the above equation simplifies to

$$\tilde{c}_{xx,N}(\tau^\circ) = \left(\frac{N - |\tau^\circ|}{N}\right) \hat{c}_{xx}(\tau^\circ) + \frac{|\tau^\circ|}{N} \hat{c}(N - |\tau^\circ|) \qquad (3.98)$$

$\hat{c}_{xx}(\tau^\circ)$, of course, is just the average of products of the form $\tilde{x}(t^\circ)\tilde{x}*(t^\circ + \tau^\circ)$. This means that the circular acvf estimator is a combination of two estimators of the acvf, one for τ° and the other for $N - |\tau^\circ|$. These two are inseparable from one another in this method of estimation. Interpretation of the estimated acvf can therefore be a problem. Of course, this is of no consequence when the data really do arise from a process with period T. However, this is not usually the case. Consequently, it is desirable to look for acvf estimation procedures that are free of this problem. We need not seek far for one. All we need do is adopt another periodicity artifice, one that begins by padding out the original sequence of N samples with a sequence of samples of 0 amplitude, let us say L of them. Then the data may be considered to arise from a specimen of a periodic process whose period is $N' = N + L$. We consider this for the simplest situation, when $L = N$ and $N' = 2N$.

In our new sequence, $\tilde{x}(t^\circ)$ of length $2N$, data samples $\tilde{x}(N)$ through $\tilde{x}(2N - 1)$ are 0. Because of this, at each time lag τ° there can be only $N - |\tau^\circ|$ nonzero products in the acvf estimate formed from the sequence. The acvf is then estimated as the average of these products with, however, the averaging factor being taken as $1/N$, N being the number of nonzero products when $\tau^\circ = 0$ rather than $1/(N - |\tau^\circ|)$. The reason for using the former is that the variance of the resulting estimator turns out to be smaller at larger values of τ° than when using the factor $1/(N - |\tau^\circ|)$. (See Jenkins and Watts, 1968.) This gives for the estimator

$$\tilde{c}_{xx,2N}(\tau^\circ) = \frac{1}{2N} \sum_{t^\circ=0}^{2N-1} \tilde{x}(t^\circ)\tilde{x}^*(t^\circ + \tau^\circ)$$

$$= \frac{1}{N} \sum_{t^\circ=0}^{N-|\tau^\circ|-1} x(t^\circ)x^*(t^\circ + \tau^\circ) = \hat{c}_{xx}(\tau^\circ) \qquad (3.99)$$

The tilde over the data samples is unnecessary. We have also returned to the circumflex notation for the acvf estimate because circularity has been eliminated in the computation even though we have arrived at $\hat{c}_{xx}(\tau^\circ)$ by an argument involving a periodicity of $2N$. This estimate does not have the difficulty exhibited by the circular acvf estimate with period N as given in Eq. (3.96). It is therefore to be preferred to $\tilde{c}_{xx}(\tau^\circ)$ in most instances.

The statistical properties of $\hat{c}_{xx}(\tau^\circ)$ are of interest. When the data $x(t)$ arise from a specimen function of random process x, we have

$$E[\hat{c}_{xx}(\tau^\circ)] = \frac{1}{N} \sum_{t^\circ=0}^{N-|\tau^\circ|-1} E[x(t^\circ)x^*(t^\circ + \tau^\circ)] \qquad (3.100)$$

This means that $\hat{c}_{xx}(\tau^\circ)$ is a biased estimate of $c_{xx}(\tau^\circ)$ because, as shown earlier, $E[\hat{c}_{xx}(\tau^\circ)] - c_{xx}(\tau^\circ) = -|\tau^\circ|c_{xx}(\tau^\circ)/N$. Use of the averaging factor $1/(N - |\tau^\circ|)$ would eliminate this problem, but only, as noted above, at the expense of increasing the variance of the estimate as τ° becomes large. This is generally thought to be undesirable.

The variance of $\hat{c}_{xx}(\tau^\circ)$ may be calculated from its definition in Eq. (3.99). The result depends upon the statistical properties of the process. In the Gaussian case, the one of most general interest, it can be shown (Jenkins and Watts, 1968) that

$$\text{var}[\hat{c}_{xx}(\tau^\circ)] \simeq \frac{1}{N} \sum_{k^\circ=-\infty}^{\infty} [c_{xx}^2(k^\circ) + c_{xx}(k^\circ + \tau^\circ)c_{xx}(k^\circ - \tau^\circ)]$$

$$(3.101)$$

This means that the variance of the acvf estimate of a Gaussian process depends upon the acvf itself, something we generally do not know beforehand. For the particular situation in which the process is white noise with variance σ_x^2, $c_{xx}(\tau^\circ) = \sigma_x^2 \delta(\tau^\circ)$ and $\text{var}[\hat{c}_{xx}(\tau^\circ)] = \sigma_x^4/N$ for all τ° except $\tau^\circ = 0$, in which case the variance is $2\sigma_x^4/N$. Note that when x is an aperiodic process with no dc component, $c_{xx}^2(\tau^\circ)$ becomes small as τ° becomes large. This means that the summation on the right-hand side of Eq. (3.101) will be finite so that when we divide it by N to obtain the variance of $c_{xx}(\tau^\circ)$, the result becomes small as N increases, indicating the estimator to be a consistent one. This also can be shown to hold when the process is non-Gaussian. Further scrutiny of Eq. (3.101) seems to indicate that difficulties are encountered when $x(t)$ has a periodic component in it, which can occur when there is residual interference from 60 Hz power lines. In this case, $c_{xx}^2(\tau^\circ)$ does not become small as τ° increases and the summation becomes infinite. Does this mean that the variance of the estimate is infinite regardless of N? The answer is no. The difficulty arises in the formulation leading to Eq. (3.101). When proper account is taken of the pure frequency component in $x(t)$, the variance of the estimate turns out to be the same as before.

The statistical relationship between estimates of the acvf made at neighboring time points is also of some interest. This refers to the fluctuations of the estimate about the estimated mean of the acvf. What we are in effect discussing is the covariance of the estimation errors. The problem is a thorny one, but some results exist for the Gaussian stationary process. In particular, the covariance between acvf estimates at τ_1° and τ_2° is given by (Jenkins and Watts, 1968)

$$\text{cov}[\hat{c}_{xx}(\tau_1^\circ), \hat{c}_{xx}(\tau_2^\circ)] \simeq \frac{1}{N} \sum_{r^\circ=-\infty}^{\infty} [c_{xx}(r^\circ)c_{xx}(r^\circ + \tau_1^\circ - \tau_2^\circ)$$

$$+ c_{xx}(r^\circ + \tau_1^\circ)c_{xx}(r^\circ - \tau_2^\circ)] \tag{3.102}$$

This equation, from which the previous one was derived, points out some useful features of the acvf estimate. First, the estimates are uncorrelated only when the x process is a white noise with $c_{xx}(\tau°) = \sigma_x^2 \delta(\tau°)$. Second, for any process which has an acvf with nonzero values extending over K successive intervals, there will be a nonzero covariance between acvf estimates that are closer than $2K$ apart, that is, for which $|\tau_1° - \tau_2°| < 2K$. Narrow band processes have covariance functions of this type. The covariance between estimates becomes smaller as $|\tau_1° - \tau_2°|$ approaches $2K$. But the major fact is that when the process is a narrow band one, a larger N is required to obtain an acvf estimate in which the covariance between estimates is to be kept beneath a given maximum. This can be of importance in dealing with acvf estimates of the EEG. An EEG with a marked alpha component will, for a fixed N, have a greater amount of covariance between acvf estimates than will an estimate of the covariance function obtained when the alpha component is small or lacking. Another aspect of the covariance function of narrow band processes is that there is little, if anything, to be gained by smoothing the acvf estimates because this does not reduce the covariance between neighboring estimates.

B. *ESTIMATION OF THE ACVF*

The functional form of the estimator in Eq. (3.99) suggests the obvious "brute force" way of calculating the estimates: averaging for each value of $\tau°$ the $N - |\tau°|$ products obtained from the N samples sequence. Computationally, the procedure is a lengthy one since complete evaluation of $\hat{c}_{xx}(\tau°)$ requires that there be $N(N + 1)/2$ multiplications and $N(N - 1)/2$ additions, a total of N^2 arithmetic operations. When N is large, the time required to complete this task becomes excessive. While some short cuts have been found for these time domain procedures, the net time savings has not been impressive. What has brought about a significant reduction in computation time has been the fast Fourier transform algorithm. Its use makes it possible to obtain estimates of the acvf by first estimating the periodogram of the data and then taking the inverse discrete Fourier transform. Since there are about $N \log_2 N$ operations involved in estimating the periodogram and about another $2N \log_2 (2N)$ in taking the inverse DFT, the great computational savings are apparent. For example, when $N = 1000$, the method of Eq. (3.99) requires about 10^6 operations, while the DFT method requires about 4×10^4 operations. The reduction in the number of operations is by a factor of over 25, a factor that increases as N increases. Because the DFT is such an efficient approach to acvf estimation when N is large, we shall describe it further.

We have already noted that the acvf estimate of Eq. (3.99) can be considered to arise from a periodicized process whose initial N samples are the $x(t°\Delta)$ and whose final N samples are all zeros. To guard against spectral leakage effects of the dc component, we subtract out the average value of the N samples before padding the sequence with zeros. We may also de-trend the data if that seems warranted. The resulting sequence of $2N$ points then possesses the acvf we are interested in. An alternative way of arriving at this acvf is to first obtain the periodogram of the padded sequence. The periodogram of an unpadded sequence of N data points has been given in Section 3.10, Eq. (3.60). When the sequence is padded to length N' by adding L consecutive zeros such that $N' = N + L$, the periodogram of the padded sequence is

$$P_{xx,N'}(n) = \frac{1}{N'} \left| X_{N'}(n) \right|^2$$

$$= \frac{1}{N'} \left| \sum_{t°=0}^{N-1} x(t°) \exp(-j2\pi n t°/N') \right|^2 \tag{3.103}$$

The upper limit in the summation is $N - 1$ rather than $N' - 1$ because the last L values of the sequence are zero. When $N' = 2N$, we have

$$P_{xx,2N}(n) = \frac{1}{2N} \left| \sum_{t°=0}^{N-1} x(t°) \exp(-j2\pi n t°/2N) \right|^2 \tag{3.104}$$

163

Notice that because the fundamental interval is $2N$ rather than N in length, there are twice as many frequencies present in the $2N$ periodogram. These additional frequency components are required to express the fact that the second half of the sample sequence is constrained to be zero. They afford no additional information about the original data but only serve as a computational vehicle to arrive at the acvf estimate. Note also that the presence of $2N$ rather than N in the denominator does not increase the number of operations involved in the computation.

Having once obtained $P_{xx,2N}(n)$, its inverse DFT can be taken and it yields the estimated acvf:

$$\hat{c}_{xx}(\tau^\circ) = \frac{1}{N} \sum_{n=-(N-1)}^{N-1} P_{xx,2N}(n) \, \exp(j2\pi n \tau^\circ/2N) \tag{3.105}$$

Use of the factor $1/N$ rather than $1/2N$ in the above equation might, at first glance, appear to be an error. It can be verified to be correct by taking the DFT of the padded sequence $\tilde{x}(t^\circ)$ and substituting this into Eq. (3.99, top). After carrying out the summations and using Eq. (3.103), we arrive at Eq. (3.105). Furthermore, because $c_{xx}(\tau^\circ)$ is an even function, the computation need only be carried out for positive values of τ°. Another way of writing Eq. (3.105) takes advantage of the fact that $P_{xx,2N}(n)$ is real. Using this, we have

$$\hat{c}_{xx}(\tau^\circ) = \frac{P_{xx,2N}(0)}{N} + \frac{2}{N} \sum_{n=1}^{N-1} P_{xx,2N}(n) \, \cos(2\pi n \tau^\circ/2N) \tag{3.106}$$

The derivation of the estimated acvf from the periodogram has just been shown to be valid for all values of τ° up to N. In practice, there is usually little need to carry this out to such large lag values. Usually, lags that are less than 10% of N are only of interest. Because of this there are further savings to be obtained in the use of the DFT. Let us assume that the acvf is of interest up to a lag of $L < N$. Then when we pad the original sequences of N data samples, we need to add L zeros to get an overall sequence of length $N' = N + L$. This guarantees that any estimation of $c_{xx}(\tau°)$ at values of $\tau° < L$ will be free from wrap-around or overlap effects with the next period of the periodicized data. The effect of padding the data with L zeros is shown in Fig. 3.10 when the lag is L. It can be seen that there are $N - L$

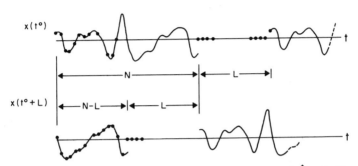

Fig. 3.10. Computation of the estimated acvf $\hat{c}_{xx}(t°)$ at lag L from a periodicized sequence of N data points padded with L zeros. Only $N - L$ products can differ from zero.

products which are nonzero and L which are forced to be zero, and that none of the nonzero products arises from the overlap of one period with the next. The N' periodogram of the padded data is given (after average values and possible trends have been removed) by Eq. (3.104) rewritten here

$$P_{xx,N'}(n) = \frac{1}{N'} \left| \sum_{t°=0}^{N-1} x(t°)\,\exp(-j2\pi n t°/N') \right|^2,$$

$$-(N' - 1) \le n \le (N' - 1) \qquad (3.107)$$

where $N' = N + L$. As before, we have a larger range of n to deal with, but the additional frequency terms in the periodogram only serve to take the padding with zeros into account. The inverse DFT then yields our estimate of the acvf:

$$\hat{c}_{xx}(\tau°) = \frac{1}{N'} \sum_{n=-(N'-1)}^{N'-1} P_{xx,N'}(n)\,\exp(-j2\pi n \tau°/N'),\; 0 \le |\tau°| \le L$$

$$(3.108)$$

Because L is usually small compared to N, the inverse transform involves not many more operations than does the computation of the periodogram.

C. CROSS COVARIANCE FUNCTION ESTIMATION

The computation of the ccvf for two N length data sequences $x(t°\Delta)$ and $y(t°\Delta)$ follows the same principles that hold for the acvf estimate. Again, we assume $\Delta = 1$. The use of the direct and inverse DFT facilitates these computations when N is large. If we are interested in estimating the ccvf for lags up to L, then padding the x and y sequences with L zeros each eliminates the possibility of an overlap in the computation. The procedure to be used, therefore, after padding the sequences, is to obtain their respective DFTs, $X_{N'}(n)$ and $Y_{N'}(n)$. From them we obtain the raw cross-spectrum estimate $P_{xy,N'}(n) = \frac{1}{N} X_{N'}(n) Y_{N'}^*(n)$ and then the estimated ccvf:

$$\hat{c}_{xy}(\tau°) = \frac{1}{N'} \sum_{n=-(N'-1)}^{N'-1} P_{xy,N'}(n) \; \exp(j2\pi n\tau°/N'), \; -L \leq \tau° \leq L$$

(3.109)

It will be remembered that $c_{xy}(\tau°)$ is not an even function of $\tau°$ and so its ccvf is to be estimated at both positive and negative values of $\tau°$. This means a doubling of the length of the last step of the computation, but when N is large, the FFT still produces a substantially shorter computation than the brute force method.

The statistical properties of the ccvf are close enough to those of the acvf so that a full development of them would in the main be repetitious. Consequently, we bring out only the highlights of the development and move quickly to the results. The most common form of the ccvf estimator is the biased version

$$\hat{c}_{xy}(\tau°) = \frac{1}{N} \sum_{t°=0}^{N-|\tau°|-1} x(t°) y^*(t° + \tau°)$$

(3.110)

166

$\hat{c}_{xy}(\tau^\circ)$ can be considered to be one period of a $2N$ periodic function, and, as already shown, this is especially important when it is obtained by Fourier methods. The biased version of the estimator is preferred for the same reason as is the biased version of the acvf, that it tends to yield a smaller variance in the estimate when τ° becomes large. The variance of the ccvf estimator is derivable from its definition. When both processes are Gaussian, it is given by (Jenkins and Watts, 1968),

$$\text{var}\,[\hat{c}_{xy}(\tau^\circ)] \simeq \frac{1}{N} \sum_{r^\circ=-\infty}^{\infty} [c_{xx}(r^\circ)c_{yy}(r^\circ) + c_{xy}(r^\circ + \tau^\circ)c_{yx}(r^\circ - \tau^\circ)] \tag{3.111}$$

This shows that the variance is calculable only when we know what the ccvf and both acvfs are. If both processes are white and uncorrelated, the second term drops out and we have

$$\text{var}\,[\hat{c}_{xy}(\tau^\circ)] = \frac{\sigma_x^2 \sigma_y^2}{N} \tag{3.112}$$

The principal fact about the ccvf estimator is that it is a consistent one. Also in common with the acvf estimator, the covariance between estimates at two different lag times depends upon the difference between the lags and the covariance properties of the processes. The covariance of the estimator is a generalization of Eq. (3.111) which we show here for the special case when x and y are uncorrelated:

$$\text{cov}\,[\hat{c}_{xy}(\tau_1^\circ), \hat{c}_{xy}(\tau_2^\circ)] \simeq \frac{1}{N} \sum_{r^\circ=-\infty}^{\infty} c_{xx}(r^\circ)c_{yy}(r^\circ + \tau_2^\circ - \tau_1^\circ) \tag{3.113}$$

Equation (3.113) can be seen to be a discrete convolution of the two acvfs, the separation variable being $\tau_2^\circ - \tau_1^\circ$. Among other things, this means that when X and Y are uncorrelated narrow band (nearly sinusoidal or pacemakerlike) processes centered at about the same frequency, the covariance between estimates can rise and fall cyclically over an extensive range of time separations. This in turn can lead to spurious indications of covariance between processes unless special measures are taken, beyond merely increasing N, to reduce the magnitude of the estimated covariance between estimates. One such measure is prefiltering the X and Y data to individually "whiten" them before the covariance testing is carried out. The details of such a procedure are beyond the scope of this presentation and may be found in Jenkins and Watts (1968). However, the net import is that the use of the ccvf estimator as a means for measuring dependency between processes is beset with difficulties. These should be carefully assessed before experimentation designed to exploit ccvf estimation is entered into. There is a distinct danger of arriving at erroneous conclusions, especially in the case of pacemakerlike processes.

3.19. COHERENCE FUNCTIONS

The difficulties associated with ccvf estimation have brought about the development of an alternative method for evaluating the relationship between continuous processes, the coherence function. The coherence function is a measure based upon the auto- and cross-spectral properties of the processes, not upon their cvfs. It closely resembles the square of a correlation coefficient between the spectral components of the processes at a particular frequency f. Thus the coherence function, or squared coherence, is defined as

$$\kappa_{xy}^2(f) = \frac{\left|C_{xy}(f)\right|^2}{C_{xx}(f)C_{yy}(f)} \tag{3.114}$$

Because the $\left|C_{xy}(f)\right|^2$ ranges in absolute value from 0 to $C_{xx}(f)C_{yy}(f)$, $\kappa_{xy}^2(f)$ can be seen to be a normalization of the square of the cross spectrum by the product of the autospectra. The normalization is important because it compensates for large values in the cross spectrum that may have been brought about not by an increase in the coupling between the processes at frequency f but by an inherently large concentration of power at that frequency in either the X or Y process. If the X and Y processes are identical, then $C_{xy}(f) = C_{xx}(f) = C_{yy}(f)$ and $\kappa^2_{xy}(f) = 1$ at all frequencies. At the opposite extreme, if X and Y are independent processes, $C_{xy}(f) = 0$ and $\kappa^2_{xy}(f) = 0$ at all frequencies. Between these two extremes there lies a wealth of possible relationships between the processes that can often be measured usefully by the coherence function. It may be, for example, that X and Y are closely related but only over a limited range of frequencies. This would be the case if X and Y each represented a noisy "locked in" response to a sinusoidal signal of frequency f_0. In this case the coherency would be nearly unity at f_0 and zero elsewhere. Similar situations may exist when the processes are not driven ones. They may be highly coherent over certain ranges of frequency and incoherent elsewhere. Note should be taken here of the fact that the coherence function suppresses any phase information concerning the two processes--it considers their relationship only in terms of power at a given frequency. Later in the chapter we discuss the use of phase measures to detect process interrelationships. It is also worth noting that when one of the processes is a well-defined stimulus, coherency measures are inferior to average response or cross-correlation techniques. Coherency measures find their major application when the processes are substantially random ones.

The coherence function exemplifies a change in emphasis from temporal to frequency measures. It can bring a certain amount of clarification to interprocess relationships. In this regard the estimator of the coherence function has properties that seem to be superior to those of the ccvf estimator. It is these properties which we consider now. The estimator $\kappa^2_{xy}(f)$ for the coherence function needs to be defined carefully. A meaningful estimate cannot be obtained directly from the raw auto- and cross-spectra of the processes. To see this, it is only necessary to examine what would happen if this were the case, viz.,

$$\frac{\left|P_{xy}(f_n)\right|^2}{\left|P_{xx}(f_n)\right|\left|P_{yy}(f_n)\right|} = \frac{\left|X_N(f_n)Y_N^*(f_n)\right|^2}{\left|X_N(f_n)\right|^2\left|Y_N(f_n)\right|^2} = 1, \quad \text{for all } f$$

$$(3.115)$$

Clearly, this is a useless quantity. To be useful, a coherence function estimator must be formed from smoothed spectral estimates of the processes. The smoothing operations, however, necessitate consideration of the same issues that were dealt with in the estimation of auto- and cross-spectra, resolution, and bias. Their effect on the coherence function estimator is more difficult to determine, simply because of the way the coherence function has been defined. Though formal solutions for the bias and covariance of coherence function estimates have not been obtained for all the situations of interest involving (a) different kinds of processes, (b) different spectra, and (c) different smoothed spectral estimators, it has been possible by the use of simulation techniques to develop useful relationships for the bias and variance in many situations of interest. A property of major interest is that the coherence function estimator obtained from smoothed spectral estimates appears to be a robust one. That is, it is insensitive to whether the processes are Gaussian or not. This means that one can employ coherence function estimation without having to be particularly concerned about whether the results of the analysis are sensitive to the amplitude distributions of the particular processes involved.

As a rule, it is the small values of coherence that are especially important to deal with. They are the ones that are normally encountered in dealing with the EEG, for example. Electrode sites that are not close usually produce data in which clear correlations are not obvious. And if they were, there would be little reason to perform a coherence function analysis. To see how large the coherence function might be in a not too unreal situation, let us consider a simple model in which the data sources X and Y consist of a common signal process S embedded in independent noise processes N_1 and N_2. The temporal representation of this situation is

$$x(t) = n_1(t) + s(t)$$

$$\text{(3.116)}$$

$$y(t) = n_2(t) + s(t)$$

The power spectrum representation of this situation is

$$C_{xx}(f) = C_{n_1 n_1}(f) + C_{ss}(f)$$

$$C_{yy}(f) = C_{n_2 n_2}(f) + C_{ss}(f) \qquad \text{(3.117)}$$

$$C_{xy}(f) = C_{ss}(f)$$

The last relationship follows from the Fourier transform of the ccvf between X and Y. We must have $c_{xy}(\tau) = c_{ss}(\tau)$ because the only correlation between X and Y is that caused by the presence of S in both. The coherence function is then

$$\kappa_{xy}^2(f) = \frac{c_{ss}^2(f)}{[C_{n_1 n_1}(f) + C_{ss}(f)][C_{n_2 n_2}(f) + C_{ss}(f)]} \qquad \text{(3.118)}$$

If we assume n_1 and n_2 to have identical spectra, this can be simplified to

$$\kappa_{xy}^2(f) = \frac{1}{[1 + C_{nn}(f)/C_{ss}(f)]^2} \qquad \text{(3.119)}$$

Let us now consider the signal process to have strength equal to the noise processes at frequency f. Then $\kappa_{xy}^2(f) = 1/4$, a rather small coherence. A signal-to-noise ratio of the order of unity tends to be large in comparison to that encountered in a number of interesting neurological situations, and so our major concern insofar as coherence function estimation is concerned must be with the behavior of $\hat{\kappa}_{xy}^2(f)$ when coherency is low.

The behavior of the coherence function estimator is best known when it is derived from smoothed spectral estimates having

20 or more degrees of freedom. This means, for example, smoothing over 10 neighboring frequencies with a rectangular spectral window or using 10 data sequences when Bartlett smoothing is employed. Under these circumstances it has been found (Enochson and Goodman, 1965) that when the squared coherence is between 0.3 and 0.98, its estimator $\hat{z}$, expressed in terms of the Fisher z variable, has a nearly Gaussian distribution. $\hat{z}$ is given by

$$\hat{z} = \tanh^{-1} \hat{\kappa}_{xy} = \frac{1}{2} \log \frac{1 + \hat{\kappa}_{xy}}{1 - \hat{\kappa}_{xy}} \tag{3.120}$$

The mean and variance of $\hat{z}$ are given by

$$\mu_{\hat{z}} = \tanh^{-1} \kappa_{xy} + \frac{1}{d.f. - 2}$$

$$\sigma_{\hat{z}}^2 = \frac{1}{d.f. - 2} \tag{3.121}$$

d.f. is the degrees of freedom associated with the spectral smoothing window and has been discussed previously. A rectangular window covering 10 neighboring frequencies has 20 degrees of freedom. The second term in the mean is a bias which becomes small as the degree of smoothing increases. The variance of the estimate also becomes small as the width of the spectral window increases, but obviously one does not wish to widen the window too much and thereby lose spectral resolution. One may surmise, however, that the covariance of coherence function estimates at nearby frequencies increases with the degree of smoothing. When the squared coherence is less than 0.3, one can continue to deal with the z transformed version of $\hat{\kappa}_{xy}$, but the bias and the variance of the estimator need to be modified. Benignus (1969) has shown by using simulation techniques that a better estimate for κ_{xy}^2, small or large, is

$$\tilde{\kappa}_{xy}^2 = \hat{\kappa}^2 - \frac{2}{d.f.} \left(1 - \hat{\kappa}_{xy}^2 \right) \tag{3.122}$$

The same techniques also show that a better estimate of the variance of $\hat{z}$ is given by

$$\tilde{\sigma}_{\hat{z}}^2 = \sigma_{\hat{z}}^2 \left[1 - 0.004^{(1.6\ \hat{\kappa}_{xy}^2 + 0.22)} \right]$$
(3.123)

Further refinements to the estimator have been made by Lopes da Silva *et al.* (1974). Confidence limits for $\hat{\kappa}_{xy}^2$ may be constructed using these results. They are shown in Fig. (3.11). N is the

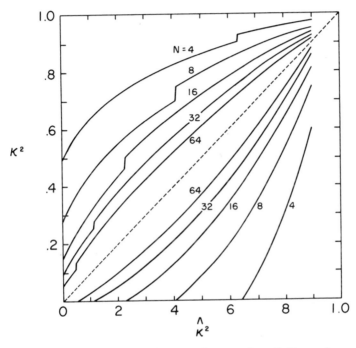

Fig. 3.11. The 95% confidence intervals of the coherence function, plotted for the number of data segments used in smoothing. The discontinuities in the upper bounds reflect the change to a one-tailed interval when the lower confidence limit descends to 0. [Benignus, V. A., IEEE Trans. Audio Electroacoust. AU-17, 145 (1969).]

number of segments used in Bartlett smoothing, and therefore is twice the number of degrees of freedom of the spectral estimate. The discontinuities in the upper bounds result from the method of computation and are of no special significance. The curves are instructive. Suppose we perform Bartlett smoothing with 16 segments of data. Only when $\hat{\kappa}_{xy}^2 > 0.23$ can we then say with about

95% confidence that the two processes have some coherence at the frequency tested. The expected value of the squared coherence is 0.23 but the confidence limits are 0 and 0.46. The figure clearly shows that rather large estimation errors will be the rule rather than the exception when the squared coherence is low. In view of these considerations, it is not surprising that nearly all who discuss the use of the coherence function recommend extreme caution in its use. Even large coherence function estimates may not justify the interpretation that there is dependency between the processes.

Several interesting applications of the coherence function to the study of the EEG have been made. We mention only two. Lopes da Silva *et al*. (1973) used the coherence function to study the relationship between cortical alpha rhythms and thalamic generators. They found instances of significant coherence between the two regions as well as cortico-cortical coherences which were high over large regions of the cortex. Another interesting application of the coherence function has been given by Gersch and Goddard (1970). They used it to test for the location of an epileptic focus in terms of its nearness to one of a number of electrode sites within the brain. This involved dealing with the coherence function for pairs of data sources (electrode sites) before and after possible coherence with a third site had been taken into account. By showing that the activity of two sites was coherent in the important frequency range of 4-12 Hz when the effects of a third site were present and then became incoherent when the effects of that site were computationally removed, they were able to infer that the third site was near the epileptic focus.

3.20. PHASE ESTIMATION

Another method for determining the existence of correlation between two processes is to use the information in the phase of the two processes rather than their power. The phase spectrum is derived from the cross spectrum by the relationship

$$F_{xy}(f) = \arctan[-Q_{xy}(f)/L_{xy}(f)] \tag{3.124}$$

The denominator is the real part of $C_{xy}(f)$ and the numerator the imaginary part. If the processes X and Y are uncorrelated, then no particular phase relationship is to be expected at any frequency. $F_{xy}(f)$ will be a random variable with mean 0 uniformly distributed over the range $-\pi/2$ to $\pi/2$. On the other hand, if there is a correlation between the two processes, this will show up in the phase spectrum in the form of a preferred phase angle related to frequency. For example, when X and Y both contain a signal process S as in Eq. (3.116), the phase spectrum will be 0 for all f. If X contains S, and Y contains a linearly filtered version of S, $F_{xy}(f)$ can take on any real value. The estimator $\hat{F}_{xy}(f)$ of the phase spectrum is a random variable defined by

$$\hat{F}_{xy}(f) = \arctan[-\hat{Q}_{xy}(f)/\hat{L}_{xy}(f)] \tag{3.125}$$

where $L_{xy}(f)$ and $Q_{xy}(f)$ are, respectively, the real and imaginary parts of $X(f)Y^*(f)$. The phase estimator, like the squared coherence estimator, is useful only when it is preceded by smoothing of the cross spectrum. Under these circumstances the variance of the estimate decreases with increasing squared coherence and the number of degrees of freedom of the smoothed spectral estimate. The relationship is

$$\text{var}[\hat{F}_{xy}(f)] \simeq \frac{1}{\text{d.f.}}\left(\frac{1}{\hat{K}_{xy}^2} - 1\right) \tag{3.126}$$

Decreasing the variance of the phase estimator obtained from a fixed length sample by increasing the degrees of freedom brings about, as before, a decrease in the spectral resolution and a lessened ability to detect correlations that may exist only over narrow frequency bands. Discussion of further properties of the phase estimator may be found in Jenkins and Watts (1968). Thus far it has not been widely applied to the study of EEG activity.

REFERENCES

Benignus, V. A., *IEEE Trans. Audio Electroacoust.*, AU-17, 145 (1969).
Bergland, G. D., *IEEE SPECTRUM* 6, 41 (1969).
Enochson, L. D. and Goodman, N. R., AFFDL TR-65-57, Res. and Tech. Div., AFSC, Wright-Patterson AFB, Ohio (1965).
Gersch, W. and Goddard, G. V., *Science* 169, 702 (1970).
Jenkins, G. M. and Watts, D. G., "Spectral Analysis and Its Applications," Holden-Day, San Francisco, 1968.
Lopes da Silva, F. H., van Lierop, T. H. M. T., Schrijer, C. F. and Storm van Leeuwen, W., *Electroenceph. Clin. Neurophysiol.* 35, 627 (1973).
Lopes da Silva, F. H., van Lierop, T. H. M. T., Schrijer, C. F. and Storm van Leeuwen, W., in "Die Quantifizierung des Electroencephalogramms" (G. K. Schenk, ed.), p. 437. AEG Telefunken, Kunstanz, 1973.
Oppenheim, A. V. and Schafer, R. W., "Digital Signal Processing," Prentice-Hall, Englewood Cliffs, 1975.
Otnes, R. K. and Enochson, L., "Digital Time Series Analysis," Wiley, New York, 1972.
Welch, P. D., *IEEE Trans. Audio Electroacoust.* AU-15, 70 (1967).

Chapter 4

EVOKED POTENTIALS:
AVERAGING AND DISCRIMINANT ANALYSIS

4.1. INTRODUCTION

An evoked response is defined to be the sum of (a) the stimu-lus-evoked activity of the brain, (b) the brain noise which is brain activity not related to the stimulus, and (c) the nonbrain noise which is electrical activity originating outside the brain. It includes instrumentation noise and electronic artifacts of all types. In our context signal is synonymous with the stimulus-evoked activity and noise, with the remainder of the response. Since stimulus-evoked activity is not generally discernible in a single response to a stimulus, it is desirable to find some way to separate this activity from the noise. Although in some types of experiments this can be done by adjusting the site of the recording electrode, in many other experiments this is not feasible, *e.g.*, the scalp recordings of the human EEG. Other analytical methods must be employed to permit separation of the stimulus-evoked activity from the interfering noise. Under appropriate conditions, a simple averaging procedure will allow such a separation (Rosenblith, 1959).

As an example, consider the following type of experiment. Sensory stimulation of the nervous system evokes a neuroelectric response. However, the evoked responses are obscured by the brain and nonbrain noises. Consequently, repetitive stimulation usually results in recording dissimilar evoked response waveshapes despite identical experimental conditions, due to the background noise. Even the mere presence of a response to the stimulus may be diffi-cult to discern in any single waveform.

Averaging the recorded waveforms together will attenuate the noise but not the signal if the following conditions approximately hold:

1. The signal and noise linearly sum together to produce the recorded waveform;

2. The evoked signal waveshape attributable solely to the stimulus is the same for each repetition of the stimulus;

3. The noise contributions to the observed data appear sufficiently irregular so that they can be considered to constitute statistically independent samples of a random process.

Response averaging and its related data analysis procedures are valid for both T-continuous and T-discrete data. Without loss of generality, we shall use continuous waveform notation.

The averaging procedure consists of adding together the set of recorded response waveforms associated with each stimulus delivery The addition is initiated by a timing signal which occurs either when the stimulus is presented, or by a fixed time interval before or after stimulus presentation. Initiation of averaging prior to stimulus presentation allows analysis of the prestimulus activity in the structure being observed. The average of the prestimulus activity can serve as a baseline for evaluation of the averaged evoked activity. Since the common signal waveform is synchronized with the stimulus while the interfering noise waveforms are asynchronous, the signal waveforms will sum in direct proportion to the number of stimuli used while the net noise waveform will increase less rapidly due to cancellation effects. When completed, the sum of response waveforms is divided by the number of stimuli delivered. This normalizes the result to the average response. Stated analytically, let each recorded waveform be denoted by

$$x_i(t) = s(t) + n_i(t); \quad i = 1, 2, \dots N; \quad 0 \le t \le T \qquad (4.1)$$

Where N is the number of stimuli, $x_i(t)$ the response to the ith stimulus, $s(t)$ the signal (evoked response), $n_i(t)$ the noise during the time epoch associated with the ith stimulus, and T the duration of the time epoch over which each waveform is recorded.

The average over the sample of N waveforms is used to estimate $s(t)$. The sample average, the average evoked response, is
denoted by $\hat{s}(t)$, where

$$\hat{s}(t) = \frac{1}{N} \sum_{i=1}^{N} x_i(t) = s(t) + \frac{1}{N} \sum_{i=1}^{N} n_i(t) \qquad (4.2)$$

Equation (4.2) is a complete analytic description of the
averaging procedure. The remainder of this chapter is concerned
with the questions of how good is the estimate of $s(t)$ provided by
averaging, and how relaxation of the three assumptions affects the
results.

Equation (4.2) indicates that the quality of the estimator
$\hat{s}(t)$ depends upon the relative magnitudes of $s(t)$ and the average
of the noise waveforms. Before proceeding further, some notations
will be introduced. The variance of the noise $E[n^2_i(t)]$ will be
denoted by σ^2 and as a result of the assumed independence of noise
samples, $E[n_i(t)n_k(t)] = 0$ for all $i = k$. Without loss of generality, it is also assumed that the expected value of $n_i(t)$ will
be zero. Thus the expected value of $\hat{s}(t)$ is

$$E[\hat{s}(t)] = E\left[\frac{1}{N} \sum_{i=1}^{N} x_i(t)\right] = s(t) + \frac{1}{N} \sum_{i=1}^{N} E[n_i(t)] = s(t) \qquad (4.3)$$

Equation (4.3) indicates that the averaging procedure is an
unbiased estimator of the evoked signal. It holds out the possibility that, with a sufficiently large number of stimuli, $\hat{s}(t)$
will approximately equal $s(t)$. However, it does not state how
effectively the noise is attenuated for a given number of stimulus
repetitions, or how many such repetitions are required for a desired level of noise attenuation. A computation of the *standard
deviation of the average*, referred to as the standard error *(SE)*,
provides an estimate of the expected magnitude of the noise
residual.

$$(SE)^2 = E[\hat{s}(t) - s(t)]^2 = E\left[\frac{1}{N}\sum_{i=1}^{N} n_i(t)\right]^2$$

$$= \frac{1}{N^2}\sum_{i=1}^{N}\sum_{j=1}^{N} E[n_i(t)n_j(t)] = \frac{1}{N^2}\sum_{i=1}^{N} E\, n_i^2(t)$$

$$= \frac{1}{N^2} \cdot N\sigma^2$$

Thus

$$SE = \sigma/\sqrt{N} \tag{4.4}$$

Equation (4.4) states that averaging attenuates the noise to a residuum that is directly proportional to the intensity of the background noise and inversely proportional to the square root of the number of evoked waveforms used. In theory, if a sufficient number of stimuli are presented, the residual noise can be made arbitrarily small. In practice, there are limits upon the amount of data available, and so a nonzero standard error will always be encountered.

The essential assumptions in the above discussion were that the evoked signal waveforms be identical for all stimuli and that the noise waveforms be uncorrelated random variables. If the noise waves are not uncorrelated, then expression (4.4), the standard error may not be valid. If the signals are not identical, then neither expression (4.3), the expected sample average, nor expression (4.4) are valid. In practice, the conditions for this model will only be approximately valid, so that Eq. (4.3) and Eq. (4.4) will apply to a limited extent.

4.2. ESTIMATION OF VARIABILITY

It is often of interest and importance to obtain a measure of the variability of the set of waveforms associated with responses to a given stimulus. Such knowledge allows one to determine the degree of reliance that can be placed upon the waveshape of the average. If the average is computed from a sample of waveforms with low variability, then the fine detail of the average waveform may be considered to be a reflection of the underlying evoked response and not due to random fluctuations. Conversely, if the variability of the set of waveforms in the sample is high, then, at best, only the broad outline of the underlying evoked response may be discerned in the average waveform. Much of the detail, and in some instances the entire waveform, may be due primarily to the residue of the random noise.

A technique for appraising the variability of the average response is to subdivide the set of available waveforms into subsets, compute an average for each subset, and compare, usually by plotting all averages on the same graph. The degree of reproducibility of the averages is a measure of background noise. This technique readily lends itself to visual inspection. It is possible to arrive at a qualitative judgment of how much reliance to place in the average evoked waveforms. However, if statistical tests of significance or hypothesis testing are desired, such a procedure will be inadequate. A more quantitative measure of variability is required.

An estimate of σ the standard deviation of the background noise is needed. Equation (4.4) is an example of the advantage of knowing σ. Knowledge of σ and the number of waves in the average provide a direct, quantitative estimate of the amount of residual noise. The estimate of the standard deviation is computed as follows:

$$
\hat{\sigma} = \left[\frac{1}{N-1} \sum_{i=1}^{N} [x_i(t) - \hat{s}(t)]^2 \right]^{1/2}
$$

$$
= \left[\frac{1}{N-1} \sum_{i=1}^{N} [x_i(t)]^2 - \frac{N}{N-1} [\hat{s}(t)]^2 \right]^{1/2}
$$

$\hat{\sigma}$ denotes the estimate of the standard deviation. Division by $N-1$ rather than N is necessary for an unbiased estimate (Mood and Graybill, 1963). Note that σ (and $\hat{\sigma}$) can be a function of time if the noise statistics are nonstationary. For notational simplicity, this will not be made explicit.

4.3. CONFIDENCE INTERVALS

Utilizing the standard deviation of the noise, a measure of the variability of the data can be computed. The measure is a statement that the true mean value lies within a certain range of amplitudes with a given probability. First, the probability level is chosen; then the corresponding range of amplitudes, centered about the estimate of the mean, are computed. The range of amplitudes is known as a confidence interval.

Determination of the probability level requires some care. It is desirable to select a level close to unity, so that one may be reasonably confident that the corresponding range of amplitudes contain the true mean. However, if the probability level is too high, then the corresponding amplitude range will be uselessly large.

As an example, consider a process where the noise has a normal distribution, the noise samples are independent and the standard deviation σ is known. The mean of the responses s is estimated by $\hat{s}$, the average of N samples. Form the expression*

$$t = (\hat{s} - s)/(\sigma/\sqrt{N}) \qquad (4.6)$$

where t is related to the unknown mean s by Eq. (4.6). Since the expected value of $\hat{s}$ is s, $\sigma/\sqrt{N}$ is the standard deviation of $\hat{s}$ and the noise has a normal distribution, t is a normal random variable with zero mean and unity standard deviation. Hence the distribution of t is known. Thus it is possible to compute the probability that t lies between any two amplitudes; use Eq. (4.6) to find the probability that the unknown mean lies within a corresponding range of amplitudes. The probability density of t is

$$f(t) = (1/\sqrt{2\pi}) \exp(-t^2/2) \qquad (4.7)$$

Suppose that we wish to obtain the limits of the interval

---

* Note that t does not denote time in the remainder of this section. It denotes a statistic for which the symbol customarily is t.

which has 0.95 probability of containing s, the true mean. This is equivalent to finding the range of t which corresponds to the probability 0.95. Thus

$$p(-1.96 < t < 1.96) = \int_{-1.96}^{1.96} \frac{1}{\sqrt{2\pi}} \exp(-t^2/2) \, dt = 0.95 \qquad (4.8)$$

From Eq. (4.6). the inequalities

$$-1.96 < [(\hat{s} - s)/(\sigma/\sqrt{N})] < 1.96$$

are equivalent to the inequalities in Eq. (4.8). These inequalities can be arranged so that

$$p[(\hat{s} - 1.96 \, (\sigma/\sqrt{N}) < s < \hat{s} + 1.96 \, (\sigma/\sqrt{N})] = 0.95 \qquad (4.9)$$

The limits of $(\hat{s} - 1.96 \, \sigma/\sqrt{N})$ to $(\hat{s} + 1.96 \, \sigma/\sqrt{N})$ specify the confidence interval. For a fixed probability, the narrower the confidence interval, the closer the sample average $\hat{s}$ is likely to be to the true mean s. When applying the method of confidence intervals to average evoked responses, the object is to obtain two waveforms between which the true evoked waveform lies with a specified probability at each point in time. This may be done by selecting a probability level and simply computing at each time point the confidence interval.

Usually the standard deviation is unknown, so that Eq. (4.6) cannot be used. However, there is a method which utilizes $\hat{\sigma}$, the estimate of the standard deviation instead of the exact value. In this instance

$$t = (\hat{s} - s)/(\hat{\sigma}/\sqrt{N}) \qquad (4.10)$$

Under certain conditions the distribution of t is known to be the Student's t distribution with $N - 1$ degrees of freedom (Mood and Graybill, 1963). It has been shown analytically that if the process has a normal distribution, the distribution of t will be Student's t. Empirical studies have demonstrated that for a sufficiently large number of samples, t for other distributions will also have a Student's t distribution (Boneau, 1959; Havlicek and Peterson, 1974). The Student's t is a well known and commonly tabulated distribution. For large N, it approaches a normal distribution with zero mean and unity standard deviation.

As an example, suppose $\hat{s}$ and $\hat{\sigma}$ have been computed, using 30 waveforms. The 0.90 confidence interval is desired. From a table of the Student's t distribution, we obtain

$$p(-1.70 < t < 1.70) = \int_{-1.70}^{1.70} f(t, 29) \, dt = 0.90 \qquad (4.11)$$

degrees of freedom. Note that the density is a function of the sample size N. The above inequality is rearranged to obtain

$$p[\hat{s} - 1.70 \ (\hat{\sigma}/\sqrt{30}) < s < \hat{s} + 1.70 \ (\hat{\sigma}/\sqrt{30})] = 0.90$$

4.4. COMMENTS ON ASSUMPTIONS

It was assumed above that the actual stimulus evoked responses (signals) in a set of data were all identical and that the differences between the observed waveforms were due to the associated noise. The noise statistics were assumed to be constant and the noise associated with each evoked response was assumed to be independent of the noise from all other evoked responses. An elementary averaging technique was then described and analyzed. Unfortunately, in some instances the above mentioned assumptions upon which it was based do not hold.

The assumptions of homogeneity for the set of evoked responses or uncorrelated noise may be oversimplifications. When the data are gathered over a relatively long period of time, there is the possibility that the subject's state will vary, and so may the signal waveshape. A variation in signal waveshape will also occur if the latency of one or more of its components is random. The responses obtained under these circumstances are termed non-homogeneous. Techniques have been devised for dealing with them and may have to be utilized if meaningful averages are to be obtained.

In practice, it is desirable to minimize the experiment time required to obtain a satisfactory estimate of the signal. With short periodic interstimulus intervals, there is a distinct possibility that the noise will be correlated, and hence the standard error will not be inversely proportional to the square root of the number of evoked responses in the average. In such situations there may also be interference in the form of overlap between the late components of one evoked response and the early components of the next. Consequently there can be a problem of trade off between the amount of noise reduction and length of experiment.

The noise reduction produced by averaging is a phenomenon based largely in part upon the noise process being stationary, with each noise sample reasonably typical of the set of likely noise samples. If the noise occasionally contains a large, atypical component such as may be due to an artifact, then the cancellation effect seen with stationary noise will not apply to its reduction. Procedures that are reasonably impervious to such events may be required.

4.5. ALTERNATIVE MEASURES OF VARIABILITY

The standard deviation of a sample of evoked responses can provide a basis for assessing the effects of noise and the adequacy of the sample average as an estimate of the true average. However, in some situations computation of the standard deviation may not be feasible or most appropriate. We discuss some alternative means for assessing noise effects in these situations.

A. *SPLIT SWEEP ASSESSMENT OF SIGNIFICANCE*

Since it is often desirable to minimize the time duration over which a set of evoked responses is recorded, the need arises of extracting from the data a clear estimate of the signal with the least possible number of evoked responses. Lowy and Weiss (1968) have devised a method for dealing with this problem. It is based upon the split-half technique for assessing the effects of random noise. Two averages are computed, one from the responses evoked by the odd-numbered stimuli, the other from the responses to the even-numbered stimuli. At the end of the response to each even-numbered stimulus, the two averages are compared. If they are reasonably alike, it is assumed that the effects of noise have been sufficiently attenuated and that no more data need be gathered.

Two empirical techniques were developed for making real-time comparisons between the averages, using a small laboratory computer. One technique, called the Max-Min method, is based upon the assumption that if a sufficient number of evoked responses has been used, the latencies of the peaks and troughs in the two concurrent averages will be approximately the same. It is a feature such as this that an experimenter intuitively monitors when using visual inspection to assess the reproducibility of evoked response waveforms.

The comparison is made in the following manner. The time span (e.g., 256 points) of the averages is subdivided into batches (e.g., 16 points). The mean amplitude for each batch is computed and then the batches containing the maximum and minimum are located. It is assumed that the two averages are sufficiently alike and thus a sufficient number of evoked responses are obtained when the latencies of the maximum and minimum batches, respectively, correspond for the two averages, as illustrated in the upper portion of Fig. (4.1). When they do, data gathering halts and the two average waveforms are displayed.

The second comparison technique, called the random-shuffle method, utilizes a nonparametric sign test (Siegel, 1956). This test imposes no restrictive assumptions about the noise statistics and attaches a probability level of significance to the decision that the averages represent the signal waveform rather than a noise-obscured waveform. The points that constitute each average are independently and randomly mixed or shuffled so that they are no longer in their original temporal sequence. As in the Max-Min procedure, batches are formed for both the actual averages and the randomly shuffled averages. The absolute differences are computed

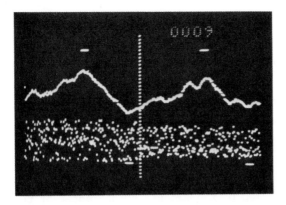

Fig. 4.1. Display of the results of a split-half comparison of average evoked potentials. The left-hand waves are for the odd-numbered evoked potentials, the right-hand waves for the even-numbered evoked potentials. The short upper bars are positioned over the maxima and the lower bars, under the minima of the two averages. The display of dots represents the same average waveform after random shuffling. The number of pairs of evoked potentials required for maxima and minima to coincide is in the upper right of the display. (From Lowy and Weiss, 1968.)

between the batches for the pair of actual averages and between the batches of the pair of shuffled averages. If, for a predetermined number of batches, the absolute difference between the pair of actual averages is less than the absolute difference between the corresponding pair of shuffled averages, then the actual averages are considered to have a sufficiently large signal-to-noise level so that they may be used as adequate estimates of the signal process. Thus data gathering is halted, and both the actual waveforms and the shuffled waveforms are displayed. Figure (4.1) illustrates the pair of shuffled waves associated with the pair of averages. The predetermined criterion number of batches involved in the decision of signal versus noise is determined by the probability level of significance that one selects for the test. For example, if 13 out of 16 differences between the actual pair of waves are less than the corresponding differences for the pair of randomized waves, then, using the sign test, this is equivalent to a significance level of 0.01 being reached for acceptance

187

of the hypothesis that the averages represent the signal waveform rather than a noise-obscured waveform.

The Lowy-Weiss methods are well suited for real-time implementation on a small laboratory computer. The computational procedures are faster and simpler to execute than the conventional tests of significances such as the well-known Student's t test and are equivalent to a test of this type.

B. PLUS-MINUS REFERENCE METHOD

Schimmel (1967) has devised a procedure which provides a visual indication of the amount and character of the residual noise associated with the average evoked response. This method is based upon the assumption that each individual evoked response consists of an invariant signal plus an independent random noise wave. If an even number of evoked responses are alternately added and subtracted, then the signal component will vanish leaving a residual noise wave with the same statistical properties as the residual noise wave associated with the conventional average. An illustration is presented in Fig.(4.2). This procedure can be implemented on real-time computers and on conventional multichannel average

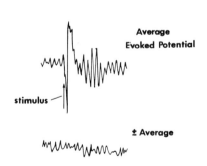

Fig. 4.2. An example of the use of Schimmel's plus-minus method. The upper waveform is the average evoked potential. The lower waveform is the plus-minus average, which provides an indication of the noise level. [Adapted from H. Schimmel, Science 157, 92 (1967). Copyright 1967 by The American Association for The Advancement of Science. Reproduced by permission.]

response computers in conjunction with some ancillary switching circuitry. It is a particularly apt method for visual assessment of residual noise.

4.6. CORRELATED NOISE, OVERLAP AND STIMULUS SPACING

If the time intervals between stimuli are sufficiently large, then the noise activity associated with each epoch following a stimulus will be uncorrelated with noise from other epochs. Also, there will be no interaction between the late components of one evoked response and the early components of subsequent evoked responses. It is then reasonable to assume that the rms noise associated with the average evoked response will be attenuated in inverse proportion to the square root of the number of evoked responses and that in this regard the exact timing of the stimuli is not critical. However, in some instances it may be necessary to use relatively short interstimulus periods. The occasion can arise if the state of the subject is likely to change over a long data gathering session. For short interstimulus intervals, the exact timing may be of critical importance.

Consider periodic timing of the stimuli. Periodic stimuli may be used because the instrumentation is relatively simple. Also, in some experimental designs the stimulus frequency is a discriminandum; however, periodic evoked responses can be particularly susceptible to interference due to their overlap and to rhythmic noise. Rhythmic noise can be caused by artifacts such as interference from a power line or by the locking-in of an on-going bioelectric rhythm. The noise attenuation characteristics for averaging with periodic stimuli will be examined first, followed by those for aperiodic stimuli.

Denote the number of evoked responses by N and represent the kth recording of the evoked response, consisting of a signal plus noise by

$$x_k(t) = s(t) + n_k(t) \qquad 0 \le t \le T \tag{4.12}$$

where $s(t)$ is the invariant signal, $n_k(t)$ the noise during the kth response, and t represents the time elapsed with reference to the stimulus time in each epoch. T is the interstimulus period. The sample average will be

$$\bar{x}(t) = s(t) + \frac{1}{N} \sum_{k=1}^{N} n_k(t) \tag{4.13}$$

Assume that the noise is wide-sense stationary and has zero mean. Then the expected value of Eq. (4.13) is $s(t)$. The noise power is the expected variance of Eq. (4.13) and is

$$\text{var}[\bar{x}] = E\left[\frac{1}{N^2} \sum_{k=1}^{N} \sum_{m=1}^{N} n_k(t) n_m(t)\right] \tag{4.14}$$

The time between $n_k(t)$ and $n_m(t)$ is $(k - m)T$. Thus

$$\text{var}[\bar{x}] = \frac{1}{N^2} \sum_{k=1}^{N} \sum_{m=1}^{N} R_n[(k - m)T] \tag{4.15}$$

where $R_n(t)$ is the autocovariance function of the noise. The Fourier transform of $R_n(t)$ is the power spectrum of the noise $W_n(f)$. Then Eq. (4.15) can be written

$$\text{var}[\bar{x}] = \frac{1}{N^2} \sum_{k=1}^{N} \sum_{m=1}^{N} \int_{-\infty}^{+\infty} W_n(f) \exp[j2\pi f(k - m)T] \, df \tag{4.16}$$

Interchanging the order of integration and summation and recognizing that the two summations are complex conjugates:

$$\text{var}[\bar{x}] = \int_{-\infty}^{+\infty} W_n(f) \left|\frac{1}{N} \sum_{k=1}^{N} \exp j2\pi fTk\right|^2 \, df \tag{4.17}$$

The summation is a simple power series of the form $a + a^2 + a^3 + \cdots + a^N = a(1 - a^N)/(1 - a)$. After some manipulations, this can be expressed as

$$\text{var}[\bar{x}] = \int_{-\infty}^{+\infty} W_n(f) \left(\frac{\sin N\pi Tf}{N \sin \pi Tf}\right)^2 \, df \tag{4.18}$$

Equations (4.17) and (4.18) make it explicit that averaging is equivalent to a particular form of linear filtering since $\sin N\pi Tf/(N \sin \pi Tf)$ can be considered to be the magnitude of the averaging filter's transfer function. Thus the sequence of responses $x_k(t)$, passed through a linear filter with this transfer function, yields an output whose average already known to be $s(t)$

has a variance given by Eq. (4.18). An illustration of the square of the magnitude of the transfer function for $N = 5$ is provided in Fig. (4.3). The transfer function is a function with peaks of unity amplitude at frequencies k/T and troughs near frequencies $(k + 1/2)T$. The broadness of the peaks is proportional to $1/N$.

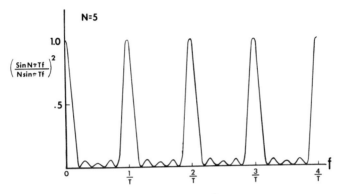

Fig. 4.3. $[\sin N\pi Tf/(N \sin \pi Tf)]^2$ versus f for $N = 5$.

The power of broad band noise, of bandwidth $1/T$ or greater will be roughly attenuated by a factor of approximately $1/N$. This is similar to the attenuation characteristic of uncorrelated noise, a result to be expected since the autocorrelation function of such broad band noise is small for times greater than T. Narrow band noise, with spectra centered about zero frequency (a slowly changing noise) or about k/T (a rhythmic noise at the stimulus frequency or one of its harmonics), will not be attenuated as much and hence may contribute significantly to $\bar{x}(t)$. A plot of variance versus number of evoked responses for narrow band noise centered at k/T and a bandwidth of f_x Hz is presented in Fig. (4.4). It can be seen that for narrow band noise centered near zero frequency or at a stimulus harmonic, attenuation can be significantly less than for uncorrelated, broad band noise. The variance due to narrow band noise centered near $(k + 1/2)T$, a trough of the transfer function, will be attenuated by a factor of approximately $1/N^2$,

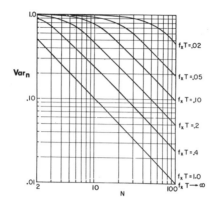

Fig. 4.4. Normalized variance, var$_n$, of an average response versus the number of stimuli N for periodic stimuli. Var$_n$ is obtained by dividing the variance of the average response var $[\bar{x}]$ by the variance of the evoked potentials var $[x_k(t)]$. (From Ruchkin, 1965.)

as contrasted to the $1/N$ reduction of uncorrelated broad band noise. This property can be used to advantage in reducing the interference due to 60 Hz pickup, the stimulation rate being adjusted so that $60 = (k + 1/2)T$.

An evoked response may persist beyond the time of occurrence of the subsequent stimulus. If the stimuli are periodic, then the overlapping late components will be time locked to the subsequent evoked response. Consequently, such overlapped components will appear in the average response without attenuation and thus interfere with the desired data (Kinney *et al.*, 1973). Other than lengthening the interstimulus duration, there is no way in which the overlap can be removed short of changing from the method of periodic stimulation.

A. APERIODIC STIMULI

The preceding discussion noted that averages based upon periodic stimuli will not effectively attenuate interference due to overlap or to background rhythms whose frequencies are near the stimulation rate or a harmonic. Intuitively, it is reasonable to suppose that if the stimuli are sufficiently aperiodic, such disturbances would be adequately attenuated. The overlapping components and rhythmic noise will then be asynchronous with respect to the stimuli and evoked responses. Thus neither will necessarily add directly in proportion to the number of stimuli during averaging; instead, there will be a tendency for cancellation to occur.

First, we consider the effects of stimulus aperiodicity upon overlap. To simplify the analysis, we neglect background noise. The unvarying signal is represented by

$$s(t) = e(t) + L(t)$$

where $L(t)$ denotes the late components that can interfere with the early components $e(t)$ of subsequent evoked responses. For simplicity it is assumed that the duration of $L(t)$ is such that it persists into the time epoch of the immediately following stimulus but not into subsequent ones. It is further assumed that the physiological processes are such that in the time interval following the kth stimulus the recorded activity $x(t)$ is represented by

$$x_k(t) = s(t) + L(t + T_{k-1})$$

where T_k is the time between the kth and $(k + 1)$th stimulus and $L(t + T_{k-1})$ is the interfering overlap from the preceding response. For aperiodic stimuli, T_k can be represented by $T + \theta_k$, where T is the average interstimulus interval and θ_k is a random time variable with zero mean. The θ_k are statistically independent of each other. For notational convenience, represent $L(t + T + \theta_{k-1})$ by $\lambda(t + \theta_{k-1})$. Then the observed average response will be

$$\bar{x}(t) = s(t) + \frac{1}{N} \sum_{k=1}^{N-1} \lambda(t + \theta_k) \tag{4.19}$$

Since the response to the first stimulus will not be affected by overlap, the summation is from 1 to $N - 1$. Averaging over θ_k, the expected value of the average is

$$E[\bar{x}(t)] = s(t) + (1 - \frac{1}{N}) \int_{-\infty}^{+\infty} p(\theta) \, \lambda(t + \theta) \, d\theta \tag{4.20}$$

where $p(\theta)$ is the probability density of θ. Equation (4.20) indicates how the overlap interferes with the true average evoked response waveshape $s(t)$: It introduces a bias. This bias is essentially independent of the number of stimuli when N is large; however, it is a function of the probability density of the interstimulus periods. From Eq. (4.20) it can be seen that the probability density function acts somewhat similarly to the impulse response of a linear filter whose input is $\lambda(t)$. Thus, it may be possible to develop a $p(\theta)$ which effectively attenuates the main components of $\lambda(t)$. Details for designing $p(\theta)$ are presented by Ruchkin (1965). A related approach that deals with the relationship between single unit events and slow waves is given in Chapter 8. In general it is possible to devise $p(\theta)$ which will attenuate high frequency overlap activity such as rhythmic activity after discharges. However, low frequency activity, such as slow shifts, cannot be attenuated by aperiodic presentation of the stimuli. As a rough rule of thumb, the effective time span of $p(\theta)$ should be greater than the period of the lowest frequency overlap component to be attenuated.

B. NARROW BAND NOISE AND APERIODIC STIMULI

The utilization of aperiodic stimuli can also increase the degree of attenuation of narrow band rhythmic noise. For simplicity, we now neglect overlap interference. It can be shown that for a suitable aperiodicity, the average response variance due to noise will be attenuated by $1/N$ whether or not the noise is broad or narrow band. The only exception is low frequency noise whose bandwidth is narrow relative to the average rate of occurrence of the stimuli. Such noise cannot be effectively attenuated.

Consider a train of aperiodic evoked responses. The $(k + 1)^{th}$ evoked response is denoted by

$$x(t - kT - \sum_{\nu=1}^{k} \theta_{\nu})$$

where as before, θ_{ν} is the zero mean, random time increment of the period between the kth and $(k + 1)$th stimuli. The average of N such evoked responses is represented by

$$\bar{x}(t) = s(t) + \frac{1}{N} \sum_{k=0}^{N-1} n\left(t + kT + \sum_{\nu=1}^{k} \theta_\nu\right) \qquad (4.21)$$

The expected value of $\bar{x}(t)$ is $s(t)$ and the variance is

$$\mathrm{var}[\bar{x}] = \frac{1}{N^2} \sum_{k=0}^{N-1} \sum_{m=0}^{N-1} E\left[n\left(t + kT + \sum_{\nu=1}^{k} \theta_\nu\right) n\left(t + mT + \sum_{\mu=1}^{m} \theta_\mu\right)\right]$$

$$(4.22)$$

The operator E symbolizes the joint average over all θ_ν and $n(t)$. If the noise from each trial is uncorrelated with the noise from all other trials, Eq. (4.22) reduces to

$$\mathrm{var}[\bar{x}] = \frac{1}{N} E[n^2(t)]$$

as was shown in Eq. (4.4). If the noise power spectrum is narrow in bandwidth compared with the frequency of the periodic stimulus, then the noise from each trial may be correlated with noise from other trials. This will certainly be true if the noise is a low frequency process. In such a case the amplitude of the noise changes slowly from trial to trial, and cancellation when averaging will be negligible. Aperiodic stimulation will not produce the $1/N$ noise reduction factor for such low frequency noise; only by using long intertrial intervals will produce this. If the narrow band noise is a high-frequency rhythmic process, there is no need to use long intertrial intervals. Aperiodic stimulation can ensure that averaging will reduce the variance of $\bar{x}$ by about $1/N$, as in the case of uncorrelated noise. To see how this occurs, consider a narrow band noise whose spectrum is near the frequency or a harmonic of the stimulation rate. Similar values of noise amplitude will tend to recur in each trial at the same latency with respect to the stimulus time. Thus, the noise amplitudes will not cancel when the data are averaged. However, if the stimulus times are suitably randomized, then the noise will be asynchronous with respect to the stimulus times, similar noise amplitudes will not tend to recur, and hence cancellation may occur when the data are averaged. A detailed discussion of how aperiodic stimulation can attenuate variance due to narrow band noise and design of appropriate probability density functions of θ is presented by Ruchkin (1965). As a rough rule of thumb, for a $1/N$ reduction in variance, the effective time span of $p(\theta)$ should be greater than the lowest frequency component of the narrow band noise.

4.7. THE MEDIAN EVOKED RESPONSE

An implicit assumption of average response computing is that the response waveforms each consist of invariant stimulus-evoked activity (signal) plus ongoing electrical activity of the brain. The ongoing activity (noise) obscures the signal. It is usually further assumed that the noise activity is random and not time locked to the stimulus, that the noise samples associated with each evoked response have zero mean value, are statistically independent of one another, and have similar statistical properties. Then the signal waveform corresponds to the mean of the evoked response waveforms. Thus, when a sufficiently large number of evoked responses is averaged, the noise contribution will tend to become small and the resulting average evoked response provides a good estimate of the signal waveform. These assumptions are usually not entirely satisfied in a real experiment, as has already been pointed out with respect to the independence of noise samples. Other departures from these assumptions also occur. Occasionally, perhaps due to an artifact, an atypically large noise wave will occur. That is, it occurs more often than the usual assumptions of Gaussian statistics would indicate. This departure degrades the performance of the linear averaging technique. The effect of such occasional large noise waves will be to produce an average that differs significantly from the actual signal.

Borda and Frost (1968) have devised a nonlinear technique for coping with the problem of atypically large artifactual disturbances. Instead of the average, they compute the median response at each time point. The median evoked response is then used as the estimate of the signal waveform. The rationale for using the median can be understood by considering the differences between the average and median computational procedures at a fixed latency point with respect to stimulus onset. The average is computed by summing the data and dividing by the number of responses. The median response is derived from the rank ordering of the data and is the amplitude value which half of the responses are greater than and the other half less than.

As an example, consider a case where both the median and mean are zero. Replace one of the positive data amplitudes by a spurious, very large positive amplitude. The average will change, perhaps significantly, but the median will not change since its position in the rank ordering of the data is not affected by the spurious datum. As a second example, suppose that a large noise peak causes a negative sample to be replaced by a large positive one. In this case the rank order of the original median will change. However, the change in magnitude will only amount to the difference between the original median and the amplitude of the nearest positive datum.

Figure (4.5) from Borda and Frost (1968) illustrates the use of the mean and median for a small sample of data. Waveforms A and A' are the average and median, respectively, of nine evoked responses. A large random noise waveform was added to the data as a tenth response to produce waveforms B and B' as the resulting average and median. Waveforms C and C' illustrate how the average and median are affected by the addition of a long duration square wave to the set of evoked responses.

Usage of the median leads to questions concerning the goodness of the sample median as an estimator of the signal waveform under typical experimental conditions. The above example empirically demonstrates that the median can be much less susceptible than the average to large occasional artifactual noise

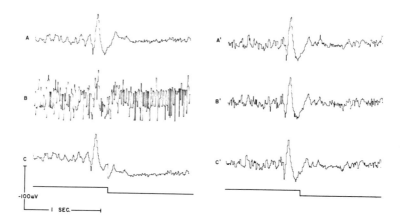

Fig. 4.5. A: Plot of the average evoked potential from nine trials. A': Median of the same nine evoked potentials. B: Average of the nine evoked potentials used in A plus a tenth waveform consisting of high amplitude random noise. B': Median of the same ten waveforms used in B. C: Average of the nine evoked potentials used in A plus a tenth waveform consisting of a 300 μV square wave of one second duration. C': Median of the same ten waveforms used in C. (From Borda and Frost, 1968.)

waveforms. However, the question of the comparative performances of the average and median as estimators of the signal in the absence of this type of noise is also of interest. It raises the question, is the price paid for the greater insensitivity of the median to larger artifactual noise a substantially poorer (higher standard deviation) estimate of the signal compared to the average in those cases when the noise is artifact free? Ruchkin (1974) has shown that for noise with Gaussian statistics, the standard deviation of the sample median is approximately 25% larger than the standard deviation of the sample average. Thus, there is only a small degradation in the estimate of the signal by the median in the absence of large occasional artifactual noise.

Confidence limits for evaluating the goodness of a sample median estimate can be determined using the sign test (Ruchkin, 1974). Since the sign test is nonparametric, there are no restrictive assumptions concerning the noise statistics. Given N independent amplitude samples of data and a specified probability level P_L, an amplitude interval can be found at each time point within which the signal amplitude is contained with probability P_L. Denote the ranked amplitudes at a single time point of the N data samples

$$x(1) < x(2) < \ldots x(k-1) < x(k) < \ldots x(N-1) < x(N)$$

The index k indicates the rank order of the datum amplitude. The probability that the interval between the Lth ranked sample and the $(N + 1 - L)$th ranked sample contains the median is

$$P_L = 1 - 2 \sum_{k=0}^{L-1} \binom{N}{k} (0.5)^N \qquad (4.23)$$

A tabulation of $2 \sum_{k=0}^{L} \binom{N}{k} (0.5)^N$ is provided in Table VIII by Bradley (1968). Thus, to find the P_L confidence limits for a given N, find the limits corresponding to P_L and then, from the ranked tabulation of the data, find $x(L)$ and $x(N + 1 - L)$. These two amplitudes are the P_L confidence limits.

The median has a clear advantage over the average with respect to its insensitivity to atypically large artifactual disturbances (although rigorous proof is lacking). For purely Gaussian noise, the statistical stabilities of the median and average are comparable. However, the median has two disadvantages; one is that if the noise is quasi-sinusoidal, the inherent nonlinearity of the median computation can exhibit spurious harmonics of the noise components. It may be possible to remove these harmonics by filtering the median waveform if the signal and noise harmonic frequencies are sufficiently disparate. Unfortunately, little is known about how the harmonic distortion interacts with the signal. Some discussion may be found in Cooper (1972) and Ruchkin and Walter (1975).

The second disadvantage of the median lies with the procedures for computing it. An exact computation of the sample median requires that all data be stored. This may not be practical for a large number of samples, although a histogram of the evoked response amplitudes at each time point may suffice. However, substantially more locations of computer memory may be required than for the average.

For the large N case Walter (1971) has devised an approximation to the sample median which requires about the same amount of computer memory as an average. It utilizes the fact that when N is large, the evoked response amplitudes $x_k(t)$ will be above the median about as often as they are below. Denoting the sample median of the k earliest evoked responses by $Mer_k(t)$, Walter suggests for stationary data the algorithm

$$Mer_k(t) = Mer_{k-1}(t) + \text{sgn} \ [x_k(t) - Mer_{k-1}(t)] \qquad (4.24)$$

where sgn $[y]$ is $+1$ if y is positive, zero if y is zero, and -1 if y is negative.

The rationale for this is as follows. Assume for a large k that $Mer_{k-1}(t)$ will be a good estimate of the sample median, and thus $x_k(t)$ is as likely to be greater than $Mer_{k-1}(t)$ as it is likely to be less than $Mer_{k-1}(t)$. Thus the probability of adding a one to $Mer_{k-1}(t)$ is the same as the probability of subtracting a one. Consequently, with successive data samples, $Mer_k(t)$ will tend to fluctuate about the true median and ultimately be within about one amplitude unit of it. The initial value, $Mer_0(t)$ is arbitrarily set to zero, the median value for noise only, and so $Mer_k(t)$, may be a poor estimate to the median when k is small and signal is present. However, $Mer_k(t)$ will tend to converge to the true median since sgn$[x_k(t) - Mer_{k-1}(t)]$ will more frequently be $+1$ as long as $Mer_{k-1}(t)$ is less than the median [or -1 more frequently as long as $Mer_{k-1}(t)$ is greater than it]. $Mer_k(t)$ will not be a good estimate of the median until k is approximately equal to the number of units of magnitude by which the true median deviates from zero.

4.8. NONHOMOGENEOUS SETS OF EVOKED POTENTIALS

When averaging, it is usually assumed that the individual evoked reponses composing the observed sample are all of one class. The differences between individual observed waveforms are attributed to extraneous, random noise in which the evoked responses are imbeded. The noise effects presumably will be diminished by averaging. The assumption of response homogeneity is not valid if, during data gathering, the state of the subject changes. More than one type of evoked response waveshape will then be generated. Adaptation, habituation, and learning are examples of significant phenomena associated with nonhomogeneous reponses.

An average computed from a nonhomogeneous sample of data can be an imprecise and misleading representation of the evoked response phenomena if for no other reason than that the existence of more than one type of evoked response may be of great functional importance. It may be useful, if not necessary, to test the sample of evoked responses for nonhomogeneity, to classify each individual evoked response, and to compute an average for each of these evoked response classes. The latter assumes the responses can be segregated into enumerable classes and are not varying on some continuum. Various methods for analyzing nonhomogeneous sets of evoked responses have been devised. Some have general applicability with few restrictions placed upon the nature of the data. Others are intended for dealing with specific kinds of nonhomogeneities. When applicable, they may be easier and more appropriate to use. We will discuss both specific and general procedures.

4.9. CORRELATION ESTIMATION OF A CONSTANT WAVEFORM WITH VARYING LATENCY

The method of average response computation is meant to extract an invariant signal waveform from a collection of signal-plus-noise waves. Such a method will yield misleading and even erroneous results if the signal waveform varies during the course of the experiment. In some cases significant variations in the signal waveshape may be expected. For example, the shape of the signal waveform may be constant but its latency from stimulus onset may fluctuate. Simple averaging of such responses will result in an average response waveshape which is a latency blurred version of the stimulus evoked waveshape. To see this, let $g(t - \tau)$ represent the signal waveform when the latency shift is τ, and $p(\tau)$ the probability density of the latency. Assume the background noise has zero mean. Then the expected average response waveform is the waveform associated with the probability weighting of each response according to its latency.

$$g(t) = \int_{-\infty}^{+\infty} p(\tau) \, g(t - \tau) \, d\tau \qquad (4.25)$$

The effect of averaging a variable latency waveform is similar to passing the signal through a linear filter whose weighting function corresponds to the probability density function of the latency. The average waveform $g(t)$, is seen to be a smeared distortion of the actual desired signal.

Woody (1967) has developed an iterative filter algorithm which will compensate for random latency shifts and extract the signal waveshape from responses containing variable latency signal plus noise. The heart of Woody's technique is the operation of correlation detection. Consider the simple case of identification of a set of latencies for an otherwise invariant waveform in the absence of noise. Let us suppose that there is a prototypic waveform template $f(t)$ available. The data consist of the set $f(t - \tau_n)$, where $n = 1,2,\dots N$, and N is the sample size. The τ_n may be determined by cross correlating the data waveforms with the protoype to obtain the covariance function.

$$R(\Delta) = \int_{-\infty}^{+\infty} f(t) \, f(t - \tau_n + \Delta) \, dt \qquad (4.26)$$

$R(\Delta)$ will be a maximum for $\Delta = \tau_n$. Hence by computing the covariance function over the range of Δ and determining the maximum for each waveform, the latency, with respect to the time base of the stencil, can be obtained in principle.

A difficulty is that even when $f(t)$ is known beforehand, the $R(\Delta)$ associated with it may have a rather broad maximum. In the presence of significant amounts of noise, this maximum may be difficult to estimate with accuracy.

A further difficulty exists when $f(t)$ is not known, i.e., when there is no prototypic stencil. Indeed, one of the main objects of the data analysis is to obtain this waveform. Due to the noise all waveforms in the data set will differ from one another, even if latency variations are eliminated. The problem in this case is to estimate the latency variation for each wave, shift the waveforms so that they are all aligned and then sum them to obtain a *best* estimate average response waveform. Woody's method deals with this problem by using an iterative approach. It assumes that the noise is additive and an arbitrary template waveform is selected at the outset. On the basis of a prior knowledge of what the wave probably looks like, each response in the data set is cross correlated with the template to find the time of maximum corvariance T_m. The set of data waves are aligned according to their estimated latencies and then are averaged together. The resulting waveform is taken to be a better estimate of the desired signal waveform than the initial a priori one. It replaces that template and the process of obtaining the latencies and computing the average of the latency-shifted waveforms is repeated. A block diagram of this procedure is presented in Fig. (4.6).

Denote the stencil by $f(t)$ and the individual evoked response plus noise waveform by $g_n(t)$. The time epoch of the evoked response is from zero to T. Then the covariance computation yields $R(\Delta)$, where

$$R(\Delta) = \frac{1}{T} \int_0^T f(t) \, g_n(t - \Delta) \, dt \qquad (4.27)$$

and the range of Δ is some fraction of $-T$ to T. It is assumed that the value of Δ for which $R(\Delta)$ is a maximum [i.e., $g_n(t - \Delta)$

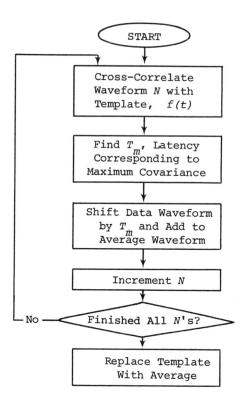

Fig. 4.6. Block diagram of Woody's iterative filter algorithm.

most similar to $f(t)$] is the negative of the latency shift of $g_n(t)$. The shifting operation of forming $g_n(t - \Delta)$ from $g(t)$ causes an edge effect to occur whereby a portion of $g_n(t - \Delta)$ lies outside the range $(0, T)$. Woody considered two methods for dealing with this problem. In one, that portion of $g_n(t)$ which was contiguous with the interval $(0, T)$ was used in the covariance computation. Thus, new data were introduced with each shift in the value of Δ. In the other, $g_n(t)$ was treated as a periodic function. Data that were shifted out of one end of the interval $(0, T)$ would be shifted into the other end. In this way, by using end-around-looping, no new data were introduced. Empirically,

Woody found that end-around-looping was the superior method.

At the completion of the computation of a new template, a computation is made to determine the *goodness* of the current stencil as a representation of the average waveshape. The cross-correlation coefficient between the stencil and each data waveform, shifted by its estimated latency, is computed. Then an average of the correlation coefficient is computed. The closer the average correlation coefficients are to unity, the better the stencil represents the signal waveform and the better are the estimates of the latencies. The iteration procedure is halted when the average correlation coefficient either exceeds a criterion level or does not change significantly with successive iterations.

Although there is no guarantee that this process will converge to the true signal waveform unless the initial estimate of the waveform is a good one, Woody found that in practice the initial choice of the stencil was not critical. The average waveform for the uncompensated data, a randomly selected data waveform, or an arbitrarily chosen waveform, so long as it is not simply a horizontal line, may suffice. Convergence to false peaks rarely occurred. However, a poor choice of the initial stencil could substantially increase the number of iterations required to converge to an acceptable final stencil. It was found empirically that the rms signal-to-noise ratio had to exceed 0.2 in order for convergence to occur, and that usually fewer than six iterations were required.

It should be noted that this technique is intended for sets of responses in which all components have the same latency behavior. It cannot work if there are two or more components which have different variations in their respective latencies.

4.10. HOMOGENEOUS SUBSETS

If a nonhomogeneous sequence of evoked responses can be subdivided into reasonably long homogeneous subsequences, then the contiguous subsequences can be separated by utilization of a cumulative sum (Cumsum) procedure developed by Burns and Melzack (1966). Implementation of the Cumsum method can be facilitated through the use of an ancillary procedure called Precum which indicates the latencies of the varying response components responsible for the nonhomogeneities. If the sequence of evoked responses is relatively short and/or fluctuations in type occur in a frequent but irregular manner, then the subsequences will not be entirely contiguous and the Precum and Cumsum methods will not be effective. Another method, Sort (Ruchkin, 1971) can then be used. It operates upon the amplitude histograms of the evoked responses at each latency point and is independent of the temporal order in which the various response types occur. It will detect the nonhomogeneities, identify the dissociated response subsequences, sort the data into homogeneous response subsets, and estimate the waveshape associated with each response type.

4.11. THE CUMSUM PROCEDURE

The Cumsum technique utilizes the amplitudes of the evoked responses at a particular latency to construct a cumulative sum (Cumsum). The Cumsum is defined by

$$\text{Cumsum}_t(k) = \sum_{i=1}^{k} x_{it} \qquad k = 1,\ 2,\ \dots\ N \qquad (4.28)$$

where x_{it} represents the amplitude of the ith observed evoked response at latency t. The solid line in Fig. (4.7) illustrates a hypothetical Cumsum curve for a response sequence which subdivides into two consecutive homogeneous subsequences. The initial evoked response amplitudes at latency t are relatively large so that the initial slope of the Cumsum curve is correspondingly steep. Later in the response sequence there is a decrease in amplitude of the responses at latency t and the corresponding slope of the Cumsum decreases as a result. The dashed straight line is the Cumsum graph expected from the average if a homogeneous response was involved.

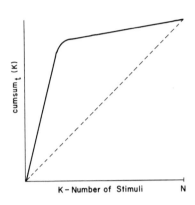

Fig. 4.7. Hypothetical Cumsum.   (From Ruchkin, 1968.)

Visual inspection of a Cumsum graph will determine whether
the component of the evoked response at the given latency is nonhomogeneous and where in the sequence of responses the changes
occur. Separate averages can then be computed for each subsequence.
How to test the departures of Cumsum from a straight line for its
significance is discussed below.

A.   THE PRECUM METHOD

When a large number of average evoked responses are to be
analyzed, it may not be feasible to compute and examine the Cumsums
for all latencies. The precumulative sum analysis (Precum) is then
useful. The Precum, which is computed at all latencies, measures
the extent to which a sequence of evoked responses breaks down
into different contiguous subsequences and indicates the latencies
of such nonhomogeneous components. It does not indicate when in
the evoked response sequence the changes occur. That information
is obtained from computing Cumsum at the latencies where Precum
reaches significant values.

Intuitively, the area between the actual Cumsum curve and
the straight line obtained in the homogeneous case (Fig. 4.7) is
a measure of the nonhomogeneity of the evoked response sequence.

Since random fluctuations will also cause the Cumsum graph to deviate from a straight line, the measure should be normalized with respect to the intensity of random fluctuations. This normalized measure is Precum and has been defined as follows:

$$Precum = \frac{6}{N+1} \frac{\frac{1}{N} \sum_{k=1}^{N} [\, Cumsum_t(k) - \frac{k}{N} Cumsum\ (N)\,]^2}{var_t} \quad (4.29)$$

where t is the response latency, usually from stimulus onset, and ranges from 0 to T, the maximum time for which the average is computed. Note that $(k/N)\ Cumsum_t(N)$ is the formula for the straight line from the origin to the final value of Cumsum. The numerator is seen to be a measure of the deviation of the Cumsum curve from this straight line. The variance estimate is determined in the usual manner.

Substituting x_{it} into Eq. (4.29) and canceling the 1/N terms gives the computationally useful expression

$$Precum = \frac{6}{N+1} \frac{\sum_{k=1}^{N} \left[\sum_{i=1}^{k} x_{it} - \frac{k}{N} \sum_{i=1}^{N} x_{it} \right]^2}{\sum_{k=1}^{N} \left[x_{kt} - \frac{1}{N} \sum_{i=1}^{N} x_{it} \right]^2} \quad (4.30)$$

The $6/(N+1)$ term normalizes the Precum measure so that it will have an expected mean of unity in the homogeneous case. Its exact distribution depends upon the noise and the length of the response sequence considered. See the subsequent section.

Figure (4.8) illustrates the use of Precum and Cumsum. The data were obtained by recording during a behavioral experiment from electrodes implanted in the brain of a cat (John and Shimokochi, 1966). Precum, as a function of latency t, is plotted in the upper portion of Fig. (4.8). The Cumsum for $t = 40$ msec, the latency at which Precum is maximum ($Precum_{40} = 7.1$) is plotted in Fig. (4.8). The Cumsum curve does not indicate an abrupt change of type at any point, rather, it suggests a gradual decrease

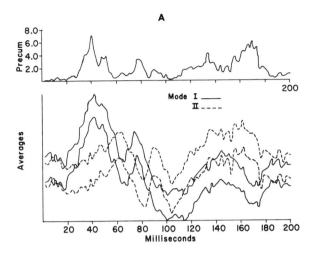

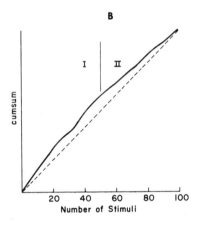

Fig. 4.8 Precum, Cumsum, and averages for a sequence of 100 evoked potentials. (A) Average from Mode I computed from potentials 2-49, for Mode II from potentials 50-100. The paired curves for each mode enclose the region of the average plus or minus one standard error. Precum reached a maximum of 7.1 at 40 msec. This value most probably indicates a multimodal sequence. (B) Cumsum is illustrated at the latency of 40 msec. (From Ruchkin, 1968.)

in evoked response amplitude and an arbitrary division of the sequence into two types. An average response and standard deviation are computed for each. Average evoked responses, correspond-

ing to the two types indicated on the Cumsum curves, are plotted
in the center portion of Fig. (4.8). Each average is represented
by a pair of curves, which are the average plus or minus the
standard error. The Student's t for the differences between the
two averages for the two types was computed at all latencies.
The maximum value occurs at 40 msec, the point of maximum Precum,
and is 3.79 (DF = 97).

B. DISTRIBUTION OF PRECUMS FOR HOMOGENEOUS RESPONSES

Since it is important to know when a Precum value is large
enough to qualify the sequence for being nonhomogeneous, some
guide lines for determining the values of Precum that correspond
to this situation can be given. The distribution of Precum for
the homogeneous case was investigated by means of a computer simulation (Ruchkin, 1968). The Precum values were computed and their
distribution was obtained for the case of an uncorrelated noise
with zero mean and constant variance. For the homogeneous case,
Precum does not depend upon the constant component in the response.
Two thousand Precums were computed for each sequence length. Results were quite similar for both Gaussian and uniformly distributed noise. Table (4.1) contains the mean, standard deviation and
level l_p which was exceeded by p% of the homogeneous Precum for
six sequence lengths when the noise was Gaussian.

Table (4.1) and examinations of experimentally obtained
Precum data suggest the following rules of thumb: Precum below
about 1.0-1.5 seems to correspond to a homogeneous sequence, and
when it is above 4.0, to a nonhomogeneous sequence. The relationship of Precum to the average response waveshape can be helpful
in deciding whether intermediate values of Precum correspond to
nonhomogeneous sequences. Both waveforms are available since
computation of Precum requires computation of the average response. If the Precum wave consists of sharp irregularly spaced
peaks in comparison with the average response, then its peak

TABLE 4.1

Distribution of Precum for Homogeneous Sequences

Length of Sequence N	Mean	SD	$p = 50\%$	20%	10%	5%	2%	1%
5	1.0	.5	.8	1.5	1.8	2.1	2.3	2.5
10	1.0	.7	.8	1.4	2.0	2.6	3.2	3.6
20	1.0	.8	.7	1.4	2.0	2.6	3.4	3.9
50	1.0	.8	.7	1.4	2.0	2.6	3.5	4.2
100	1.0	.9	.7	1.5	2.1	2.8	3.6	4.4
200	1.0	.9	.7	1.5	2.1	2.8	3.7	4.5

levels may be attributable to random fluctuations. However, if the Precum waveform consists of relatively broad components, then it may indicate that segments of the evoked response are covarying and this may be indicative of a nonhomogeneous process.

When Precum contains more than one significant component, the corresponding subsequences of evoked responses may have different patterns of mode change. That is, different components of the response may undergo change at different times in the sequence. It may be necessary to compute separate Cumsums at each latency and possibly separate the averages as determined by these patterns.

A limitation of Precum and Cumsum is that only nonhomogeneous sequences consisting of long and consistent homogeneous subsequences of evoked responses will be recognized. The longer the subsequences, the more certainly will they be detected by Precum and Cumsum analyses. But it is possible that type changes will occur from response to response (*e.g.*, for slow rates of stimulus presentations). Cumsum plots for such sequences will not systematically deviate from a straight line. Other techniques for dealing with response sequences of this kind need to be employed and are described below in the section on Sort.

C. AN ALGORITHM FOR COMPUTING PRECUM

It is possible to compute Precum without prior computation of the average. For notational convenience represent $Cumsum_t(k)$ by the symbol S_{kt}. Substitution of S_{kt} into Eq. (4.29) yields

$$Precum_t = \frac{6}{N(N+1)} \frac{\sum_{k=1}^{N} (S_{kt} - \frac{k}{N} S_{Nt})^2}{var_t} \tag{4.31}$$

Expanding the quadratic and reducing summations to closed form where possible

$$Precum_t = \frac{6}{N(N+1)} \frac{\sum_{k=1}^{N} S_{kt}^2 - \frac{2S_{Nt}}{N} \sum_{k=1}^{N} kS_{kt} + \frac{(N+1)(2N+1)S_{Nt}^2}{6N}}{var_t} \tag{4.32}$$

The three sums in the numerator of Eq. (4.32) can be computed concurrently since S_{kt} is the running sum of the x_{it} and S_{Nt} is the final value of that sum. For large N, the sums $\sum kS_{kt}$ and $\sum S_{kt}^2$ may become very large so that care may be required to avoid overflow when using Eq. (4.32) on a computer with small word size.

4.12. THE SORT METHOD

Sort (Ruchkin, 1971) is a method for sorting a nonhomogeneous sample of evoked responses into homogeneous subsets. It is not dependent upon the contiguity of the various evoked response types. It can be used in situations where Cumsum will not detect and separate nonhomogeneous data. Sort was originally developed for use with a laboratory computer system where the data analyst could interact with the computer, rapidly obtaining results, changing parameters if necessary, and focusing upon features in the data that may be of particular interest to him.

The Sort method entails four consecutive stages of operations:

(1) Initially, it determines the nonhomogeneous components

of the evoked responses by examination of the amplitude histograms.

(2) It then divides the amplitude ranges of those histograms which indicate the presence of nonhomogeneous components into subranges designed to separate the nonhomogeneities.

(3) It classifies each evoked response at the selected time points according to the amplitude subrange to which it belongs. These three steps crudely quantize the set of evoked responses into a simple representation in which various combinations of amplitude levels represent presumably homogeneous subsets of data.

(4) It computes the average and standard deviation waveshapes for each subset.

The above procedures are implemented as follows. Initially, for all of the data, the average evoked response, standard deviation waveform, and the amplitude histograms at each time point of the analysis epoch are computed. The histograms are used to indicate the presence and location of the nonhomogeneous components in the evoked response set. They provide the basis for dividing each of them into amplitude subranges that will hopefully segregate the homogeneous components from one another. The average and standard deviation are obtained primarily for the computational purpose of normalizing the histograms so that they are centered about the mean and their bin widths are a fixed fraction of the standard deviation.

The rationale and assumptions underlying the use of the histograms arise from the familiar consideration of an evoked response as the sum of signal and noise. The first is time locked to the stimulus; the second is random activity, not time locked to the stimulus. In a group of evoked responses at a given latency, the contributions due to random activity are statistically independent of one another and tend to yield Gaussian amplitude distributions (Saunders, 1963).

Consider the amplitudes of a sample of evoked responses at a single latency. If the time-locked processes are homogeneous, then the distribution of amplitudes will be governed by a single probability density function. The random fluctuations will be such that the probability density at that latency will have one mode near the mean, will be roughly symmetrical, and will tend to be Gaussian, as illustrated in Fig. (4.9a). Now suppose that while the sample of evoked responses is being recorded, the subject changes state. Associated with each state can be a different time-locked process, each having its own probability density and associated average value at the time latency. Although each density function may have a single mode, the overall probability density at the latency can be multimodal, reflecting the different states of the total sample. Figure (4.9b) illustrates a hypothetical probability density for a two-state case. Another possibility is that the change in states results in a gradual change in the

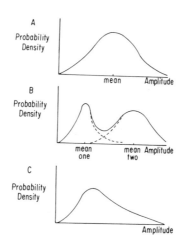

Fig. 4.9. Hypothetical probability densities. (A) Homogeneous data. (B) Nonhomogeneous data where the sample contains evoked potentials of two different types drawn from populations with different mean values. The dashed lines indicate the density functions for the two populations. (C) Nonhomogeneous data caused by a gradual time shift in the mean. (From Ruchkin, 1971.)

expected average at a given latency. Then a skewed or other non-Gaussian density, as illustrated in Fig. (4.9c) may occur.

Thus the shape of the histogram can be used to assess the homogeneity of the data. Figure (4.9b) suggests how the histograms can also be used to sort nonhomogeneous data into homogeneous groups. An amplitude threshold can be set near the minimum ordinate between two modes. All evoked responses with amplitudes below that threshold would be classified as one type; all above as a second type. Due to random fluctuations, misclassifications would occur, but some degree of response separation into homogeneous groups would be achieved, based solely upon the response amplitude at the latency examined.

A quantitative assessment of nonhomogeneity is made by computing for each time point: (1) the chi-squared measure for the fit of the histogram to a normal distribution; (2) counting the number of modes (N mode) of the broad outline of the histogram. A large value of chi-squared and/or an N mode greater than one is taken as an indication of a nonhomogeneity at a particular latency. The broad outline of the histogram is obtained by smoothing it. The smoothing routine description and the probabilities of unimodal, normal data falsely indicating more than one mode for various degrees of smoothing are presented in the Appendix at the end of the chapter.

N mode and chi-squared tend to be complementary tests. N mode readily detects the presence of histograms of the form illustrated in Fig. (4.9b) but not that of Fig. (4.9c). Chi-squared is particularly sensitive to factors such as skewness. It readily detects histograms of the type illustrated in Fig. (4.9c) but may fail to detect histograms of the type illustrated in Fig. (4.9b).

Utilizing the chi-squared and N mode waveforms the user selects a nonhomogeneous response component; then, using the histogram at the selected latency, the user divides its amplitude range into subranges, one to each assumed homogeneous group of responses. Several time points may be analyzed simultaneously. Using the amplitudes at the selected time points, the computer then classifies each evoked response according to the subranges

it falls into at these points. Then evoked responses with identical classifications are grouped together. Averages and standard
deviations computed for each group and a table of evoked response
classifications are formed.

Example 1

The Sort method was initially developed and applied to
evoked response measurements obtained from behavioral experiments
(John et al. 1969). The subject was expected to perceive a stimulus and then make and act upon a decision based upon the identification of the stimulus. It was found that there were certain
evoked response components which were characteristic of the subject's behavior rather than of the stimulus which elicited the
response. Such components tended to occur late in the behavioral

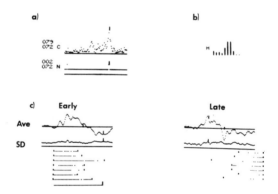

Fig. 4.10. (a) Oscilloscope displays of chi-squared (top
waveform) and N mode. Time epoch is the first 100 msec following
stimulus onset. Sampling interval is 1 msec. (b) Oscilloscope
display of the amplitude histogram at 72 msec latency. (c) Oscilloscope displays of the average and standard deviation waveforms
which tend to occur early (left) and late (right) in the trials.
The time epoch is the first 124 msec following stimulus onset.
The lower part of each display shows a set of seven trials. The
beginning and end of each trial are denoted by heavy markers.
Each dot represents an evoked potential which contributes to the
average shown above it. (From Ruchkin, 1971.)

trials and were not readily discerned in averages based upon the
entire data set. An example of the detection of the nonhomogeneity and the resulting averages for the two subsets is given in
Fig. (4.10a-c). Chi-squared and N mode are displayed in Fig.
(4.10a). The value of any ordinate of the waveforms is displayed
by placing the vertical bar (cursor) at the point of interest.
The ordinate and abscissa values are given by the upper and lower
numbers, respectively, which are to the left of the identification
letters. The histogram of amplitude at 72 msec is displayed in
Fig. (4.10b). A distinct nonhomogeneity is indicated at 72 msec
latency of the evoked responses. The histogram indicates a skew
towards negative amplitudes. An amplitude-sorting threshold was
set between the fourth and fifth bins. One hundred and twenty-
eight evoked responses had more positive amplitudes at 72 msec
latency. These evoked responses tended to occur in the early portion of the behavioral trials. Thirty-five evoked responses were
more negative, displaying a fast component at 72 msec. These
evoked responses tended to occur in the later portion of the
trials. Separate averages and standard deviations for the early
and late evoked potentials and an indication of how each evoked
potential was classified are displayed in Fig. (4.10c). In the
average for the entire set of data, the fast negative component
at 72 msec was masked by the preponderant *early* evoked responses.
The fast negative component at 72 msec latency was consistently
found in the late evoked responses from other data sets with the
same behavioral outcome. It was clearly associated with the behavioral phenomena. Without a sorting procedure it could remain
undetected due to the obscuring effect of the large number of
early evoked responses.

Example 2

Insight into possible misclassification errors of the Sort
program are provided by the following example. The data consist
of evoked responses from eight individual sequences. Four of the

sequences, consisting of 97 evoked responses, were in response to visual stimuli presented at the rate of 3.1 flashes/sec (V1). The other four sequences, consisting of 64 evoked responses, were elicited by a 7.1/sec stimulus (V2). The eight sequences were grouped together into one set of 161 evoked responses for the purpose of testing whether they could be sorted according to stimulus. Since the stimuli are known for each sequence, the computed classification can be compared to the actual conditions.

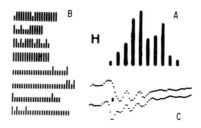

Fig. 4.11. Results of Example 2, an analysis of a set of evoked potentials elicited by one of two different stimuli (V1 or V2). A: The histogram at the sorting latency of 30 msec. B: Illustration of the evoked potential classifications. Each row of bars represents a trial. The height of each bar indicates the type of evoked potential. One unit height is Type 1; two units is Type 2. The bottom four trials are in response to V1. The top four trials are in response to V2. C: The averaged potentials for the two types—the lower is for Type 1; the upper is for Type 2. The time base is 124 msec. The heavy marker at 30 msec indicates the sorting latency. (From Ruchkin, 1971.)

The most pronounced indication of nonhomogeneity was at the latency of 30 msec, where the histogram was bimodal with a chi-squared of 20 ($DF = 9$). The results of sorting the evoked responses according to their amplitudes at 30 msec latency are presented in Fig. (4.11). The histogram of amplitudes is displayed in Fig. (4.11a). The threshold was set in the middle of the sixth bin from the left. Figure (4.11b) indicates the classification for the set of trials. A bar one unit high corresponds to a type 1 evoked response, two units high to a type 2 response. The four bottom rows represent the V1 trials, the four top rows the V2 trials. The lower waveform in Fig. (4.11c) is the average evoked response for the type 1 subset, and the upper waveform is the average for type 2 subset. The type 1 subset is composed mainly by data from the V1 trials whilst the type 2 subset is composed mainly of data from the V2 trials. If it is assumed that all of the V1 evoked responses should have been classified as type 1 and all the V2 responses as type 2, then 23 out of 161 evoked responses are misclassified.

It can be seen that the Sort program should be used with care. When a latency is selected and an amplitude threshold set, the sorting process will force the average responses of separated sets to differ. If misused, the method can say "yes" to almost any question. Using both chi-squared and N mode to indicate non-homogeneities reduces such a possibility. However, these measures are based upon assumptions which may be only partially valid. It is uncertain, for example, how statistics such as N mode and chi-squared, when used in a time series, correlate from point to point. Thus one must be cautious in relying upon strictly numerical measures of statistical significance. Instead, these waves should be considered as indicators which expedite analysis, rather than criteria for considering a result valid. Validation should be sought beyond the framework of the sorting procedure. Results should be validated by similar groups of averages obtained by operating independently upon data sets recorded under similar conditions, or by nonrandom arrangement of evoked response types in the sets of sequences. Only in cases where the chi-squared and N mode waves have especially broad, consistent components of high significance might they constitute a self-sufficient basis for considering a result valid.

Further examples of the use of the Sort method may be found in John *et al.* (1973, 1975) and Bartlett *et al.* (1975).

4.13. DISCRIMINANT ANALYSIS

The Precum-Cumsum and Sort procedures are intended for situations where little is known about nonhomogeneities in the evoked potential data. They have been primarily applied to experiments in which, in a given set of trials, stimulus conditions were held constant but changes took place in the subject's behavior (John *et al.* 1973, 1975). It was hypothesized that there were evoked potential components reflecting both exogeneous sensory registration mechanisms and endogenous cognitive processes that determine behavior. It was further hypothesized that the endogenous components changed due to changes in cognitive state that led to the behavioral response but that the exact temporal sequence of cognitive states was unknown. Hence it was not possible to directly divide the set of evoked potentials into homogeneous subgroups corresponding to the individual cognitive states. Consequently the Sort procedure was utilized in order to assign the evoked potential data into homogeneous subgroups.

In some situations there may be additional knowledge available concerning the data nonhomogeneities. Assume that we know the number of homogeneous subgroups into which the data can be divided and that for each subgroup there are some representative evoked potentials available. We will call this set of data the training set. In addition to the training set there may be a set of evoked potentials of unknown classification. They may have been obtained under experimental conditions similar to those of the training set and be known to have the same type of nonhomogeneities and statistics as the training set. The problem is how to assign each unclassified evoked potential to the proper subgroup, using for the sorting the information available in the training set. Solutions to this problem have been developed, making use of multivariate statistics (Anderson, 1958; Afifi and Azen, 1972). Linear discriminant analysis is one such approach and has been found to be feasible for classifying evoked potentials (Donchin, 1969;

Gardiner and Walter, 1969). In the remainder of this section we attempt to describe the principles and assumptions underlying its use.

We begin with two examples that illustrate how linear discriminant analysis is applied in some special cases. These cases are designed to bring out the features of the linear discriminant analysis procedure. Since discriminant methods have been formulated for time-discrete data and are implemented by digital computers, we assume that the data are in T-discrete form.

Example 1: Uncorrelated Noise with Constant Variance

Denote the evoked potentials to be classified by $x_i(t°\Delta)$, where $i = 1$, M_u, $t° = 1$, N and Δ is the time sampling interval. M_u is the number of unclassified evoked potentials and N is the number of time points used to represent each evoked potential. The training set consists of K subgroups. Denote the average of the evoked potentials in the kth subgroup by $\hat{\mu}_k(t°\Delta)$. It is assumed that

(1) The noise statistics are Gaussian and so are each subgroup;

(2) The noise at time point $t°\Delta$ is uncorrelated with noise at $u°\Delta$, for all $t° \neq u°$;

(3) The variance of the noise σ_n^2 is the same at each point (*i.e.*, the noise is stationary)

In this case it can be shown that a nearly optimum discriminant procedure, in the sense that the expected probability of misclassification is minimized, is to compute the mean square difference between the unclassified evoked potential and the average evoked potential for each group and then assign it to the group for which the mean square difference is smallest. (The sample mean is used because the true mean is unknown. Since the estimate of the mean improves as the number of samples increases, the discriminant procedure will similarly approach asymptotically optimum performance.) In analytical terms we compute for each k, $k = 1$, K, the difference measure D_{ki}.

$$D_{ki} = \sum_{t°=1}^{N} [x_i(t°\Delta) - \hat{\mu}_k(t°\Delta)]^2$$

$$= \sum_{t°=1}^{N} x_i(t°\Delta)^2 - 2 \sum_{t°=1}^{N} \hat{\mu}_k(t°\Delta) \; x_i(t°\Delta)$$

$$+ \sum_{t°=1}^{N} \hat{\mu}_k(t°\Delta)^2 \qquad\qquad (4.33)$$

D_{ki} can be interpreted as a squared distance measure between the ith response and the average response of the kth subgroup; $x_i(t°\Delta)$ is assigned to the subgroup for which D_{ki} is minimal.

The amount of computation can be reduced by noting that $\sum_{t°} x_i(t°\Delta)^2$ does not vary with k, and hence need not enter into the discriminant computation. Consequently, Eq. (4.33) can be reformulated as

$$d_{ki} = \sum_{t°=1}^{N} \hat{\mu}_k(t°\Delta) \; x_i(t°\Delta) - \frac{1}{2} \sum_{t°=1}^{N} \hat{\mu}_k(t°\Delta)^2 \qquad (4.34)$$

$x_i(t°\Delta)$ is assigned to the subgroup for which d_{ki} is largest. Note that the key operation for classification is the computation of the cross product of the $x_i(t°\Delta)$ and $\hat{\mu}_k(t°\Delta)$ waveforms. The cross product becomes larger as $x_i(t°\Delta)$ becomes more similar in shape and amplitude to $\hat{\mu}_k(t°\Delta)$. The sum over $\hat{\mu}_k(t°\Delta)^2$ is a bias term that compensates for differences in magnitude between the $\hat{\mu}_k(t°\Delta)$ waves. The larger magnitude of $\hat{\mu}_k(t°\Delta)$ waveforms will always have a tendency to result in relatively large cross products for a given $x_i(t°\Delta)$, whether or not they are similar. However, the $\frac{1}{2} \sum_{t°} \hat{\mu}_k(t°\Delta)^2$ term corrects for this, since the negative bias will be larger for the larger magnitude $\hat{\mu}_k(t°\Delta)$ waves.

Example 2: Uncorrelated Noise with Variable Variance

The conditions are the same as in Example 1, with the sole exception that the variance of the noise may differ from time point to time point (*i.e.*, the noise may be nonstationary). Denote the sample variance at time point $t°\Delta$ by $\hat{\sigma}_n(t°\Delta)^2$. In this case a nearly optimum discriminant procedure is to compute a weighted mean square difference between the unclassified evoked potential and the average evoked potential for each group. The weighting factor is the inverse of the sample variance at each time point. Thus those time points for which the noise variance is large contribute less to the discriminant function than time points for which the noise variance is small. In effect, this means that the discriminant function is based primarily upon those time points for which the more reliable measurements of evoked potential amplitude can be made. (The procedure would be optimum if the true mean and variance could be used. However, they are unknown and so their sample estimates are used instead. The discriminant procedure is asymptotically optimal if the estimates approach their true values as the sample size becomes large.)

In analytical terms, we compute for each k, $k = 1, K$

$$
\begin{aligned}
D_{ki} &= \sum_{t°=1}^{N} \frac{[x_i(t°\Delta) - \hat{\mu}_k(t°\Delta)]^2}{\hat{\sigma}_n(t°\Delta)^2} \\
&= \sum_{t°=1}^{N} \frac{x_i(t°\Delta)^2}{\hat{\sigma}_n(t°\Delta)^2} - 2\sum_{t°=1}^{N} \frac{\hat{\mu}_k(t°\Delta)}{\hat{\sigma}_n(t°\Delta)^2} x_i(t°\Delta) \\
&\quad + \sum_{t°=1}^{N} \frac{\hat{\mu}_k(t°\Delta)^2}{\hat{\sigma}_n(t°\Delta)^2}
\end{aligned}
\tag{4.35}
$$

As in the case of Eq. (4.33), the first term on the right-hand side is a constant, and we need only consider the d_{ki}:

$$
d_{ki} = \sum_{t°=1}^{N} \frac{\hat{\mu}_k(t°\Delta)}{\hat{\sigma}_n(t°\Delta)^2} x_i(t°\Delta) - \frac{1}{2}\sum_{t°=1}^{N} \frac{\hat{\mu}_k(t°\Delta)^2}{\hat{\sigma}_n(t°\Delta)^2}
\tag{4.36}
$$

The evoked potential $x_i(t°\Delta)$ is assigned to the group for which d_{ki} is a maximum.

Example 3: General Case: Correlated Noise

In practice there may be correlation of the noise component of the data between time points, *i.e.*, the noise may not be white. Hence Eq. (4.36) may not be optimal, even if the true means and variances are used. The optimum discriminant procedure for the general case of correlated noise is not far different from Eq. (4.36) and can be stated in the following general symbolic form:

$$d_{ki} = \sum_{t°=1}^{N} \alpha_k(t°\Delta) \; x_i(t°\Delta) - b_k \tag{4.37}$$

As in Examples 1 and 2, the $x_i(t°\Delta)$ will be assigned to the subgroup for which d_{ki} is maximum. Each $\alpha_k(t°\Delta)$ may be considered to be a waveform whose shape is determined by the noise variances, covariances, and subgroup average. The $\alpha_k(t°\Delta)$ will tend to resemble the subgroup average waveform $\hat{\mu}_k(t°\Delta)$, and will have characteristics that differ from those of the noise. For example, if the noise consists primarily of high frequency activity and is relatively large at certain time points, the $\alpha_k(t°\Delta)$ will tend to consist of low frequency activity and be small at those time points where the noise variance is large. In effect, the $\alpha_k(t°\Delta)$ will tend to weight heavily those time points of the data waveforms for which reliable measurements have been made. The b_k term in Eq. (4.37) plays the same role as the bias terms in Eqs. (4.34) and (4.36). The cross product of $\alpha_k(t°\Delta)$ with $x_i(t°\Delta)$ in Eq. (4.37) will generally tend to be larger for the subgroups with larger $\alpha_k(t°\Delta)$, whether or not $x_i(t°\Delta)$ is most similar to activity in these subgroups. The b_k term introduces a negative bias that compensates for this effect. A more detailed discussion of the formulation of the $\alpha_k(t°\Delta)$ and b_k terms and how they are computed is presented by Afifi and Azen (1972). A complete derivation of the general case is presented by Anderson (1958).

The linear discriminant procedures described here are optimal in the sense of least expected number of misclassification errors when the noise statistics are Gaussian and the same for each group. They may not be optimal for the non-Gaussian noise case; however, they are still likely to yield satisfactory results and are relatively simple to implement.

4.14. STEPWISE DISCRIMINANT ANALYSIS

The use of linear discriminant analysis involves two sequential steps. The first is to compute the constants of the discriminant function; namely, the $\alpha_k(t°\Delta)$ waveform and the b_k. These are obtained from the training set data used to establish the classifications. The estimates of the means of the subgroups and of the noise variances and covariances are used to compute these constants. The second step is to use these discriminant constants to classify each unknown evoked potential.

As thus far formulated, the discriminant function [Eqs. (4.34), (4.36), and (4.37)] has utilized all N time points of the data. In practice there may be significant differences between subgroups at only a few of the N time points. For example, sensory-evoked potentials typically consist of several prominent components at different latencies. A particular manipulation of experimental parameters, e.g., stimulus intensity, task etc., may cause only one or a few of the components to vary systematically. Consequently, when the data are segregated into subgroups of homogeneous experimental conditions, there will be major differences between the subgroups only at the time points corresponding to those components which varied systematically with the changing experimental conditions. These time points will be the most important for discriminating between the subgroups. Use of the other time points in the evoked potential is not likely to improve the discrimination procedure significantly, if at all, and conceivably could degrade it due to spurious noise effects. Thus it is desirable to identify those time points which best discriminate between subgroups of the training set data and only to use them to classify the unknown evoked potentials.

A linear discriminant procedure which determines a restricted set of *best discriminant* time points is available as a standard computer program (Dixon, 1970). The procedure is called stepwise discriminant analysis (Afifi and Azen, 1972). It is called step-wise because it determines the time points to be used by applying a step by step approach to the training set data. The first step is to determine the single time point which is most effective in discriminating between subgroups in the training set. The measure of effectiveness is provided by an "*F* statistic." This statistic can be interpreted as the ratio of the *across subgroups* variance of the subgroup averages to the average of the *within subgroups* vari-ance. The "*F* statistic" is the basis of the one-way-analysis of variance, a widely used statistical test of significance of dif-ferences (Mood and Graybill, 1963). Given a training set with K subgroups, denote the number of evoked potentials in the kth sub-group by m_k and further denote the ith waveform in the kth sub-group by $x_{ki}(t°\Delta)$. Then F may be expressed as

$$F(t°\Delta) = \frac{[1/(K-1)] \sum_{k=1}^{K} m_k [\hat{\mu}_k(t°\Delta) - A(t°\Delta)]^2}{[1/(M-K)] \sum_{k=1}^{K} \sum_{i=1}^{m_k} [x_{ki}(t°\Delta) - \hat{\mu}_k(t°\Delta)]^2} \qquad (4.38)$$

where

$$M = \sum_{k=1}^{K} m_k$$

and

$$A(t°\Delta) = \frac{1}{M} \sum_{k=1}^{M} \sum_{i=1}^{m_k} x_{ki}(t°\Delta)$$

$F(t°\Delta)$ will be largest for time points where the differences be-tween the averages for each subgroup are largest in comparison with the noise variance. Hence it is at these time points that the most reliable discriminations can be made and from them the one point with the largest $F(t°\Delta)$ is selected for use in the discriminant function.

Having selected the single time point with the largest $F(t°\Delta)$, partial means and variances of the evoked potential amplitudes at all other time points are computed, conditioned upon the knowledge of the amplitude at the selected time point. This is an important procedure since the behavior of the evoked potential amplitudes at some of the other time points may be highly correlated with the amplitude at the selected time point. Obviously the information provided by additional highly correlated time points will not greatly improve discrimination performance because such information is redundant to that provided by the selected time point alone. The partial means and variances for the other time points are based upon their *residual* data, that which remain after removing the components which are correlated with the data from the selected time point. The partial means and variances are used to compute the $F(t°\Delta)$ for all time points except the previously selected one. Of these remaining time points, the one with the largest partial $F(t°\Delta)$ is selected for use in the discriminant function. The data at this time point will be relatively uncorrelated with the data at the previously selected time point. Consequently, use of the second time point, determined from the partial F statistics, will provide maximum additional information for improving discrimination performance.

The above procedure for determining time points to be used in the discriminant function is iterated after each new time point is chosen to be in the selected set. In each step partial means and variances are computed for all points not previously chosen, conditioned upon knowledge of the set of previously chosen points. The partial $F(t°\Delta)$'s are then computed, and the time point with the maximum $F(t°\Delta)$ is determined. Iteration is continued until the maximum partial F statistic of the unselected time points is less than a predetermined criterion level. When this occurs, the selection of time points to be used in the discriminant function is terminated, and a linear discriminant function of the form of Eq. (4.37) is computed using the selected time points. In addition to determining at each step which new time point is to be selected for discrimination, the previously selected time points are tested to determine if any have become redundant. Redundant points are dropped from the selected set.

Stepwise discriminant analysis is a quasi-optimal procedure for selecting nonredundant, *best discriminant* time points. There is no assurance that it will find the absolutely optimal set of time points. However, it will usually yield a *satisfactory* set of time points. As an aid in assessing the goodness of the discriminant function so determined, various performance indicators are usually computed at each step. These include a classification table which indicates how the training set data would be classified by a linear discriminant function based upon the time points selected in the previous and current steps.

Stepwise discriminant analysis is useful not only for classifying waveforms but also simply for determining a nonredundant set of time points at which the training set data are most discriminable. The amplitudes at the selected time points can serve as an objectively determined, concise, quantitative set of parameters for characterizing differences between evoked potential populations. Although stepwise discriminant analysis uses the standard F statistic to select the quasi-optimal discriminant time points, it should not be relied upon to attribute statistical significance to the differences between subgroups. The F Statistic is intended to assess significance of differences for univariate data. When F values are computed for several time points, some large, apparently significant F values may occur due to chance alone. Lachin and Schactor (1974) have demonstrated that this effect can occur in a stepwise discriminant analysis. They suggest that significance of differences be assessed by other procedures, such as a multivariate analysis of variance.

Examples of the application of stepwise discriminant analysis to processing of evoked potential data may be found in the reports by Donchin and coworkers (Donchin, 1969; Donchin et al., 1970, 1973), Gardiner and Walter (1969), and Gardiner (1972). A computer simulation study of the efficacy of the application of stepwise discriminant analysis to evoked potential data has been reported by Donchin and Herning (1975). Stepwise discriminant analysis has also been used in the study of the properties of neurophysiologic waveforms other than evoked potentials. For example, Sklar et al. (1973) have used stepwise discriminant analysis to investigate the differences between the power spectra of EEG's from normal and dyslexic children.

4.15. APPENDIX: HISTOGRAMS, SMOOTHING, N MODE

Due to random fluctuations, it is possible for spurious maxima to occur in a histogram. Thus, it is desirable for the mode count to be based upon the broad outline of the histogram. This can be achieved by smoothing the histogram prior to counting the modes. The following algorithm was used to smooth the ten bin amplitude histograms used in the Sort program. It was used since it was readily implemented on a small, binary number system digital computer.

$$H_s(i) = \frac{1}{8} \left[H(i - 1) + 6H(i) + H(i + 1) \right], \quad i = 1, 10 \quad (4.39)$$

$H(i)$ represents the number of waveforms whose amplitude at the chosen latency falls into histogram bin i. $H_s(i)$ represents the ordinate of the smoothed histogram. The $H(i)$ values remain constant throughout the computation of the $H_s(i)$ values.

The smoothing algorithm can be used iteratively. Increasing the number of iterations increases the degree of smoothing, thereby reducing the probability that random fluctuations will cause a false indication of a mode. However, increased smoothing also tends to eliminate peaks and increases the probability that a genuine mode will not be detected. Table (4.2) presents the probabilities of Gaussian data falsely indicating an N mode greater than one, for up to five smoothing iterations. For each entry in the table, there were 4000 independently generated histograms. Sequences of independent, Gaussian random numbers were generated by a digital computer, and ten bin histograms were formed from them. Then the histograms were operated upon by the smoothing N mode routines. The N mode routine did not count modes due to single peaks in $H(1)$ if it was in the form of a ramp extending out to at least the third bin.

TABLE 4.2

Per Cent False Indications

Number of smoothing iterations		0	1	2	3	4	5
Number of Evoked Potentials	64	71.4	38.4	13.8	3.3	.5	.1
	128	51.7	20.1	5.0	0.9	.2	.0
	192	39.0	12.8	2.6	0.3	.0	.0
	256	29.4	8.4	1.4	0.1	.0	.0

Each histogram is centered about its average, the boundary between the fifth and sixth bins corresponding to the average value, and the bin width is one-half the standard deviation of the noise. The first and tenth bins count the number of amplitudes which deviate from the average by two or more standard deviations. Only a relatively small number of events are expected to occur in the end bins of histograms computed for samples of Gaussian and similar unimodal data. Such small numbers are particularly susceptible to random fluctuations and are likely to cause spurious modes even when smoothing is used. Consequently, the N mode routine deliberately excludes modes due only to counts in end bins. However, if one or both end bins have very pronounced peaks, they will be detected by chi-squared.

REFERENCES

Afifi, A. A. and Azen, S. P., "Statistical Analysis, A Computer Oriented Approach." Academic Press, New York, 1972.

Anderson, T. W., "An Introduction to Multivariate Statistical Analysis." Wiley, New York, 1958.

Bartlett, F., John, E. R., Shimokochi, M., and Kleinman, D., *Behav. Biol.* 14, 409 (1975).

Boneau, C. J., *Psychol. Bull.* 57, 49 (1959).

Borda, R. P., and Frost, J. D., Jr., *Electroenceph. Clin. Neurophysiol.* 25, 391 (1968).

Bradley, J. V., "Distribution-Free Statistical Tests." Prentice-Hall, Englewood Cliffs, New Jersey, 1968.

Burns, S. K., and Melzack, R., *Electroenceph. Clin. Neurophysiol.* 20, 407 (1966).

Cooper, R., *in* "Handbook of Electroencephalography and Clinical Neurophysiology" (A. Rémond, ed.), Vol. 4(B), pp. 413-15. Elsevier, Amsterdam, 1972.

Dixon, W. F., "BMD Computer Programs," Univ. California Press, Los Angeles, 1970.

Donchin, E., *Electroenceph. Clin. Neurophysiol.* 27, 311 (1969).

Donchin, E., Callaway, E., III, and Jones, R. T., *Electroenceph. Clin. Neurophysiol.* 29, 429 (1970).

Donchin, E., Kubovy, M., Kutas, M., Johnson, R., Jr., and Herning, R. I., *Percept. Psychophys.* 14, 319 (1973).

Donchin, E. and Herning, R. I., *Electroenceph. Clin. Neurophysiol.* 38, 51 (1975).

Gardiner, M. F. (ed.), "Workshop on the Applications of Stepwise Discriminant Analysis at the University of California." Brain Information Service Press, Los Angeles, 1972.

Gardiner, M. F. and Walter, D. O., *in* "Average Evoked Potentials: Methods, Results and Evaluations," (E. Donchin and D. Lindsley, eds.) p. 335. NASA, SP-191, Washington, D. C. 1969.

Havlicek, L. L. and Peterson, N. L., *Psychol. Reps.* 34, 1095 (1974).

John, E. R. and Shimokochi, M., Unpublished observations (1966).

John, E. R., Shimokochi, M., and Bartlett, F., *Science* 164, 1534 (1969).

John, E. R., Bartlett, F., Shimokochi, M., and Kleinman, D., *J. Neurophysiol.* 36, 893 (1973).

John, E. R., Bartlett, F., Shimokochi, M., and Kleinman, D., *Behav. Biol.* 14, 247 (1975).

Kinney, J. S., McKay, C. L., Mensch, A. J., and Luria, S. M., *Electroenceph. Clin. Neurophysiol.* 34, 7 (1973).

Lachin, J. M. and Schacter, J., *Psychophysiol.* 11, 703 (1974).

Lowy, K. and Weiss, B., *Electroenceph. Clin. Neurophysiol.* 25, 177 (1968).

Mood, A. M. and Graybill, F. A., "Introduction to the Theory of Statistics," 2nd ed., McGraw-Hill, New York, 1963.

Rosenblith, W. A. (ed.), "Processing Neuroelectric Data."
    M. I. T. Press, Cambridge, 1959.
Ruchkin, D. S., *IEEE Trans. Bio-Med. Eng.* BME-12, 87 (1965).
Ruchkin, D. S., *Exp. Neurol.* 20, 275 (1968).
Ruchkin, D. S., *Comm. Behav. Biol.* 5, 383 (1971).
Ruchkin, D. S., *IEEE Trans. Bio-Med. Eng.* BME-21, 54 (1974).
Ruchkin, D. S. and Walter, D. O., *IEEE Trans. Bio-Med Eng.*
    BME-22, 245 (1975).
Saunders, M. G., *Electroenceph. Clin. Neurophysiol.* 15, 761 (1963).
Schimmel, H., *Science* 157, 92 (1967).
Siegel, S., "Nonparametric Statistics for the Behavioral Sciences."
    McGraw-Hill, New York, 1956.
Sklar, B., Hanley, J., and Simmons, W. W., *IEEE Trans. Bio-Med.
    Eng.* BME-20, 20 (1973).
Walter, D. O., *Electroenceph. Clin. Neurophysiol.* 30, 246 (1971).
Woody, C. D., *Med. and Biol. Engng.* 5, 539 (1967).

Chapter 5

EVOKED POTENTIALS:
PRINCIPAL COMPONENTS AND VARIMAX ANALYSIS

5.1. INTRODUCTION

Until now we have concentrated on data analysis procedures concerned with characterizing the individual or joint properties of time functions. When the data consist of a set of several waveforms, then it is also of interest to analyze the nature of the relationships that exist between the set members, hopefully discovering attributes that they share in common.

The need for such procedures has arisen in a variety of evoked response studies (John et al., 1964; Donchin, 1966; Suter, 1970; Bennett et al., 1971; Squires et al., 1975; Donchin et al., 1975). In some of these studies average evoked responses have been recorded simultaneously from several brain sites for the purpose of analyzing the relationships between the neuroelectric activity at these locations. In other studies several average evoked responses have been recorded from a single anatomical site during controlled variations in the experimental conditions. In the latter case, there was an average response waveform associated with each experimental condition. The relationships between these waveforms provided a quantitative statement of the effect of the variation of the experimental parameters upon the evoked electrical activity of the brain.

When characterizing the nature of the relationships between individual members in a large set of waveforms, it is desirable to describe the structure of the set of waveforms by a relatively small, parsimonious number of basic parameters. One method is to represent each observed average response waveform by a linear combination of a set of basic waveforms. This set is basic in the sense that it is used to represent each observed waveform with a high degree of fidelity, a point discussed more fully later. The representation of each data waveform differs from the others only in the relative contributions to it of the basic waveforms. If the number of basic waveforms needed to represent adequately all the observed waveforms is substantially less than the number of data waves, then one can achieve both a significant degree of data reduction and simplify study of the intricacies of the waveform interrelationships.

If the basic waveforms can be given biological meaning by relating them, for example, to physiological sites of origin or specific neural pathways, then such a representation can provide direct insight into the physiological mechanisms generating the data. They may conceivably serve as a means for modelling the biological system. A necessary condition for a linear representation of the data set to serve as a legitimate and realistic framework for a model is that, to within a reasonable approximation, the biological generators which give rise to the data interact in a linear manner. However, this condition alone does not ensure that biological meaning can be attributed to the basic waveforms of any particular linear representation, no matter how concise the representation may be. It will be shown that there is no mathematically unique linear representation, and thus the choice of a particular representation is, to some extent, arbitrary. Consequently, the validity of a linear model depends upon the degree of correspondence to its biological substrate rather than its mathematical formulation. This issue will be further discussed below.

This chapter is primarily motivated by problems that arise in the analysis of sets of average evoked potentials. This means that the background noise has effectively been eliminated and that the averages are *good* estimates of the underlying evoked activity. Because random activity makes only a minor contribution to the differences among the average response waveforms, waveform differ-

ences reflect manipulations of parameters that are under the experimenter's control.

5.2. LINEAR REPRESENTATIONS OF WAVEFORMS

The general form of a linear representation of a set of N
data waveforms $s_n(t)$ where n ranges from 1 to N, is given by Eq.
(5.1)

$$s_n(t) = \sum_{m=1}^{M} c_{nm} f_m(t) \qquad (5.1)$$

(e.g., the $s_n(t)$ may be average evoked responses). There are M
basic waveforms; $f_m(t)$ denotes the mth one of them. If the data
waveforms are continuous functions of time, then the $f_m(t)$ waveforms will also be continuous. If the data waves are represented
by their sampled values at discrete instants of time, then the
$f_m(t)$ will have the same type of representation and t will be a
discrete variable. In practice, when processing data on a digital
computer, the waveforms will be sampled. Thus, in all further discussion in this chapter it will be assumed that $s_n(t)$ and $f_m(t)$
are sampled waveforms with t, the time index ranging in integer
increments from one to T, the maximum number of time points required to represent the waveforms.* c_{nm}, the weighting coefficient,
denotes the contribution of the mth basic waveform to the nth data
waveform. Since the $f_m(t)$ waveforms are common to all the data
waveforms, the array of c_{nm} coefficients provides a complete, objective, and quantitative description of the waveforms from which
all their similarities and dissimilarities can be studied.

A common example of a linear representation is the Fourier
series expansion of data waveforms. The sine and cosine functions
constitute the basic waveforms and the associated Fourier coefficients constitute the weighting coefficient array.

----

*In other chapters, the symbols $t°\Delta$ were used to distinguish
sampled time from continuous time. Such notation will not be used
here.

5.3. THE CROSS CORRELATION COEFFICIENT

Since the analysis of a set of waveforms is intrinsically a study of the similarities and dissimilarities between the members of the set, it is useful at this point to introduce a particular measure of waveform similarity, the cross correlation coefficient. It provides an objective, quantitative similarity measure. The cross correlation coefficient[*] is defined as follows:

$$\rho_{ik} = \frac{\sum_{t=1}^{T} [s_i(t) - \bar{s}_i][s_k(t) - \bar{s}_k]}{\sqrt{\sum_{t=1}^{T} [s_i(t) - \bar{s}_i]^2 \sum_{t=1}^{T} [s_k(t) - \bar{s}_k]^2}} \tag{5.2}$$

where $\bar{s}_i = (1/T) \sum_{t=1}^{T} s_i(t)$ is the mean value of wave-s_i over the time epoch T.

If the two waveforms are identical in shape, then the coefficient is unity. If the waveforms have the same shape except that they are of opposite polarity, then $\rho_{ik} = -1$. When the waveshapes are dissimilar, the magnitude of the coefficient will be less than one. A zero coefficient is indicative of maximum dissimilarity. Note that the correlation coefficient does not indicate differences in magnitude. If two waveforms have the same shape, but have different magnitudes, then the correlation coefficient is unity.

5.4. SIGNAL SPACE

Perhaps the best way to consider linear representations of signals is in terms of signal space geometry. The data waveforms can be given the geometric interpretation of vectors in a signal space that can be visualized in its three-dimensional form. Each

---

[*] For the sake of brevity, in this chapter the terminology cross correlation coefficient and correlation coefficient will be synonymous.

waveform can be thought of as a vector, radiating from the origin, in a space of T dimensions, where the τth reference axis corresponds to the amplitude at time $t = \tau$. A simple illustration of a three time point waveform and its corresponding geometric representation is given in Fig. (5.1). The orientation and length of the signal vector is specified by the three amplitude samples.

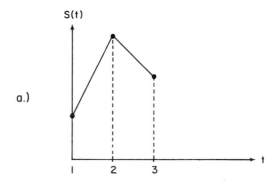

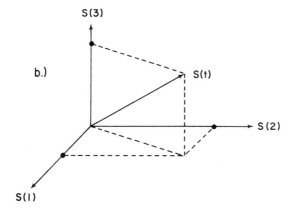

Fig. 5.1 An example of (a) a three time point waveform and (b) its geometric representation in signal space.

A signal space is essentially a multidimensional space in which the set of coordinates of a point in the space corresponds to a set of parameter values which specify the waveform of the signal to be represented. The coordinates need not necessarily be amplitude samples. Among other possibilities that may be used as the coordinates of a signal space are the coefficients of a Fourier series expansion of the waveform. In general, any complete[*] linear expansion of a waveform can constitute the framework for a signal space, with the weighting coefficients being used as the coordinates of the space and the basic[†] waveforms corresponding to the axes of the signal space. From this point of view, the amplitude sample representation of a waveform can be thought of as a particular, complete linear expansion where the basic waveforms are the set of T waveforms defined at their sample times as

$$f_1(1) = 1, \ f_1(2) = 0, \ f_1(3) = 0, \ \ldots \ f_1(m) = 0, \ \ldots \ f_1(T) = 0$$
$$f_2(1) = 0, \ f_2(2) = 1, \ f_2(3) = 0, \ \ldots \ f_2(m) = 0, \ \ldots \ f_2(T) = 0$$
$$\vdots$$
$$f_m(1) = 0, \ f_m(2) = 0, \ f_m(3) = 0, \ \ldots \ f_m(m) = 1, \ \ldots \ f_m(T) = 0$$
$$\vdots$$
$$f_T(1) = 0, \ f_T(2) = 0, \ f_T(3) = 0, \ \ldots \ f_T(m) = 0, \ \ldots \ f_T(T) = 1$$

Essentially each of these basic waveforms picks out the value of the sampled function at one integer-valued time point.

In general

$$f_n(t) = \begin{cases} 1, & n = t \\ 0, & n \neq t \end{cases}$$

and the amplitude samples are the corresponding weighting coefficients.

The shape of a waveform determines the orientation of its corresponding vector in signal space while the waveform magnitude determines the vector length. Consequently, the signal vectors

---

[*]Completeness means that the set of basic functions is capable of perfectly representing any waveform in the signal space.

[†]The basic waveforms are frequently referred to as basis functions in the literature.

corresponding to waveforms that have *similar shapes* have *similar orientations*. The correlation coefficient of a pair of waveforms is just the cosine of the angle between their corresponding signal vectors. A correlation coefficient of +1 or -1 indicates that the signal vectors are colinear. The signal waveshapes are then the same, except that when they are of opposite polarity, the correlation coefficient is -1. A zero correlation coefficient is indicative of maximal dissimilarity. Signal vectors whose correlation coefficient is zero are orthogonal. If there are T time points, then the signal vectors lie in a space of T dimensions. However, the dimensions of the subspace containing the signal vectors may be less than T. For example, if there are only two signal vectors in the set, then the set will be contained within a two-dimensional plane, no matter how large T may be. The two axes of the plane, which define its orientation in the signal space, will each consist of T dimensions, but the location of any of the signal vectors *within* their common two-dimensional plane can be specified by two coordinates.

If one wishes to describe how the two signals are related in terms of their degree of similarity, then it is not necessary to locate their respective positions in the T-dimensional signal space. Rather, it is only necessary to specify their position in the two-dimensional subspace spanned by their common plane. All information concerning their magnitudes and relative orientation can be specified by their positions within the plane. Consequently, a linear expansion of the form of Eq. (5.1) can be formulated in which there are only two basic orthogonal waveforms corresponding to the axes of the plane. Each waveform will require only two weighting coefficients, thereby reducing an originally T-dimensional representation of the waves to a two-dimensional one. Note, however, that this two-dimensional representation only specifies the similarity relationships between the two waveforms. If the original shapes are desired, then the information available in the T-dimensional representations of the basic waveforms must be used.

This reasoning can be extended to the general case of a set of N signal vectors in a T-dimensional signal space, where N is less than T. The set of signal vectors will be contained in a subspace of, at most, N dimensions. The axes of the N-dimensional hyperplane containing the signal vectors need to be specified as T-dimensional vectors in the complete signal space, but the location of each of the signal vectors within the N-dimensional hyperplane itself can be specified only by N coordinates. These convey all the information concerning the relative orientations and magnitudes of the set of N signals. Consequently, a linear expansion can be formulated having only N basic waveforms, those corresponding to the axes of the hyperplane that specifies the relationships between the N waveforms. If the original shapes are desired, then the information available in the T-dimensional representations of the basic waveforms must be resorted to.

It should be further noted that there is no unique set of axes or representation for a set of signal vectors. All that is required is that the set of axes span the N-dimensional subspace in which the data lie. As we shall see, however, other considerations indicate that some representations are to be preferred over others.

The above examples indicate that the dimensionality of the subspace containing a set of waveforms can be less than the dimensionality of the overall signal space in which they are defined. So far we have reasoned that when the number of signal vectors, N is less than the dimensionality of the signal space T, then the dimensionality of the subspace containing the signal vectors will be no more than N. However, under certain conditions there can be an even greater reduction in dimensionality.

Consider the example of two signal waveforms. When their waveshapes are identical, then their correlation coefficient will be unity. Hence the two corresponding signal vectors are colinear and are contained in a one-dimensional subspace. Generalizing from the two waveform cases, it can be shown that when the N signal waveforms meet certain criteria for similarity, they will be contained in a subspace of less than N dimensions. There need not be waveforms with identical shapes, as in the two signal waveform example, but there should be sufficient waveshape similarity so that the magnitudes of the correlation coefficients between the various signal waveforms tend to be large. For such a condition, the corresponding signal vectors will tend to have similar orientations and consequently, the set of N signal vectors will tend to lie in a subspace of less than N dimensions. The correlation coefficients between all possible pairs of signal waveforms in a data set characterize the overall degree of similarity of the data and, through suitable analytical techniques to be described below, can be used to compute the dimensionality of the data signal space. The dimensionality is a direct indication of the overall similarity of the set of waveforms and specifies the number of basic waveforms required for a linear expansion representation of the data set. In general, the upper bound of the dimensionality of a set of waveforms is less than or equal to the smaller of N and T, where N is the number of waveforms and T is the number of time points used to describe each waveform. The argument is as follows. Since the waveforms are each specified by T samples, the set lies within a signal space of T dimensions. However, the N waveforms can at most span a subspace of N dimensions. Hence the dimensionality of the set of signals can at most be the smaller of N and T.

5.5. LINEAR EXPANSION METHODS, FACTOR ANALYSIS AND OTHER TECHNIQUES

There is no unique expansion for a set of waveforms of the form of Eq. (5.1). This point is illustrated by Fig. (5.2). The c_{ij} coefficient is the projection of the ith signal $s_i(t)$ upon the jth axis. The reference axes can be oriented in any direction in signal space, and they need not be orthogonal. [See Fig.

(5.2c).] The $s_i(t)$ are the same for Fig. (5.2a-c). However, the $f_j(t)$ and the associated array of coefficients differ. It is

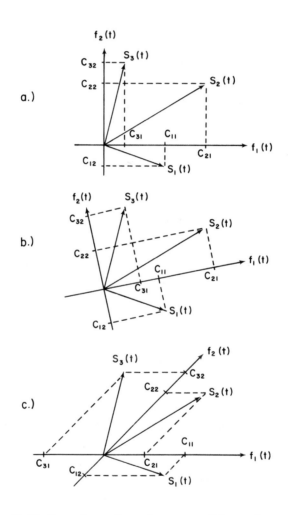

Fig. (5.2) Examples of various possible reference axes for the representation of three waveform vectors contained in a signal space of two dimensions. (a) and (b) illustrate orthogonal reference axes and (c) illustrates a nonorthogonal pair of axes.

only necessary that the number of separately oriented axes equal the dimensionality of the space spanned by the set of signal vectors. Thus it can be seen that a linear expansion scheme can be chosen arbitrarily. The choice will depend upon the computational feasibility and the degree of insight the experimenter has of the evoked responses he is dealing with.

A straightforward procedure for decomposing signal waveforms is to specify the basic waveforms directly. The Fourier series expansion of the data waveforms is an example of this approach. The sine and cosine functions are the basic waveforms and their associated Fourier coefficients are the weighting coefficient array. In some instances a Fourier series analysis may be desirable and satisfactory. However, many situations arise in the analysis of evoked potentials in which a Fourier analysis is neither most concise nor particularly physiologically meaningful. It is advantageous to find a set of basic waveforms which are physiologically meaningful.

The problem of obtaining a suitable representation of a set of evoked potential waveforms is analogous to that dealt with by Factor Analysis, a method developed largely for analyzing multivariate psychological data. In the Factor Analysis model, it is assumed that the data arise from a linear interaction of factors such that the model can be described by a linear expansion of the form of Eq. (5.1), the basic waveforms corresponding to the factors. Consequently, Factor Analysis methods have been used to obtain linear expansions of data waveforms. Their initial development occurred in the years prior to the widespread availability of digital computers and consequently the early methods were usually significantly limited by considerations of computational feasibility. Feasibility has now become less of a constraint and methods such as Principal Factors, with its associated Varimax Rotation, have been widely used. As will be described below, such methods can provide an *optimal* data representation scheme and may be readily implemented.

5.6. FACTOR ANALYSIS AND PRINCIPAL FACTORS

In Factor Analysis, the data analyst usually makes an initial estimate of (a) the extent to which each data waveform is composed of components common to other data waves, the communality, and (b) the extent to which activity is specific to each wave alone, the uniqueness. Adjustments are then made in the computational procedures so that the analysis is carried out upon the estimated common components. The problems posed by this approach have been discussed at length (Harmon, 1967). Such an approach is not often used in signal analysis applications because when the method of Principal Factors is used, the computational procedure implicitly separates common from unique activity (Watanabe, 1967).

In Factor Analysis the basic waveforms are not specified in advance as in a Fourier series expansion. Instead they are determined by the structure of the data waveforms. Usually, for reasons of computational simplicity, the basic waves, the axes of the signal space, are constrained to be an orthonormal set, as specified by Eq. (5.3).

$$\frac{1}{T} \sum_{t=1}^{T} f_i(t) f_j(t) = \begin{cases} 0, & i \neq j, \quad \textit{orthogonality} \\ 1, & i = j, \quad \textit{normality} \end{cases} \qquad (5.3)$$

In terms of signal space geometry, the axes of the space will be orthogonal and their orientation in the space will depend upon the particular distribution of the data signal vectors. It should be recalled that there is no unique set of basic waveforms. However, most factor analysis procedures attempt to orient the axes along main groupings of the data vectors, with the intent of identifying common components by as parsimonious a coordinate system as possible. The basic waveforms associated with such orientations can lend themselves to meaningful interpretation of the data at hand.

5.7. MATRICES AND SIGNAL ANALYSIS

Since a set of data waveforms can be sizeable, the application of signal analysis/factor analysis procedures can involve extensive computational operations. Under these circumstances, it is important to have a symbolism and conceptual framework that lends itself to the manipulation of large amounts of data. The concept of matrices can be useful, especially if the data interactions are to be described by sets of linear algebraic equations.

A matrix is an array of NT numbers, arranged into N rows and T columns, as illustrated by Eq. (5.4).

$$\underline{B} = \begin{bmatrix} b_{11} & b_{12} & \cdots & b_{1T} \\ b_{21} & b_{22} & \cdots & b_{2T} \\ \vdots & \vdots & \ddots & \vdots \\ b_{N1} & b_{N2} & \cdots & b_{NT} \end{bmatrix} \qquad (5.4)$$

The matrix element b_{ij} is located in the ith row and the jth column. As an example, the matrix $\underline{B}$ can represent a set of waveforms. Physically, b_{ij} corresponds to the amplitude of the ith response waveform of a set of N waveforms, at the jth of its T time points.

Two matrices $\underline{A}$ and $\underline{B}$ are equal if they have the same number of rows and columns and $a_{ij} = b_{ij}$ for all i and j.

A. MATRIX PROPERTIES, DEFINITIONS

The *transpose* of a matrix is a second matrix formed by interchanging all rows and columns of the first matrix. For example, suppose $\underline{A}$ is a two-row by three-column matrix

$$\underline{A} = \begin{bmatrix} a_{11} & a_{12} & a_{13} \\ a_{21} & a_{22} & a_{23} \end{bmatrix} \qquad (5.5)$$

then the transpose of $\underline{A}$ is

$$\underline{A}' = \begin{bmatrix} a_{11} & a_{21} \\ a_{12} & a_{22} \\ a_{13} & a_{23} \end{bmatrix} \tag{5.6}$$

A matrix is said to be *square* if the number of rows and the number of columns are equal.

When a matrix consists of only one row or one column, then it is referred to as a row or column vector. Examples of vector arrays are given below.

$$\underline{d} = \begin{pmatrix} d_1 \\ \vdots \\ d_T \end{pmatrix}, \quad \underline{d}' = (d_1 \cdots d_T) \tag{5.7}$$

$\underline{d}$ is a column vector and $\underline{d}'$, its transpose, is a row vector. Such arrays might represent a single waveform of T points.

For notational convenience, matrices will be denoted by un-derlined upper case letters and vectors by underlined lower case letters. Matrix operations and properties that are particularly relevant to analysis of waveform sets are briefly presented below. A fuller treatment is presented by Harmon (1967, Chapter 3).

B. MATRIX ADDITION

If two matrices have the same number of rows and columns, they may be added or subtracted to form a sum or difference matrix as illustrated below.

$$\underline{C} = \underline{A} + \underline{B}$$

where

$$c_{ij} = a_{ij} + b_{ij} \quad \text{for all } i \text{ and } j \tag{5.8}$$

246

C. SCALAR MULTIPLICATION

Scalar multiplication of a matrix is defined as follows: Let B denote the matrix and c the scalar. Then the elements of the scalar product matrix $A = c\,B$ are

$$a_{ij} = c\,b_{ij} \quad \text{for all } i \text{ and } j \tag{5.9}$$

D. MATRIX MULTIPLICATION

Matrices can be multiplied together to form a product matrix. The elements of the product matrix are related to the original matrices as follows:

$$C = A\,B$$

$$c_{ij} = \sum_{n=1}^{N} a_{in} b_{nj} \quad \text{for all } i \text{ and } j \tag{5.10}$$

where A has N columns and B has N rows. A general requirement of the multiplication operation is that the number of columns in the left-hand matrix A must equal the number of rows in the right-hand matrix B. There is no restriction on the number of rows of A or the number of columns of B. The matrix multiplication operation is not generally commutative, so that in general

$$A\,B \neq B\,A \tag{5.11}$$

5.8. MATRICES AND LINEAR EXPANSIONS OF WAVEFORMS

Many common operations in signal analysis implicitly involve matrix multiplications. For example, the linear representation of a set of N waveforms by M basic waveforms can be expressed as a multiplication of two matrices. The first matrix C is formed from the weighting coefficients of the basic waveforms and the second F, from the amplitudes of the basic waveforms at the T time points. Thus, at time point t

$$s_{nt} = \sum_{m=1}^{M} c_{nm} f_{mt} \qquad (5.12)$$

where

$$1 \le n \le N, \quad 1 \le t \le T$$

The matrix of weighting coefficients is

$$\underline{C} = \begin{bmatrix} c_{11} & \cdots & c_{1m} & \cdots & c_{1M} \\ \vdots & & \vdots & & \vdots \\ c_{N1} & \cdots & c_{Nm} & \cdots & c_{NM} \end{bmatrix} \qquad (5.13)$$

The ith row contains the M coefficients that describe the ith waveform in terms of the M basic waveforms. The matrix of basic waveforms is

$$\underline{F} = \begin{bmatrix} f_{11} & \cdots & f_{1t} & \cdots & f_{1T} \\ \vdots & & \vdots & & \vdots \\ f_{M1} & \cdots & f_{Mt} & \cdots & f_{MT} \end{bmatrix} \qquad (5.14)$$

Each row represents a basic waveform. The signal waveform matrix is thus

$$\underline{S} = \begin{bmatrix} s_{11} & \cdots & s_{1t} & \cdots & s_{1T} \\ \vdots & & \vdots & & \vdots \\ s_{N1} & \cdots & s_{Nt} & \cdots & s_{NT} \end{bmatrix} \qquad (5.15)$$

Each row represents a signal waveform. Thus (Eq. (5.12) can be expressed in matrix format as

$$\underline{S} = \underline{C} \, \underline{F} \qquad (5.16)$$

248

A. *CROSS CORRELATION*

The cross correlation coefficient, see Eq. (5.2), for a pair of waveforms can be expressed by matrix products. Let $a_t = s_i(t)$ and $b_t = s_j(t)$. First note that the cross correlation

$$R = \frac{1}{T} \sum_{t=1}^{T} a_t b_t \tag{5.17}$$

can be rewritten by considering the waveforms to be column vectors, $\underline{a}$ and $\underline{b}$:

$$\underline{a} = \begin{pmatrix} a_1 \\ \vdots \\ a_T \end{pmatrix}, \quad \underline{b} = \begin{pmatrix} b_1 \\ \vdots \\ b_T \end{pmatrix}$$

Thus

$$R = (1/T)(\underline{a}' \, \underline{b}) \tag{5.18}$$

The correlation coefficient, as defined by Eq. (5.2), can then be written in terms of matrices. Denote the mean values over time of a_t and b_t by $\bar{a}$ and $\bar{b}$. Then form the vectors

$$\underline{\hat{a}} = \begin{pmatrix} a_1 - \bar{a} \\ \vdots \\ a_t - \bar{a} \end{pmatrix}, \quad \underline{\hat{b}} = \begin{pmatrix} b_1 - \bar{b} \\ \vdots \\ b_t - \bar{b} \end{pmatrix} \tag{5.18a}$$

This permits substitution of these vectors for expressions of the form of Eq. (5.17) which occur in the numerator and denominator of Eq. (5.2). The result is that the correlation coefficient is

$$\rho_{ab} = \underline{\hat{a}} \, \underline{\hat{b}} \, / \sqrt{(\underline{\hat{a}}' \, \underline{\hat{a}})(\underline{\hat{b}}' \, \underline{\hat{b}})} \tag{5.18b}$$

5.9. TRANSPOSE OF MATRIX PRODUCTS

The transpose of the product of matrices is the product in reverse order of multiplication of the transposes of the individual

249

contributing matrices. For example,

If $\underline{D} = \underline{A}\ \underline{B}\ \underline{C}$, then $\underline{D}' = \underline{C}'\ \underline{B}'\ \underline{A}'$

5.10. SOME SPECIAL MATRICES

If the transpose of a square matrix equals the original matrix, then it is called a *symmetric matrix*. This means that the elements of a symmetric matrix satisfy the relationship $r_{ik} = r_{ki}$ for all i and k. The symmetry is about the main diagonal of the matrix, the diagonal whose elements are r_{ii}.

Symmetric matrices are encountered when cross correlations, covariances, or correlation coefficients are computed for all pairs of data in a waveform set. If there are N waveforms, the correlations, arranged suitably, will yield a symmetric $N \times N$ matrix (N rows and N columns). For example, for cross correlations we have

$$r_{ik} = r_{ki} = \frac{1}{T} \sum_{t=1}^{T} s_{it} s_{kt} \qquad (5.19)$$

A similar symmetry relationship holds for correlation coefficients. Such matrices by themselves constitute a complete, quantitative statement of similarities existing in the data set. They can be operated upon by factor analysis methods to obtain linear expansions of the data.

A special form of symmetric matrix is the *diagonal matrix*. It has zeros everywhere except along the diagonal.

$$\underline{A} = \begin{bmatrix} a_{11} & 0 & \cdots & 0 \\ 0 & a_{22} & \cdots & 0 \\ \vdots & \vdots & \ddots & \vdots \\ 0 & 0 & \cdots & a_{NN} \end{bmatrix} \qquad (5.20)$$

The *identity matrix* is a diagonal matrix whose diagonal elements all equal unity. It is denoted by $\underline{I}$. It has the property that for any matrix $\underline{B}$,

$$\underline{B}\,\underline{I} = \underline{I}\,\underline{B} = \underline{B} \tag{5.21}$$

If all members of a set of N waveforms are orthogonal to one another, then the associated cross covariance matrix will be an $N \times N$ diagonal matrix and the correlation coefficient matrix will be an $N \times N$ identity matrix

5.11. MATRIX INVERSE

A square matrix $\underline{B}$, may have an *inverse*, denoted by $\underline{B}^{-1}$. The inverse has the property that

$$\underline{B}\,\underline{B}^{-1} = \underline{B}^{-1}\,\underline{B} = \underline{I} \tag{5.22}$$

Inverses do not exist for all square matrices. Those that do not have inverses are called *singular matrices*. The nonexistence of an inverse means that at least one of the elements of the inverse is infinite.

For example, consider the solution to a set of N linear equations where there are N unknowns:

$$\begin{aligned}
W_{11}x_1 + W_{12}x_2 + W_{13}x_3 &= y_1 \\
W_{21}x_1 + W_{22}x_2 + W_{23}x_3 &= y_2 \\
W_{31}x_1 + W_{32}x_2 + W_{33}x_3 &= y_3
\end{aligned} \tag{5.23}$$

The x_i terms are unknown and the W_{ij} and y_j are known. The above set of equations can be represented in matrix form.

$$\underline{W}\,\underline{x} = \underline{y} \tag{5.24}$$

If $\underline{W}$ is nonsingular, then $\underline{x}$ may be found by premultiplying both sides of Eq. (5.24) by $\underline{W}^{-1}$

$$\underline{x} = \underline{W}^{-1}\,\underline{y} \tag{5.25}$$

If $\underline{W}$ is singular, then it has no inverse and hence no unique solution for the x_i can be obtained. In terms of Eq. (5.23), this means that the W_{ij} are such that there is a linear dependence among the three equations. With only one or two independent equations, it is not possible to solve for three unknowns. If the rows (or columns) of the W_{ij} array are thought of as vectors in a space, then in geometric terms linear dependence and hence, singularity arises when the three vectors span a space of only one (colinear) or two dimensions (coplanar).

The relationship between the inverse of a matrix product and the inverses of the individual matrices is

$$(\underline{A}\ \underline{B}\ \underline{C})^{-1} = \underline{C}^{-1}\ \underline{B}^{-1}\ \underline{A}^{-1} \tag{5.26}$$

5.12. ORTHOGONAL MATRICES

An orthogonal matrix is a square matrix whose inverse and transpose relate such that

$$\underline{U}^{-1} = \underline{U}' \quad \text{and} \quad \underline{U}\ \underline{U}' = \underline{I} \tag{5.27}$$

A matrix whose rows or columns are orthogonal basic waveform vectors is an orthogonal matrix. Orthogonal matrices play a fundamental role in the development of a principal factors expansion.

5.13. PROPERTIES OF LINEAR EXPANSIONS BASED UPON ORTHONORMAL BASIC WAVEFORMS

A commonly used measure of the size of a signal waveform is its power, defined as follows for the nth signal s_{nt} of a collection of signals whose durations are T seconds.

$$\text{power of } s_n(t) = P_n = \frac{1}{T} \sum_{t=1}^{T} s_{nt}^2 \tag{5.28a}$$

In terms of signal space, the power of s_{nt} corresponds to the square of the length of the signal vector divided by T.

The coefficients of an orthonormal set of basic waveforms have some general properties which aid in interpreting the expansion. A fundamental property is that the mth basic waveform contributes c_{nm}^2, the square of the mth expansion coefficient, to the power of the nth signal. This can be inferred by substituting the linear expansion for s_{nt} in Eq. (5.28) and showing that P_n is equal to the sum of the squared coefficients, as follows:

$$P_n = \frac{1}{T} \sum_{t=1}^{T} \left[\sum_{m=1}^{M} c_{nm} f_{mt} \right]^2$$

$$= \frac{1}{T} \sum_{t=1}^{T} \sum_{m=1}^{M} \sum_{k=1}^{M} c_{nm} c_{km} f_{mt} f_{kt}$$

$$= \sum_{m=1}^{M} \sum_{k=1}^{M} c_{nm} c_{km} \frac{1}{T} \sum_{t=1}^{T} f_{mt} f_{kt}$$

Using the orthogonality relation Eq. (5.3) for the basic waveforms, we find

$$P_n = \sum_{m=1}^{M} c_{nm}^2 \tag{5.28b}$$

A measure of the importance of a basic waveform is the power it contributes to the total power of the entire set of waveforms. This contribution is denoted by

$$P_m = \sum_{n=1}^{N} c_{nm}^2 \tag{5.29}$$

The purpose of developing the theory of linear expansions is that it permits finding expansions that hopefully will perfectly reconstruct N data waveforms utilizing significantly fewer basic waveforms M. In practice an absolutely perfect reconstruction is rarely possible with less than N basic waveforms if $N < T$, or less than T basic waveforms, if $T < N$. However, if one is willing to tolerate some error in reconstruction, then a smaller number of basic waveforms can be used. The quality of a linear expansion can be evaluated by measuring how the original data waveforms differ from their corresponding approximate constructions. One commonly used measure of the difference between two waveforms is the mean square error, defined as the average over time of the square of the difference between the two waveforms at each point in time. The mean square error corresponds to the square of the distance between the ends of the two signal vectors. The mean square error between the nth data signal s_{nt} and its approximate representation by any technique $\hat{s}_{nt}$, is denoted as

$$MSE_n = \frac{1}{T} \sum_{t=1}^{T} [s_{nt} - \hat{s}_{nt}]^2 \tag{5.30a}$$

If the approximate representation of s_{nt} is based upon an orthogonal set of basic waveforms, then the mean square difference reduces to the difference between the powers of the original waveform and its approximation.

For orthonormal basic waveforms, omission of the mth basic waveform from the representation of waveform n increases MSE_n by c_{nm}^2. If the indexing of the basic waveforms is arranged such that the higher m, the smaller the power contribution P_m to the waveform approximation, then the total mean square approximation error caused by utilizing only the first K of the set of M waveforms will be

$$MSE_K = \sum_{m=K+1}^{M} P_m \tag{5.30b}$$

Since the measured data waveforms will generally consist in part of stray, random noiselike details, it may not be necessary or even desirable to reconstruct the data waves perfectly. In a fortunate situation common in evoked potential studies, the effect of these stray events, which are uncorrelated from one data wave to the next, is to produce a large number of basic waveforms which contribute negligibly to the average responses.

5.14. PRINCIPAL COMPONENTS

A desirable property for an orthonormal waveform representation to have is that, for any fixed number of basic waveforms K, the total mean square error shown in Eq. (5.30) should be the minimum attainable by any set of orthonormal basic waveforms. Such a representation, called a principal factor expansion, can be found for any set of data waveforms. Determination of the basic waveforms and the weighting coefficients for individual data waveforms is essentially implemented by means of a least-mean-square error fitting process.

The first basic wave f_{1t}, is the least-mean-square error fit of a single waveform to the entire data set. The second basic wave, orthonormal to the first, is the least-mean-square error fit to the residual from the fit of the first wave. The process is continued until the $s_i(t)$ data signal space is completely specified by the f_{it} set.

As a simple example, consider the two data signal vectors in Fig. (5.3). It is desired to obtain a principal factors set of axes. The first axis $f_1(t)$ is oriented so that the sum of the squares of the projections $c_{11}^2 + c_{21}^2$ is a maximum. This is equivalent to minimizing

$$\frac{1}{T} \sum_{t=1}^{T} \left[(s_{1t} - c_{11} f_{1t})^2 + (s_{2t} - c_{21} f_{1t})^2 \right].$$

f_{2t} is then immediately determined since it is constrained to be orthonormal to f_{1t}. In the general case of N data waveforms, f_{1t} will be oriented so as to maximize the sum of the square of the projections on f_{1t}, $\sum_{i=1}^{N} c_{i1}^2$. Then f_{2t} will be oriented so as to maximize $\sum_{i=1}^{N} c_{i2}^2$ subject to the constraint that f_{2t} be orthonormal to f_{1t}. This process is continued until the entire data signal space is spanned by the f_{mt} basic vectors. In two dimensions, only one maximization is necessary; in M dimensions, there are $M - 1$ because of the orthogonality constraint.

Roughly speaking, the least-mean-square error property of principal factors serves to separate out the predominant waveform components common to many data waveforms from the smaller, uncorrelated events associated with individual data waveforms. The predominant events are fitted by the low index (high power contribution) basic waves, while the small, singular events are fitted by the high index (low power contribution) basic waves. The least-mean-square fit property makes principal factors particularly useful for determining the number of basic waves required for a satisfactory representation of the data since, for a fixed number of orthonormal basic waves, the principal factors expansion yields the smallest approximation error. In signal space terminology, the principal factors method establishes the effective dimensionality of the space containing the data. As will be shown below,

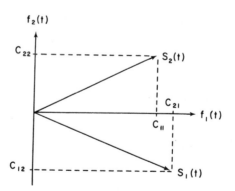

Fig. 5.3. An example of the principal component axes for the representation of a pair of signal waveforms.

once the dimensionality of the data set has been established, other expansions, which may be more useful for interpreting the results, can be derived from the principal factors representation.

Factor analysis usually involves estimating the stray, un-correlated events, the *uniqueness,* prior to the expansion and then making appropriate adjustments in the waveform powers so that only the activity common to the data set, the *communality,* is involved in the expansion. However, from the point of view of the signal analysis problem, such adjustments need not be made in advance. The unique activity will be represented by the low power basic waveforms, and so can be identified and eliminated from further analysis subsequent to the expansion. When this procedure is fol-lowed for a principal factors expansion, the procedure is referred to as a principal components analysis.

In general, principal components basic waveforms are optimal in the sense of yielding the least-mean-square fit only for the particular set of data waveforms from which they have been de-rived. They will probably not be optimal when applied to any other data set, and they may not even be sufficient to represent it.

5.15. COMPUTATION OF PRINCIPAL COMPONENTS

The data wave correlation matrix forms the starting point of a method for obtaining the basic waveforms and weighting coef-ficients of the principal components expansion. The avenue of approach to this expansion involves what are referred to as the eigenvectors and eigenvalues of the correlation matrix. To each correlation matrix there corresponds a unique set of eigenvectors and eigenvalues, and these may be obtained by straightforward, but tedious, computations. The significance of these eigenvectors and eigenvalues will be given here in an abbreviated demonstration. More details can be found in Harmon (1967, Chapter 8).

The correlation matrix will be denoted by

$$\underline{R} = \begin{bmatrix} r_{11} & \cdots & r_{1N} \\ \vdots & \ddots & \vdots \\ r_{N1} & \cdots & r_{NN} \end{bmatrix}$$

257

where the r_{nk} can be either the cross covariances or the correlation coefficients between the nth and kth waveforms in a set of N waveforms. In general the cross covariance of a pair of data waves is

$$r_{nk} = \frac{1}{T} \sum_{t=1}^{T} s_{nt} s_{kt} \tag{5.31}$$

where the mean value over the time epoch $t = 1$, T of each $s_n(t)$ is assumed to be zero. If the $s_n(t)$ are also normalized so that they each have unit power over $t = 1$, T, then the r_{nk} terms will be the correlation coefficients [see Eq. (5.2), this chapter]. The distinction between working with cross covariances or correlation coefficients will be discussed below. We now introduce the notion of eigenvalues and eigenvectors.

To the matrix $\underline{R}$ there corresponds a set of N scalars λ_i, the so-called eigenvalues of $\underline{R}$, which can be arranged in a diagonal matrix:

$$\underline{\lambda} = \begin{bmatrix} \lambda_1 & 0 & \cdots & 0 \\ 0 & \lambda_2 & \cdots & 0 \\ \vdots & \vdots & \ddots & \vdots \\ 0 & 0 & \cdots & \lambda_N \end{bmatrix}$$

Furthermore, associated with each eigenvalue is an eigenvector consisting of N elements:

$$\underline{u}_m = \begin{pmatrix} u_{1m} \\ \vdots \\ u_{Nm} \end{pmatrix}$$

Though it is by no means obvious at this point, the eigenvectors are orthogonal to each other.

$$\underline{u}'_m \cdot \underline{u}_k = \begin{cases} 1, & m = k \\ 0, & m \neq k \end{cases}$$

The N eigenvectors taken together form an N by N orthogonal matrix [see Eq. (5.27)], the eigenmatrix

$$\underline{U} = \begin{bmatrix} u_{11} & u_{12} & \cdots & u_{1N} \\ u_{21} & u_{22} & \cdots & u_{2N} \\ \vdots & \vdots & \ddots & \vdots \\ u_{N1} & u_{N2} & \cdots & u_{NN} \end{bmatrix}$$

and

$$\underline{U}' \ \underline{U} = \underline{I}$$

The eigenvectors and eigenvalues are related to their parent correlation matrix in the following way:

$$\underline{R} \ \underline{u}_m = \lambda_m \ \underline{u}_m \tag{5.32}$$

Premultiplication of vector $\underline{u}_m$ by matrix $\underline{R}$ results in another vector which is proportional to $\underline{u}_m$, with λ_m being the proportionality constant.

Equation (5.32) can be directly extended to include all eigenvectors in one expression. This is done by premultiplying $\underline{U}$ by $\underline{R}$. The result is

$$\underline{R} \ \underline{U} = \underline{U} \ \lambda \tag{5.33}$$

This relation has great significance. To illustrate, let us now introduce two diagonal matrices, one of the square roots of the eigenvalues and the other of the reciprocals of the square roots of the eigenvalues. They are, respectively,

$$\sqrt{\underline{\lambda}} = \begin{bmatrix} \sqrt{\lambda_1} & 0 & \cdots & 0 \\ 0 & \sqrt{\lambda_2} & \cdots & 0 \\ \vdots & \vdots & \ddots & \vdots \\ 0 & 0 & \cdots & \sqrt{\lambda_N} \end{bmatrix}$$

$$\sqrt{\frac{1}{\underline{\lambda}}} = \begin{bmatrix} \frac{1}{\sqrt{\lambda_1}} & 0 & \cdots & 0 \\ 0 & \frac{1}{\sqrt{\lambda_2}} & \cdots & 0 \\ \vdots & \vdots & \ddots & \vdots \\ 0 & 0 & \cdots & \frac{1}{\sqrt{\lambda_N}} \end{bmatrix}$$

Note that $\sqrt{\underline{\lambda}}\ \sqrt{\underline{\lambda}}' = \underline{\lambda}$ and $\sqrt{1/\underline{\lambda}}\ \sqrt{1/\underline{\lambda}}' = \underline{\lambda}^{-1}$. The eigenvalues relate to the diagonal elements of the correlation matrix in the following important way:

$$\sum_{m=1}^{N} \lambda_m = \sum_{n=1}^{N} r_{nn} \tag{5.34}$$

where the sum of the diagonal elements is referred to as the *trace* of the matrix. Since r_{nn} is just the power of the nth data waveform [see Eq. (5.31)], it can be seen that Eq. (5.34) is the total power of the set of data waves. Equation (5.33) can be rearranged by postmultiplying by $\underline{U}'$

$$\underline{R} = \underline{U}\ \underline{\lambda}\ \underline{U}' \tag{5.35}$$

and then factoring the matrix $\underline{\lambda}$,

$$\underline{R} = (\underline{U}\ \sqrt{\underline{\lambda}})\ (\sqrt{\underline{\lambda}}\ \underline{U}') \tag{5.36}$$

where $(\underline{U}\ \sqrt{\underline{\lambda}})' = \sqrt{\underline{\lambda}}\ \underline{U}'$. Thus, using the eigenmatrix $\underline{U}$ and eigenvalues of $\underline{R}$, $\underline{R}$ can be factored into the product of a matrix and its transpose.

We can now indicate, using Eq. (5.36), how the eigenvectors u_m and eigenvalues λ_m are related to the principal components expansion. Recall that in matrix terms, the data matrix S is made up of N signals of T dimensions each (corresponding to the T sampling times). Therefore S is an $N \times T$ matrix. It is equal to the product of the $N \times M$ coefficient matrix C and the $M \times T$ basic waveform matrix F as shown in Eq. (5.16) restated here

$$S = C F \tag{5.16}$$

Each row of F represents one vector of an orthonormal set of N basic waveforms which satisfy the relation

$$(1/T) \; F \; F' = I \tag{5.37}$$

The $N \times N$ matrix of data cross covariances can be written as

$$R = (1/T) S \; S' \tag{5.38}$$

If the data waveforms are normalized to unit power, then R is the $N \times N$ matrix of correlation coefficients. If we substitute the linear expansion (5.16) into (5.38) and take advantage of the orthonormality Eq. (5.37) of the basic functions, we obtain,

$$R = (1/T) C \; F \; F' \; C' = C \; C' \tag{5.39}$$

Hence, comparing Eqs. (5.36) and (5.39), it can be seen that the weighting coefficient matrix is given by

$$C = U \sqrt{\lambda} \tag{5.40}$$

with

$$c_{nm} = \sqrt{\lambda}_m \; u_{nm} \tag{5.41}$$

What this means is that the weighting coefficients c_{nm} which are used to reconstruct s_{nt} from the M optimal basic functions f_{mt} according to

$$s_{nt} = \sum_{m=1}^{M} c_{nm} f_{mt} \tag{5.12}$$

are determined from the eigenvalues λ_m and the components u_{nm} of the eigenvectors associated with the correlation matrix of the N data waveforms. The λ_m, u_{nm}, and the data waveforms also serve to determine the basic waveforms f_{mt}. We show this by using Eqs. (5.16) and (5.40). Premultiply Eq. (5.16) by $\underline{C}'$ and substitute for $\underline{C}'$ according to Eq. (5.40). This gives, after minor manipulations,

$$\underline{F} = \sqrt{1/\lambda} \ \underline{U}' \ \underline{S} \tag{5.42}$$

The mth basic waveform is

$$f_{mt} = \sqrt{1/\lambda}_m \sum_{n=1}^{N} u_{nm} s_{nt} \tag{5.43}$$

The value of the mth basic function at time t is a weighted sum of the n data waveforms, the weighting factors being the u_{nm}. When u_{nm} is large, the contribution of s_{nt} is accordingly large. Substitution of Eq. (5.41) into Eq. (5.29) and using the orthonormality property of the eigenvectors, $\sum_{n=1}^{N} u_{nm}^2 = 1$, indicates that the eigenvalue λ_m represents the contribution of the mth basic waveform to the total power in the set of data waveforms. It then becomes obvious that the most important basic waveforms to use in representing the experimental waveforms are those corresponding to the largest eigenvalues.

It is also true that the linear expansion of the data waveforms in terms of the basic waveforms with the k largest eigenvalues yields the least-mean-square approximation error for a set of any k orthonormal basic waves. In this sense it is the most efficient expansion; for a proof see Chapter 8 of Harmon (1967).

A further property of principal component expansions is that the column vector from the weighting coefficients matrix is orthogonal to all the other column vectors. In matrix terms, the product of $\underline{C}$ premultiplied by $\underline{C}'$ is a diagonal matrix. This can be demonstrated by substituting Eq. (5.40) for $\underline{C}$ in the matrix product and using the property that $\underline{U}$ is an orthogonal matrix.

$$\underline{C}' \; \underline{C} = \sqrt{\underline{\lambda}} \; \underline{U}' \; \underline{U} \; \sqrt{\underline{\lambda}} = \underline{\lambda} \qquad (5.44)$$

thus,

$$\sum_{n=1}^{N} c_{nm} c_{nk} = \begin{cases} 0 & \text{for} \quad m \neq k \\ \lambda_m & \text{for} \quad m = k \end{cases} \qquad (5.45)$$

Equations (5.44) and (5.45) indicate that the information each basic waveform contributes in terms of the values of its weighting coefficients is uncorrelated with the information contributed by all other basic waveforms. This is a direct consequence of the requirement that each basic wave be a least-mean-square error fit to the residuum from the least-mean-square error fit of the other basic waves. Thus only a principal components expansion has both properties that (a) the basic waveforms are orthogonal, and (b) the vectors of their weighting coefficients are mutually uncorrelated. Indeed, an alternative approach to the principal components formulation of Eqs. (5.40)-(5.43) can be based upon the absence of correlation among the weighting coefficient vectors of the basic waveforms.

5.16. COVARIANCES AND CORRELATION COEFFICIENTS

The principal components expansion is implemented by factoring the correlation matrix and so will depend upon the particular correlation measure used. Either the covariance on the correlation coefficient can be useful. In the latter case, all data waveforms are effectively normalized to unit power. This in effect makes all data waves of equal importance in determining the basic waveform set since the basic waveforms will tend to provide similar mean square approximation errors for each data waveform. If the covariances are used, then the larger amplitude waveforms will predominate in determining the principal components because the

basic waveforms will tend to give a better mean square approximation to the high power waveforms. In signal space terms, the normalization effect of correlation coefficients sets all signal
vectors to unit length, and so the orientation (shapes) of the
basic wave vectors will depend only upon the orientations of the
data vectors. When using covariances, the basic wave vectors will
depend more upon (i.e., they are biased by) the orientations of the
longer (higher power) data vectors.

When waveshape alone is of importance, normalized data are
desirable, but when the analysis is designed to reflect differences
in signal intensity, nonnormalized data are more appropriate to
use. A procedure for circumventing the bias of covariance matrix
based representation towards the large amplitude data waves is to
first normalize the data and obtain basic waveforms which fit the
normalized data waves equally well. Then scale each weighting coefficient c_{nm} by $[(1/T) \sum_{t=1}^{T} s_{nt}^{2}]^{1/2}$, the rms strength of the
data waveform which it represents. Thus the basic waveform shapes
will depend only upon the shapes of the data waveforms, but the
scaled weighting coefficients will also depend upon the data waveform amplitudes.

5.17. DIMENSIONALITY AND EIGENVALUES

In Eq. (5.28b) it was pointed out that the contribution of
the mth basic waveform to the power of the nth waveform was c_{nm}^{2}
and that $\sum_{n=1}^{N} c_{nm}^{2}$ was the contribution of the mth basic waveform
to the total power of the entire data set. Using Eq. (5.41), the
contribution of a principal components basic factor to the power
of the set of data waveforms is $\lambda_m (\sum_{n=1}^{N} u_{nm}^{2})$. Since each vector
$\underline{u}_m$ is of unit length, due to the orthonormality property,
$\sum_{n=1}^{N} u_{nm}^{2} = 1$ and the eigenvalue λ_m corresponds to P_m, the power
contribution of the mth basic waveform to the data set. Thus the
eigenvalues can be used to infer the dimensionality of the signal
space. If the sum of the K largest eigenvalues approximately
equals the total signal power, the remaining $N - K$ eigenvalues

being relatively small, then K is a reasonable estimate of the dimensionality of the signal space. Needless to say, the value of K will depend upon the criterion level the data analyst sets for the goodness of an approximation, e.g., 90%, 95%, 98%.

5.18. VARIMAX ROTATION OF THE WEIGHTING COEFFICIENTS

The conciseness of a principal components representation can be an obstacle to making a meaningful, physiological interpretation of the basic waveforms and weighting coefficients. The difficulty lies paradoxically in the fact that the basic waveform set is a best-mean-square fit to the data. The consequences of this property are illustrated in Fig. (5.4a) for a simple example of four data waveforms.

The data waveforms are normalized an represented by vectors $\underline{S}_1$, $\underline{S}_2$, $\underline{S}_3$, and $\underline{S}_4$ in a two-dimensional signal space. The vector corresponding to the first basic wave of the principal components representation $\underline{f}_{p1}$ is oriented midway among the four signal vectors, thereby maximizing the total signal power represented by $\underline{f}_{p1}$. The $\underline{f}_{p2}$ vector is perpendicular to $\underline{f}_{p1}$. Both basic waveforms are composites of the original data waveforms, and consequently, the weighting coefficients for each data signal will indicate substantial contributions from both basic waveforms. This undesirable result occurs despite some marked differences in orientation among the data vectors. The principal components analysis fails to express such orientation differences clearly. It is desirable when dealing with multidimensional signal vectors to have an expansion which provides the minimum number of orthonormal basic waveforms necessary for a preselected approximation accuracy but which is so oriented in signal space that differences between waveforms are not obscured. A technique called the "varimax" method can meet these requirements (Harmon, 1967, Chapter 14).

The varimax method is applied to the weighting coefficients associated with an orthonormal basic waveform set already obtained from the data. It need not be a principal compnents expansion but

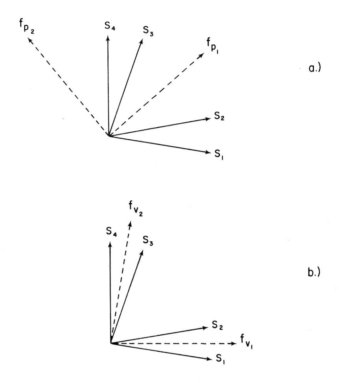

Fig. (5.4)   (a) Four data signal vectors, contained within a two-dimensional signal space, and their associated principal components axes $\underline{f}_{p1}$ and $\underline{f}_{p2}$.   (b)   The same four signal vectors and their reference axes $\underline{f}_{v1}$ and $\underline{f}_{v2}$ obtained after a varimax rotation.

usually is in practice and this is what we deal with here. One first obtains a principal components expansion and then operates upon the weighting coefficients of the M basic waveforms contributing most to the desired level of approximation accuracy. In the varimax rotation, these coefficients are adjusted to yield a new set of weighting coefficients with a simpler structure. The simplicity is in the sense that the weighting coefficients are as close to unity or zero as possible. This all or none expansion assumes that the data are normalized to unit strength. For such an expansion, the basic waveforms can be interpreted as primarily characterizing clusters of signal waveforms in the data. The data waves also become easier to interpret in that there will be a tendency for each data wave to be represented primarily by one basic waveform. As an example, see Fig. (5.4b). The purpose of a varimax rotation is to obtain a set of basic waveforms whereby each signal is represented by primarily one basic waveform and each basic waveform can be interpreted as corresponding closely to a particular signal process. However, while the orthonormality property of the basic waveforms is preserved, the properties of least-mean-square error fit and orthogonality of the weighting coefficients are lost when a varimax rotation is applied to a principal components representation. The advantages of the varimax rotation usually outweigh these losses.

The "simplicity" SI_m associated with basic wave $f_m(t)$ is defined as the variance of its squared weighting coefficients, c_{nm}^2 being the power contributed to the nth waveform by $f_m(t)$.

$$SI_m = \frac{1}{N} \sum_{n=1}^{N} c_{nm}^4 - \frac{1}{N^2} \left[\sum_{n=1}^{N} c_{nm}^2 \right]^2 \tag{5.46}$$

The "total simplicity" of the set of weighting coefficients is

$$S_{total} = \frac{1}{M} \sum_{m=1}^{M} SI_m \tag{5.47}$$

The varimax way of providing the form of signal representation we desire is to maximize Eq. (5.47) by rotating the vectors defined by the columns of weighting coefficients iteratively until S_{total} no longer increases significantly. This procedure tends to drive the magnitude of the weighting coefficients c_{nm} to either zero or one, thereby simplifying interpretation of the weighting coefficient matrix and the basic waveforms. The more closely the coefficients equal either zero or one, the larger will be the variance and average variance given by Eqs. (5.46) and (5.47) and hence, the "simpler" the matrix of weighting coefficients. The data waves are assumed to be individually normalized to unit rms amplitude. If the data are not normalized, then each c_{nm} term in Eq. (5.46) should initially be scaled by dividing it by the rms amplitude of the corresponding nth data wave.

5.19. VARIMAX ROTATION OF THE BASIC WAVEFORMS

There is an alternative varimax procedure for a principal component analysis that can be applied to the basic waveforms instead of the weighting coefficients. The basic waveforms are simplified in the sense that their magnitudes tend to be either zero or one. The varimax rotation preserves the orthonormal property of the basic waveforms while the orthogonal property of the weighting coefficient columns is lost. It may be advantageous to use this approach when it is expected that each underlying basic waveform is restricted to a specific time region with minimal overlap into other regions.

5.20. PRINCIPAL COMPONENT ANALYSIS AND THE KARHUNEN-LOEVE EXPANSION

In the preceding sections we have presented the method for obtaining a principal components expansion from the eigenvalues and eigenvectors of an $N \times N$ matrix of correlation coefficients or covariances between N data waveforms, Eq. (5.31). There is an alternative approach whereby the $T \times T$ matrix of cross correlations between the T time points of the data, as defined by Eq. (5.48), is used.

$$z_{t_1 t_2} = \frac{1}{N} \sum_{n=1}^{N} s_{nt_1} s_{nt_2} \tag{5.48}$$

In matrix notation, the equivalent of Eq. (5.48) is

$$\underline{Z} = (1/N) \, \underline{S}'\underline{S} \tag{5.49}$$

The mean value over the time epoch $t = 1, T$ of each $s_n(t)$ is assumed to be zero. Note that the covariance matrix $\underline{R}$ of Eq. (5.38) and the Z matrix are based upon the same data. The covariance matrix R of Eq. (5.38) is $N \times N$ and arises from covariances obtained by first summing over the T time points according to Eq. (5.19). The Z matrix here is a $T \times T$ covariance matrix obtained by first summing over the N waveforms at time points t_1 and t_2 according to Eq. (5.48). We now show how the principal components basic waveforms and weighting coefficients may be obtained from the Z matrix. We substitute the product C F for S in Eq. (5.49) to obtain Eq. (5.50) and utilize the fact that the basic waveforms are orthogonal and that their weighting coefficients are uncorrelated. Thus,

$$Z = (1/N) \; F'C'C \; F \tag{5.50}$$

For a principal components expansion, $C'C = \lambda$. Thus Eq. (5.50) reduces to

$$Z = (1/N) \; F' \; \lambda \; F \tag{5.51}$$

Now compare Eq. (5.51) with Eq. (5.35), restated below, in which the matrix R is expressed in terms of its matrices of eigenvectors and eigenvalues

$$R = U \; \lambda \; U' \tag{5.35}$$

Recall that λ is the diagonal matrix of eigenvalues and that the matrix of eigenvectors U has the property $U'U = I$. Now then, Eq. (5.51) is of the same format, since $(1/T)F \; F' = I$. Thus we can identify the eigenvalues and eigenvectors of Z from Eq. (5.51) by suitably scaling the F and λ matrices, as indicated in Eq. (5.52).

$$Z = (F'/\sqrt{T}) \, (T/N)\lambda \; (F/\sqrt{T}) \tag{5.52}$$

Since the matrix $(T/N)\lambda$ is diagonal and the matrix product $(F/\sqrt{T}) \, (F'/\sqrt{T})$ is an identity matrix, $F'/\sqrt{T}$ is the eigenvector matrix and $(T/N)\lambda$ is the eigenvalue matrix of Z. Thus F can be obtained by multiplying each element of the transpose of the eigenvector matrix of Z by $\sqrt{T}$. Using Eq. (5.16), restated here, the weighting coefficients can be computed by postmultiplying $\underline{S}$ by $\underline{F}'$ and scaling by $1/T$

$$\underline{S} = \underline{C}\ \underline{F} \tag{5.16}$$

$$(1/T)\underline{S}\ \underline{F}' = \underline{C}\ \underline{F}\ \underline{F}'/T = \underline{C} \tag{5.53}$$

Thus the mth coefficient of the nth data wave is

$$c_{nm} = 1/T \sum_{t=1}^{T} s_{nt} f_{mt} \tag{5.54}$$

This alternative approach to collections of signal waveforms is known as the Karhunen-Loeve (K-L) expansion, a technique used widely in the field of communication signal analysis (Davenport and Root, 1958).

While the K-L and principal components methods are equivalent, there are practical advantages of numerical computation in using one instead of the other, depending upon the situation. If the number of data waves N is less than the number of time points T, then less computation time will be required to obtain the eigenvectors and eigenvalues from the $N \times N$ data wave cross correlation matrix than from the $T \times T$ time correlation matrix. Conversely, if T is less than N, then the computations will be more rapid when the time correlation matrix is used. Recall that when the $N \times N$ data wave correlation coefficient matrix is used, all data waveforms are effectively normalized to unit power and thus all data waves are of equal importance in determining the basic waveform set. If such normalization is desired when using the $T \times T$ time correlation matrix, then the data waves must be explicitly scaled to unit power prior to computing the cross time covariances.

5.21. PRINCIPAL COMPONENTS-VARIMAX ANALYSIS OF DEVIATION WAVEFORMS

Thus far we have described factor analysis procedures based upon the original data waves. Since factor analysis and principal components analysis are concerned with determining differences among waveforms, they can be applied equally well to the set of deviation waveforms, the waveforms obtained by subtracting the average data waveform from each of the original data waves (Donchin, 1966; Suter, 1970). Though the average waveform is of no use for discrimination purposes, it can be reinserted to produce the original data waveforms after the analysis is complete. The average waveform a_t is computed across all data waves in the set as follows:

$$a_t = \frac{1}{N} \sum_{n=1}^{N} s_{nt} \qquad (5.55)$$

The deviation waveforms d_{nt} are then obtained as follows:

$$d_{nt} = s_{nt} - a_t \qquad (5.56)$$

The matrix of deviation waveforms, consisting of N rows of waveforms and T columns of time points, is denoted by $\underline{D}$.

$$\underline{D} = \begin{bmatrix} d_{11} & d_{12} & \cdots & d_{1T} \\ \vdots & \vdots & \cdots & \vdots \\ d_{N1} & d_{N2} & \cdots & d_{NT} \end{bmatrix}$$

The deviation waveforms serve to emphasize activity in those time epochs where relatively pronounced variations in waveforms are to be found. Consequently, a principal component and its subsequent varimax analysis of the deviation waveforms will tend to yield basic waveforms which particularly fit activity in the time epochs of pronounced change.

The computational procedures are similar to those previously described for analysis of the original data waveforms. A matrix of either covariances or cross correlations [see Eq. (5.17)] is computed. Correlation coefficients are not used, since their use would implicitly scale all deviation waveforms to unit rms level, thereby tending to minimize differences between waveforms. Either an $N \times N$ matrix of cross correlations or covariances between wave-forms or a $T \times T$ matrix of covariances between time points can be used. In practice a $T \times T$ matrix of covariances between time points has been used (Donchin, 1966; Suter, 1970). The covariances between time points of the deviation waveforms $z_{t_1 t_2}$ may be computed directly from the original data waves as follows:

$$
\begin{aligned}
z_{t_1 t_2} &= \frac{1}{N} \sum_{n=1}^{N} (s_{nt_1} - a_{t_1})(s_{nt_2} - a_{t_2}) \\
&= \frac{1}{N} \sum_{n=1}^{N} s_{nt_1} s_{nt_2} - a_{t_1} a_{t_2}
\end{aligned}
\tag{5.57}
$$

Note that Eq. (5.57) makes no adjustment for the baseline (dc value) of the deviation waveforms. If it is desired to center each waveform about its average over time, then the time average must be computed for each wave and be explicitly subtracted from the wave prior to using Eq. (5.57). It is not mandatory to use the time averages as baselines, and it may not even be desirable. For example, Suter (1970) used the average of the initial three time points for each individual wave to define the baseline for that wave. He reasoned that the initial activity level was more likely to reflect a real physiological baseline.

If an $N \times N$ matrix of cross correlation or covariances between waveforms is used, the average wave must first be explicitly subtracted from each data wave to obtain the deviation waves. Then, cross correlations between the deviation waves are computed as specified by Eq. (5.58). Principal components factorization of the resulting correlation matrix will yield basic waveforms and weighting coefficients that are identical to those obtained from the $T \times T$ matrix whose elements are defined by Eq. (5.57).

$$
r_{ik} = \frac{1}{T} \sum_{t=1}^{T} (s_{it} - a_t)(s_{kt} - a_t)
\tag{5.58}
$$

If it is desired to center each deviation waveform about its time average, then the covariances between the deviation waveforms rather than the cross correlation defined in Eq. (5.58) should be utilized. If some other perhaps more physiological baselines are desired, they must be explicitly computed and subtracted from the deviation waves prior to computation of the cross correlation.

A set of principal component basic waveforms and weighting coefficients can be obtained using the procedures described in Sections 5.15 or 5.20. A varimax rotation can be applied to either the matrix of basic waves or the matrix of weighting coefficients; in practice it has been applied to the basic waves (Donchin, 1966; Suter, 1970).

The weighting coefficients and basic waveforms apply only to the deviation waveforms and not to the original data waves. Under some circumstances it may be possible to "perfectly" represent the average waveform a_t with a linear expansion based upon the basic waveforms obtained for the deviation waves. If so, it is equally valid to apply the same set of basic waveforms to the original data waves and compute the weighting coefficients through the use of Eq. (5.54). Suter (1970) found that this was possible for his data.

5.22. COVARIANCES, CORRELATION COEFFICIENTS,
      AND IMPLIED BASELINES

When a principal components-varimax analysis is performed using an $N \times N$ data wave covariance (or correlation coefficient) matrix as formulated in Section 5.15, the average over time (dc value) of each waveform implicitly becomes the baseline (zero ordinate) of the waveform. Consequently, the weighting coefficients which are obtained from the eigenvalues and eigenvectors of the covariance (or correlation coefficient) matrix apply only to the waveform obtained by subtracting the dc value from the original data wave. Thus, when Eqs. (5.42) and (5.43) are used to compute the basic waveforms, the s_{nt} should consist of the original data wave minus its dc value.

If some other more physiological baseline is desired (such

273

as the prestimulus level), then it must be explicitly subtracted from the data wave. The matrix of cross correlations [Eq. (5.17)] is then used, instead of a covariance matrix, so that we do not reset the data waveforms to their dc-free levels.

When a principal components-varimax analysis is performed using the $T \times T$ time covariance matrix formulated in Section 5.20, the analysis is implicitly applied to the deviation waveform. If it is desired to analyze the original data waves (or the original data waves minus some specified baselines), then a matrix of cross correlations [Eq. (5.17)] instead of covariances should be used.

5.23. PRINCIPAL COMPONENT-VARIMAX ANALYSIS BASED UPON ORTHONORMAL WEIGHTING COEFFICIENTS

Thus far we have considered linear representations of sets of waveforms based upon orthonormal basic waveforms. This orthonormality property is expressed by Eq. (5.37), restated here.

$$(1/T) \ \underline{F} \ \underline{F}' = \underline{I}$$

$$\frac{1}{T} \sum_{t=1}^{T} f_{mt} f_{kt} = \begin{cases} 1, & m = k \\ 0, & m \neq k \end{cases} \tag{5.59}$$

The general properties of weighting coefficients associated with a set of orthornormal basic waveforms were described in Section 5.13. Then in Section 5.15, Eqs. (5.44) and (5.45), we demonstrated that for the special case of a principal components representation, each column vector of weighting coefficients associated with each basic waveform is orthogonal to (i.e., uncorrelated with) all other columns of weighting coefficients. We further pointed out that after a varimax rotation the orthonormality property of the basic waveforms was retained but the orthogonality property of the weighting coefficients was lost. While in some cases it may be advantageous for the set of basic waveforms to be orthonormal, in other cases it may be more useful for the columns of weighting coefficients to be orthogonal. The latter property may be particularly advantageous if there is reason to expect that variations in the weighting coefficients associated with each basic waveform are essentially independent of one another. It is possible to formulate a principal components representation in such a manner that the columns of weighting coefficients remain orthogonal after a varimax rotation. However, for such a representation the rotated versions of the basic waveforms will not be orthogonal.

In order for the weighting coefficient columns to remain orthogonal, it is necessary for them to constitute an orthonormal set. This constraint is expressed by Eq. (5.60), in which the notation b_{nm} and $\underline{B}$ are used to denote the weighting coefficients and their matrix. We use this notation to distinguish sets of orthonormal weighting coefficients from the previously defined coefficients, c_{nm}, which are not orthonormal.

$$\frac{1}{N} \sum_{n=1}^{N} b_{nm} b_{nk} = \begin{cases} 1, & m = k \\ 0, & m \neq k \end{cases}$$

$$(1/N)\ \underline{B}'\ \underline{B} = \underline{I} \tag{5.60}$$

It is possible to obtain the b_{nm} coefficients by scaling the c_{nm} coefficients as follows:

$$b_{nm} = \sqrt{N/\lambda_m}\, c_{nm}$$

$$\underline{B} = \sqrt{N}\ \underline{C}\ \sqrt{1/\lambda} \tag{5.61}$$

We can readily demonstrate that the columns of b_{nm} terms are orthonormal by substituting Eq. (5.61) for $\underline{B}$ in Eq. (5.60) and using Eq. (5.44), $\underline{C}'\ \underline{C} = \underline{\lambda}$.

$$(1/N)N\sqrt{1/\lambda}\ \underline{C}'\ \underline{C}\ \sqrt{1/\lambda} = \sqrt{1/\lambda}\ \underline{C}'\ \underline{C}\ \sqrt{1/\lambda} = \underline{I} \tag{5.62}$$

The basic waveforms that correspond to the b_{nm} coefficients can be obtained directly by scaling the f_{mt} terms of the previously developed principal components representation. We denote these scaled basic waveforms by h_{mt} and their matrix by $\underline{H}$ in order to distinguish them from the orthonormal basic waveforms, f_{mt}.

$$h_{mt} = \sqrt{\lambda_m/N} \ f_{mt}$$

$$\underline{H} = (1/\sqrt{N}) \ \sqrt{\underline{\lambda}} \ \underline{F} \tag{5.62}$$

That $\underline{H}$ is orthogonal but not orthonormal can be shown as follows:

$$\underline{H} \ \underline{H}' = (1/N) \ \sqrt{\underline{\lambda}} \ \underline{F} \ \underline{F}' \ \sqrt{\underline{\lambda}} \tag{5.63}$$

From Eq. (5.59) $\underline{F} \ \underline{F}'/T = \underline{I}$, hence

$$\underline{H} \ \underline{H}' = (T/N) \ \underline{\lambda} \tag{5.64}$$

Thus, we can represent the data waveforms in either of two expansions based upon principal components:

$$\underline{S} = \underline{C} \ \underline{F} = \underline{B} \ \underline{H} \tag{5.65}$$

It should be noted that the shapes of the basic time waveforms, f_{mt} and h_{mt}, are the same in both representations. The shapes of the weighting coefficients, c_{nm} and b_{nm}, as functions of n, are also the same in both representations. However, since the h_{mt} waveforms are not orthonormal, the properties described in Section 5.13 for the c_{nm} coefficients do not apply to the b_{nm} coefficients.

A further, major difference between the two expansions arises when a varimax rotation is utilized. In one case the basic waveforms f_{mt} remain orthonormal, but the associated columns of weighting coefficients c_{nm} are not orthogonal. In the other case, the columns of weighting coefficients b_{nm} remain orthonormal, but the associated basic waveforms h_{mt} are not orthogonal. These results occur whether the varimax rotation is applied to either the weighting coefficients or the basic waveforms.

Using Eqs. (5.35) and (5.40), it can be seen that the principal components c_{nm} coefficients can be obtained directly from the eigenvectors $\underline{U}_R$ and eigenvalues $\underline{\lambda}_R$ of the $\underline{R}$ matrix as follows:

$$\underline{C} = \underline{U}_R \sqrt{\underline{\lambda}}_R \qquad (5.66)$$

An analogous relationship holds for the principal components basic waveforms h_{mt} and the eigenvectors $\underline{U}_Z$ and eigenvalues λ_Z of the $\underline{Z}$ matrix.

$$\underline{H}' = \underline{U}_Z \sqrt{\underline{\lambda}}_Z \qquad (5.67)$$

Utilization of a principal components expansion based upon orthonormal weighting coefficients b_{nm} is particularly useful when it is intended to apply statistical tests, such as analysis of variance, to the variations of the weighting coefficients associated with each basic waveform. Since the columns of weighting coefficients are orthogonal to each other, each may be subjected to a separate analysis of variance.

5.24. EXAMPLES

Principal components have been used for the analysis of evoked potential data in a number of studies (John *et al.*, 1964, 1972; Donchin, 1966; Suter, 1970; Bennett *et al.*, 1971; Donchin *et al.*, 1975). In most instances a varimax rotation was employed. Three examples which illustrate the data reduction and quantification properties of principal components analyses are presented below.

A. *AUDITORY EVOKED RESPONSES AND MASKING EFFECTS*

Suter (1970) studied the variation in evoked potentials produced by tone bursts masked by variable frequency bands of noise. The data were obtained from the auditory cortex of awake cats. The stimuli consisted of either unmasked or masked tone bursts. How the evoked response waveform varied with the noise band center frequency was of primary interest. Variations produced by tone intensity and tone-to-noise intensity ratio were also studied. Average evoked potentials for each stimulus condition were obtained and represented by 64 time points 2 msec apart starting from the

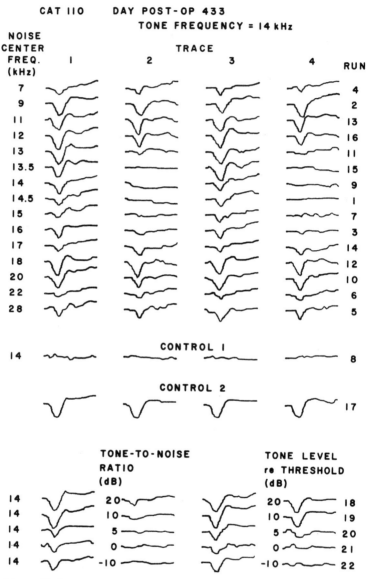

Fig. (5.5) Average evoked responses to tone bursts from a typical experimental session (cat 110). During the first 16 runs the responses in columns 2 and 4 were to tone burst marked by acoustic noise. No tone was present during control 1 run and no noise was present during control 2 run. FM masking noise was present in the second column of rows 18-22. No noise was present in the 4th column of these runs. The time base for each evoked response is 128 msec. (From Suter, 1970).

onset of the tone burst. There were 88 average evoked potentials from each experimental session. A typical example of such a set is shown in Fig. (5.5). Typically, data from 12 experimental sessions were pooled to yield a total of 1056 average evoked potentials. In signal space terms, the data consisted of 1056 vectors lying within a space of no more than 64 dimensions.

Manual measurement of the data would have been enormously time-consuming and would have introduced subjective factors in the characterization of the waveshapes. To circumvent these difficulties and to provide a suitable means of defining the evoked potential components, a principal components-varimax analysis of deviation waveforms was employed. It was hoped that these basic waveforms would also correspond sufficiently to physiological response components so as to make meaningful a study of the variation of the concomitant weighting coefficients with the stimulus parameters.

Suter performed the principal components analysis of deviation waveforms on unnormalized data waveforms, using a 64 × 64 time correlation matrix ($\underline{Z}$ matrix). He utilized a varimax rotation of orthonormal basic waveforms. He found that each set of 1056 data waveforms could be effectively represented by four basic waves. The basic waves for the data set partially shown in Fig. (5.5) are illustrated in Fig. (5.6). These four basic waveforms accounted for 88% of the total power of the data set. They also tend to be in correspondence, in terms of latency and polarity, with the physiological components recorded from this area of the brain. The variation of the weighting coefficients (for the original data waveforms) corresponding to the second basic waveform with the noise band center frequency is illustrated in Fig. (5.7). A tuning effect is clearly visible, with the minimum magnitude occurring when the noise band center frequency coincides with the frequency of the tone burst. Suter's results demonstrate that an orthogonal set of basic waveforms in some circumstances can correspond markedly to physiological defined components.

279

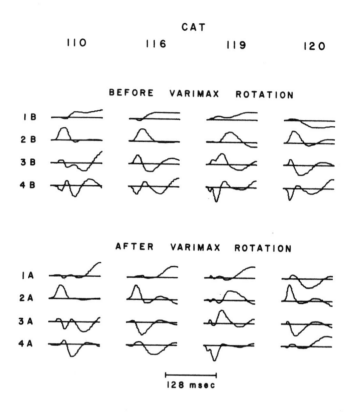

Fig. (5.6)   The four basic waveforms before B, and after A,
varimax rotation for each of four cats.   The time base is 128 msec.
(From Suter, 1970).

B.   EFFECTS OF DRUGS UPON EVOKED RESPONSES

John et al. (1972) investigated the effect of certain drugs
upon the behavior of unrestrained cats and upon concurrently recorded evoked potentials.   Principal components-varimax analysis
procedures were employed for purposes of data reduction and to delineate the relationships between the evoked potential waveshapes
recorded during different brain states induced by the drug actions.
In this study the character of the basic waveform shapes was not
of main interest; of primary interest was the array of weighting
coefficients itself.   This provided a quantitative statement of

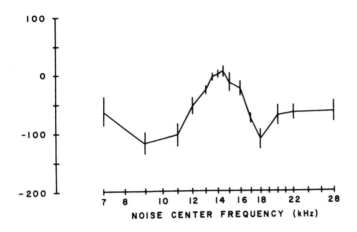

Fig. (5.7) *The mean and standard error of the weighting co-efficients of the second basic waveform after varimax rotation [Fig. (5.6), row 2A, cat 110]. These are plotted as a function of noise center frequency. The results were obtained by averaging across four sessions the coefficients obtained from each of the sessions. The average potentials from one such session are illus-trated in the first 15 rows of column 4 of Fig. (5.5). (From Suter, 1970).*

similarities and dissimilarities among the set of data waves. A varimax rotation of the weighting coefficients and orthonormal basic waveforms were utilized.

The results were expressed in terms of the matrix of squared weighting coefficients. Recall that for orthonormal basic wave-forms c_{nm}^2 is the power contribution of the mth basic wave to the nth data wave. Squaring the weighting coefficients emphasizes the differences between large and small coefficients. It was felt that polarity information was not of primary importance while the magnitude of the contribution from each basic wave to each data wave was.

Well-trained cats performed differential conditioned approach and avoidance responses. The stimuli were repetitive flashes of light at rates of two or five flashes per second. After training, the cats were injected with one of four drugs and then tested for conditioned responses. The drugs were chlorpromazine, sodium pentabarbital, methamphetamine, and an experimental tranquilizer. A representative set of 24 average evoked potentials recorded in predrug controls, after drug injection (when there was maximal interference with behavior) and saline control injections, is illustrated in Fig. (5.8) for data recorded from the visual cortex.

A principal components-varimax expansion, using a 24 × 24 correlation coefficient data wave matrix was computed. Normalization was used so that data waveshape alone determined the basic waveforms. It was found that five basic waveforms accounted for 97% of the total energy in the data set. The matrix of squared weighting coefficients is presented in Table 5.1. The matrix indicates that the predrug and saline controls tend to form a distinct cluster in the signal space and the drug actions introduce departures from the control state, each drug tending to have its own characteristic pattern. Thus it can be seen that a principal components-varimax analysis can delineate and quantify differences and similarities among waveforms recorded for different experimental conditions.

C. INDEPENDENCE OF COMPONENTS RECORDED FROM SCALP OF HUMANS

Donchin et al. (1975) investigated interactions between evoked potential components preceding and following a brief tone pip stimulus that was usually preceded by a warning flash one second earlier. A principal components-varimax analysis with orthonormal weighting coefficients was utilized. The varimax rotation was applied to the basic waveforms. The analysis was based upon a 50 × 50 time correlation matrix of deviation waveforms.

The pre- and posttone pip activity were found to be represented by different basic waveforms. The basic waveforms and the average of all the data waveforms are illustrated in Fig. (5.9). Component 1 reflects the pretone state of the subject but overlaps into the posttone epoch. There are two clearly defined post-

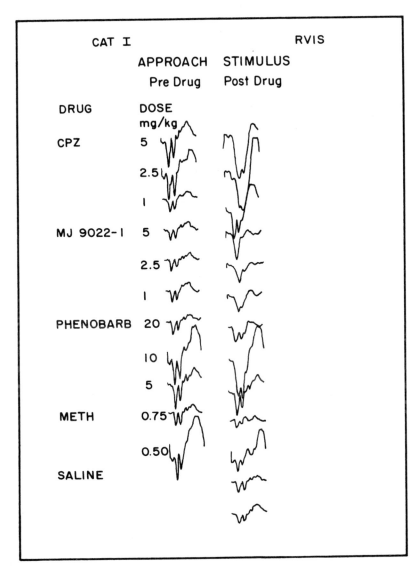

Fig. (5.8) A representative set of average evoked potentials obtained from monopolar recordings from visual cortex of a cat in response to the approach stimulus. (From John et al., 1972.)

tone components, 2 and 5 especially, which are small in the pre-tone epoch. Figure (5.9) suggests that a principal components analysis with a varimax rotation applied to the basic waveforms yields a temporally well separated set of components. Since the

TABLE 5.1

Weighting Coefficients After Varimax Rotation for the Set of
Average Evoked Potentials Illustrated in Fig. 5.8[a]

Conditions		Basic Wave	1	2	3	4	5
DRUGS	(mg/kg)						
CPZ	5		0.1	0.93	0.03	0.01	0.00
	2.5		0.01	0.77	0.01	0.19	0.00
	1		0.40	0.10	0.17	0.31	0.00
MJ	5		0.09	0.00	0.83	0.06	0.00
	2.5		0.10	0.30	0.58	0.00	0.00
	1		0.14	0.06	0.77	0.00	0.00
PHENO	20		0.52	0.02	0.37	0.07	0.00
	10		0.16	0.17	0.30	0.35	0.00
	5		0.52	0.05	0.07	0.33	0.00
METH	0.75		0.02	0.00	0.00	0.00	0.96
	0.5		0.15	0.08	0.00	0.75	0.00
SALINE	#1		0.82	0.00	0.06	0.10	0.00
	#2		0.76	0.00	0.10	0.13	0.00
CONTROLS							
Pre-CPZ	5		0.70	0.00	0.04	0.24	0.00
Pre-CPZ	2.5		0.42	0.03	0.06	0.47	0.00
Pre-CPZ	1		0.78	0.00	0.08	0.12	0.00
Pre-MJ	5		0.88	0.00	0.05	0.04	0.00
Pre-MJ	2.5		0.90	0.00	0.01	0.06	0.00
Pre-MJ	1		0.80	0.07	0.11	0.00	0.00
Pre-PHENO	20		0.85	0.00	0.06	0.06	0.00
Pre-PHENO	10		0.42	0.06	0.03	0.46	0.00
Pre-PHENO	5		0.63	0.03	0.04	0.28	0.00
Pre-METH	0.75		0.89	0.00	0.08	0.01	0.00
Pre-METH	0.5		0.50	0.01	0.04	0.43	0.00

[a]From John *et al.* (1972)

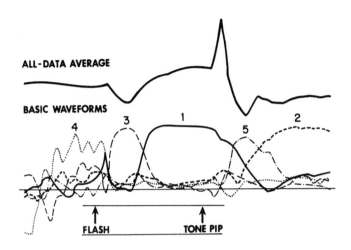

Fig. (5.9) The average of all the data waveforms (upper curve) and the five basic waveforms (lower curve). Note that basic wave 1 is associated primarily with pretone activity and basic waves 2 and 5 with post-tone activity. (From Donchin et al., 1975.)

overlap is small, only a few components contribute to the response waveform at any particular time.

Donchin *et al.* then subjected the weighting coefficients associated with basic waveforms 1 (pretone) and 5 (posttone) to separate analyses of variance. The results indicated that these two components were affected by different experimental variables, thus providing further evidence that posttone activity is, at least to some extent, independent of pretone activity.

5.25. SOME GENERAL REMARKS ON LINEAR EXPANSIONS

Linear expansion procedures such as principal components-varimax are used to best advantage when the structure of the data is to some extent known in advance. The expansion renders precise such loosely defined concepts as "similarity" and "change", quantifying them in terms of basic waveforms and their associated coef-

cients. The evaluation of the meaningfulness of an expansion depends upon the prior knowledge of the data and must make sense in
terms of what is already known. The effects of changes in experimental parameters should be isolated with each effect upon a response accounted for by a few (hopefully only one) factors. The
results should be replicated by expansions of independent sets of
data recorded under the same conditions. Suter's ability to deal
with the tuning effect present in some of his data exemplify these
points. The problem was to express in a quantitative manner an
effect that was not present in the entire waveshape. The use of
an arbitrary selection of a single or few time points for analysis
would raise the possibility of neglect of relevant information.
The principal components-varimax analysis resolved the problem in
that the analysis conformed to the approximately known behavior,
with the basic waveforms tending to correspond to previously
physiologically identified components. The point here, and in
general, is that such analyses are not expected to lead to totally
new discoveries but rather, to quantify and render precise an objective description of previously partially understood phenomena.

When one wishes to represent a set of data waveforms by a
linear expansion of basic waveforms, it is necessary to know in
advance the general properties of the data set. The aptness of
the expansion in revealing the structure of the waveforms depends
upon the set of basic waveforms. Selecting basic waveforms arbitrarily is largely an intuitive matter subject to all the weaknesses and strengths of intuition. A judicious choice of basic
waves can perhaps result in a meaningful expansion whose components
may be readily interpreted and related to the physiological phenomena. A poor choice of basic waves can result in an expansion
which is nothing more than another array of numbers, providing
little, if any, insight into the data.

An advantage of the principal components-varimax expansion
is that it removes intuition by having the basic waveforms algo-
rithmically determined by the data. This procedure meets an ex-

plicit criterion of concision and therefore is likely to provide a meaningful expansion. The feature of complete dependence upon the data at hand can also be a shortcoming, however, when expansions of separate sets of data are to be compared. The basic waveforms may well be different for each set, so that a direct comparison of weighting coefficients would be meaningless. In some instances it may be feasible to combine data sets to be compared into a single set, and a principal factors-varimax expansion can be computed for the pooled data, thereby allowing meaninful comparisons of weighting coefficients.

The development of a principal components expansion usually utilizes either the correlation coefficient or the cross covariance as the similarity measure. A drawback to them as such is that any strong components within the waveforms will have more effect upon the value of the correlation than weak components which may, in fact, be of greater interest. This can be undesirable when comparing a pair of waveforms which exhibit a clear cut, significant difference in a weak component. For example, consider Fig. (5.10). There is a distinct difference for component III of the waveform pair. However, due to the strength of components I, II and IV, which are invariant, the correlation coefficient will give little indication of the distinct difference between the two waveforms at component III. This shortcoming is passed on to principal component analyses. The basic waveforms and weighting coefficients emphasize the strong components of the data, and thus there is a danger that important but low magnitude details may be obscured or disregarded by a principal component analysis.

From what has been said above, it is clear that although methods such as principal components-varimax expansions are quantitative and objective, they cannot be applied in a stereotyped manner. One should have a concept of what one is looking for and should be prepared to exercise judgement and imagination in applying such methods.

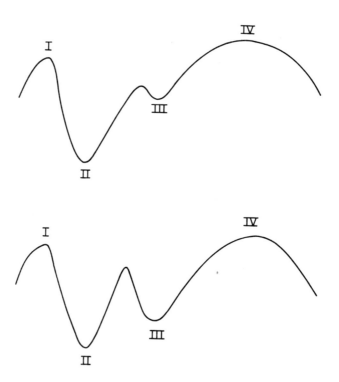

Fig. (5.10) *Hypothetical example of two waveforms with a relatively small but distinct difference.*

It was mentioned in Section 5.1 that linear expansions are not suitable for modelling processes whose data interact in a non-linear manner, but they can still be of utility as a method for data reduction and quantification. As an example, consider how variable latency data may be treated by a linear expansion. Suppose that each data wave has similar shape but different latency and amplitude as defined:

$$s_i(t) = c_i f(t - \tau_i), \qquad i = 1, N$$

The c_i expresses the variable amplitudes and the τ_i denotes the variable latencies. If the shape $f(t)$ and the distribution of latencies are such that the waveforms $s_i(t)$ occur over different time intervals, then a principal component-varimax analysis will result in several basic waveforms, spanning the time intervals over which the data waveforms occur. It would be misleading to give functional significance to such basic waveforms for the data are not due to a set of several waveform generators but rather to the variation of the delay parameter of a single generator.

Problems raised by nonlinearities or the shortcomings of correlation measures can sometimes be dealt with by preprocessing the data waves prior to expansion. For example, Bennett *et al.* (1971) studied the interactions between amplitudes and latencies of average evoked potentials by first reducing each data waveform to a tabulation of the amplitudes and latencies of its six major components as defined by the waveform's maxima and minima. Thus each waveform was represented by twelve parameters in an amplitude-latency signal space. Using these twelve point data vectors, a principal components-varimax analysis was performed. The resulting expansion delineated the interplay of amplitudes and latency of the components. In terms of the original data waveshapes, relationships between waveform amplitudes and latencies are highly nonlinear. However, by recognizing this at the outset, the authors were able to arrange their data so that a relatively simple, compact expansion was obtained.

The problem of obtaining functionally significant representations of "nonlinear" data has been explored by Shepherd (1962a,b) Bennett (1969), Kruskal (1964a,b), Trunk (1972) and Kruskal and Shepherd (1974). Their methods are not restricted to correlation coefficient similarity measures. Instead it appears possible to reduce the data to its "intrinsic dimensionality," recognizing that the observed variations may arise from but a few generator parameters rather than a large collection of generators. Application of these methods to evoked potential analysis have not yet been reported. They have been utilized in the analysis of some psychophysical data and in some engineering problems. They are called to the reader's attention since the concepts they employ have the potential to deal effectively with a broad class of biological signal processes which cannot be adequately treated by linear data analysis.

REFERENCES

Bennett, R. S., *IEEE Trans. Info. Theory* IT-15, 517 (1969).
Bennett, J. R., MacDonald, J. S., Drance, S. M., and Uenoyama, K., *IEEE Trans. Bio-Med. Eng.* BME-18, 23(1971).
Davenport, W. B., Jr., and Root, W. L., "An Introduction to the Theory of Random Signals and Noise." McGraw-Hill, New York, 1958.
Donchin, E., *IEEE Trans Bio-Med. Eng.* BME-13, 131 (1966).
Donchin, E., Tueting, P., Ritter, W., Kutas, M., and Heffley, E., *Electroenceph. Clin. Neurophysiol.* 38, 449 (1975).
Harmon, H. H., "Modern Factor Analysis," 2nd ed. Univ. Chicago Press, Chicago, 1967.
John, E. R., Ruchkin, D. S., and Villegas, H., *Ann. N.Y. Acad. Sci.* 112, 362(1964).
John, E. R., Walker, P., Cawood, D., Rush, M. and Gehrmann, J., *in* "Int. Rev. Neurobiology," (C. C. Ffeiffer and J. R. Smytheis eds.), Vol. 15, p. 273, Academic Press, New York, 1972.
Kruskal, J. B., *Psychometrika* 29, 1(1964a).
Kruskal, J. B., *Psychometrika* 29, 28(1964b).
Kruskal, J. B., and Shephard, R. N., *Psychometrika* 39, 123(1974).
Shephard, R. N., *Psychometrika* 27, 125(1962a).
Shephard, R. N., *Psychometrika* 27, 219(1962b).
Squires, N. K., Squires, K. C., and Hillyard, S. H., *Electroenceph. Clin. Neurophysiol.* 38, 387 (1975).
Suter, C. M., *Exp. Neurol.* 29, 317(1970).
Trunk, G. V., *IEEE Trans Info. Theory* IT-18, 126(1972).
Watanabe, S., *in* "Transactions of the Fourth Prague Conference on Information Theory, Statistical Decision Functions and Random Processes." Czech. Acad. Sci., Prague, (1967).

Chapter 6

SPONTANEOUS AND DRIVEN
SINGLE UNIT ACTIVITY

6.1. INTRODUCTION

The kinds of dynamic neurobiological processes treated in
the previous chapters were characterized by the particular kinds
of waveforms that they generate. The waveforms themselves were
of prime interest since their shape or their shape variations
under different experimental conditions can be interpreted to yield
some understanding of the underlying processes. There are other
biological processes in which the major data of importance are the
specific sequence of time points denoting the occurrence of signal
events. Little or no basic importance may be associated with the
particular waveforms which the signals exhibit. Point process is
the mathematical name attached to processes of this type. The
principal example of such a process is represented by the generation of neural action potentials or "spikes" from an individual
neuron. The information transmitted by a neuron is assumed, according to current principles, to be contained only in the sequence of
time points when the neuron generates its action potentials. Consequently, one ignores the detailed structure of the action potential unless one is concerned with the intracellular spike generating
mechanism or, as we shall discuss later, with distinguishing the
activity of one neuron among many. The study of unitary postsynaptic potentials and miniature end plate potentials, two other
phenomena in which the time of event occurrence is of paramount
importance, is closely related to the study of spike activity.
All have the common property that the sequence of events appears to
be fundamental to an understanding of how the signal relates to
neural function. This holds true as well for the activity of

concurrently observed units--their messages are coded somehow in the time intervals between their individual spikes.

To understand how the nervous system functions, one must first understand the spike activity of the individual neuron and then how this activity is related to that of others in its network. This means that the importance of the point process to an understanding of neuronal interactions and transactions can hardly be overstressed And yet it must be said that this is an area in which relatively meager analytical support has yet been supplied to the experimental biologist by mathematical statisticians. The mathematical diffi- culties inherent in formulating and solving the problems are great and there are comparable difficulties in practical data analysis techniques. However, the situation is improving as the problems provoke more widespread interest. In this chapter we present those aspects of the point process data analysis that are applicable to single and multiple unit activity. Both real-time and nonreal-time techniques are covered.

6.2. POINT PROCESS--AN IDEALIZATION OF NEURONAL SPIKE ACTIVITY

A random point process is one which generates a sequence of events occurring at times t_1, t_2, t_3, ... measured from the start of an observation, t_0. The intervals between the successive events are z_1, z_2, z_3, ... All events in the sequence are generated by the same probabilistic mechanism. The simplest type of random point process is one in which the intervals between successive events are independent of one another and identically distributed. In this case, the process is called a renewal process. The Poisson process is a further specialized renewal process. In general, the intervals between successively occurring events are not independent. This would be the situation, for example, if the occurrence of an event depended upon the times of occurrence of the n events immediately preceding it. As an example, in certain circumstances the proba- bility that an event will occur in a given small time interval is dependent upon the time between the last and the next to last event. This is equivalent to saying that the length of the present interval is dependent upon the length of the preceding interval. A process having these properties is referred to as a Markov process and more will be said about it later. The dependency of the present interval duration can also be on intervals earlier than the preceding one. However, the renewal and the Markov processes are probably the two point processes most referred to in the study of randomly occurring events in the nervous system. It is important to be able to discern from the data whether either of them provides a suitable description of the neural process under study. The dimensions of this problem increase when one studies the concurrent activity generated by several neurons.

The characterization of an experimentally observed process depends upon the outcome of a variety of statistical tests which are performed on its event-time sequences. The choice of these tests is further dependent upon the experimental design. The two basic types of experiments performed on single units are those which deal with (a) spontaneous activity, and (b) driven activity. Both types may be performed on a single unit or group of units, and their results indicate different but related aspects of neural function.

A. SPONTANEOUSLY ACTIVE PROCESSES

Spontaneous processes are also referred to as ongoing or continuous or undriven processes, those in which the observed events occur in the absence of any deliberately delivered external stimulus. Thus the process is a manifestation of some sustained activity within the nervous system, activity that can be observed essentially within any time span. Sometimes the process may be stationary, but this is not always the case. Some of the most important statistical tests made on point processes are those concerned with ascertaining whether a spontaneously active process is stationary or not. One usually hopes for a positive answer, for the bulk of the statistical studies of point processes deals with the stationary situation.

Also, model representations and computer simulations often become more tractable when they deal with the relatively simple structure of a stationary process. A negative answer, on the other hand, need not lead one to abandon this form of approach for there are aspects of the process that can be revealed without considerable involvement in the mathematical tribulations of nonstationary point processes. See Smith and Smith (1965), for example.

B. *DRIVEN PROCESSES*

A process which is spontaneously active may, when subjected to the delivery of an external stimulus, exhibit dependency upon the stimulus. If it does, during this mode of its behavior it is spoken of as a driven process and its properties can be studied in relationship to the various temporal, spatial and intensive properties of the parameters of the stimulus. The temporal interrelationships between the stimulus and the event times of the driven component of the process are the data to be dealt with. Sometimes it may happen that only by stimulation can a particular neuronal process be observed because it manifests no spontaneous activity. This is then a purely driven process. The study of a purely driven process is no different from one with spontaneous activity except that there are no relationships to explore between its driven and spontaneous components. The driven component of a process is nonstationary because it is characteristic for it to exhibit some change in activity shortly after the delivery of a stimulus. As time goes on, the driven activity subsides and the overall unit activity assumes more and more of the properties of the spontaneous activity (silence, if there is none) until only the spontaneous component remains. This transitory feature of driven point processes is similar to that of evoked continuous processes. For this reason they share a common method of analysis--the averaging of responses to a sequence of repeated identical stimuli.

The difficulties that are encountered in the analysis of single unit point processes are somewhat different from those met in dealing with continuous evoked responses. With the latter, as we have noted previously, it is often convenient and useful to assume that the data are produced by at least two independent processes, response and noise, whose effects on the observed data are additive. Thus, in Chapter 4 we considered the observed data to be the sum of a pure evoked response and a background noise that was in part biological and in part instrumental. It was shown that the simple procedure of averaging the continuous responses to consecutive stimuli proves to be very effective in minimizing much of the noise. Unfortunately, the same conceptual approach has limited validity in dealing with driven point processes. It is unrealistic to assume that the observed neural spike events represent the effects of two independent processes acting in such a way that one subset of spikes can be considered to be produced by a signal-related process and the other by some noise process. The reason is that whatever the signal and noise processes are that generate neural spikes, they tend to interact in a nonlinear manner insofar as the generation of spike event times is concerned. An example of this is the sequence of action potentials which are produced when a neuron's continuously varying membrane potential, representing approximately the sum of a response component and a noise component, crosses the spike-generating threshold. There is a nonlinear relationship between the rate at which spikes are generated and the fluctuations in the amplitude of the membrane potential.

Point process analysis has available to it a variety of analysis methods of varying complexity. For example, one may be concerned with the distribution of all events in the time interval after the stimulus or perhaps with just the distribution of occurrence times of the ith event following each stimulus. The decision depends, of course, upon the nature of the experiment. As the subtlety of the experiment increases, so may the analysis. As we shall see, each alternative analysis may differ substantially from the others in technique of performance and interpretation.

Though point processes require different analysis methods than continuous processes, both have probabilistic descriptions. In continuous processes these are made explicit in the power spectra, correlation functions, probability distributions, average responses, and so on, measures that are based upon the amplitude of the response as a function of time. In point processes, contrastingly, the descriptions relate solely to the times between events within the process and between these events and the external stimuli. The differences in the types of data that are obtained from continuous and point processes lead to somewhat different methods of data analysis. Fortunately, the differences are not so great as to require entirely new points of view and analysis techniques. Here we present the techniques used for analyzing single unit activity and point out their relationship to those used with continuous processes.

6.3. CLASSIFICATION OF
SPONTANEOUSLY ACTIVE PROCESSES

An idealized version of a point process is shown in Fig. 6.1.

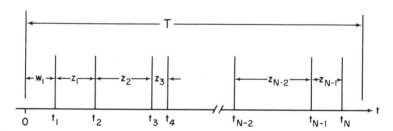

Fig. 6.1. *The event times and intervals in a T sec
segment of a point process.*

It shows a T sec segment of a sequence of N events. The events generated by the process occur at times t_i which are measured from the start of the segment. The interval w_1 between the start of the segment and the first event is the waiting time. z_i is the interval between the ith event and the $(i + 1)$th event. The properties of the process which interest us are (a) its stationarity, i.e.,

296

whether the stochastic properties of the N events in the selected segment of the sequence differ from those of other equal length segments occurring earlier or later in time; (b) its event dependencies, i.e., how the occurrence of one event is influenced by the occurrence of events preceding it and/or by the time since the process started.

(a) Stationarity. In a stationary point process, the distribution of the number of events occurring in an epoch or span of time T does not depend upon where this epoch starts. This facet of stationarity can be extended to joint distributions of a stationary process. The joint distribution of the number of events in two separate epochs of T sec duration depends only upon the time separation between the start of the two epochs, not their absolute location in time. Similar statements can be made about the higher order joint distributions of events but we will deal here only with second order or covariance stationary processes just as we did with continuous processes.

(b) Interval and event dependencies. The length of a given interval z_i is in general influenced by the lengths of the intervals preceding it, $z_{i-1}, \cdots, z_{i-0}, \cdots$. The dependency of the length of an interval upon all those preceding it can be expressed in terms of a conditional probability:

$$P[z_i | z_{i-1}, z_{i-2}, \cdots, z_{i-k}] \tag{6.1}$$

The functional notation is meant to indicate that the probability distribution of interval z_i is dependent upon or conditioned by the lengths of the k previous intervals starting with z_{i-1}. Obviously it becomes increasingly difficult to deal with such a dependency when k is large. It is more reasonable to see whether the dependency may, in fact, be restricted to only the more recent intervals and to study what the properties of such processes are. One may be able then to fit satisfactorily the experimental data by a process in which the dependency of the interval upon the past extends only over the previous several intervals. Processes which are governed by such dependencies are called kth order Markov processes. Since by choosing some low value for k we tend to reduce the model to an approximation of the real spike process, it is important that this choice be made carefully lest the model and the data analysis lose significance. Nakahama *et al.* (1972, 1974, 1975) have described some techniques for estimating the order of a Markov process, the simplest of which is the first-order Markov process.

The first-order Markov process occurs when $k = 1$, so that the length of an interval depends only upon the length of the immediately preceding one. The past history of the process affects the present interval only through the length of the interval immediately preceding it. We can write the conditional probability of the present interval as

$$P[z_i|z_{i-1}, z_{i-2}, \ldots, z_{i-k}] = P[z_i|z_{i-1}] \tag{6.2}$$

Alternatively stated in terms of events, the probability of an event occurring in any small interval of time depends only upon when the two preceding events occurred. This dependency is schematically illustrated in Fig. 6.2. To say that in a Markov process the

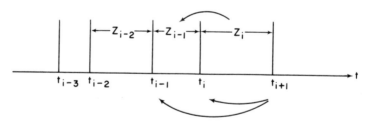

Fig. 6.2. In a Markov process the length of an interval depends only upon the length of the preceding interval. The occurrence of an event depends only upon the occurrences of the two preceding events.

present interval is dependent only upon the preceding one is not, however, to imply that there is a lack of correlation between the present interval duration and those earlier than the previous one. The contrary is true. To see this, consider what is called a stationary autoregressive process, perhaps the simplest kind of Markov process. In it, while z_i may be correlated with all the previous intervals, knowledge of z_{i-1} and the behavior of a random increment y_i completely specifies the z_i statistic. In effect, knowledge of z_{i-1} subsumes all knowledge of the previous intervals:

$$z_i - \mu_z = \alpha(z_{i-1} - \mu_z) + y_i, \qquad |\alpha| < 1 \qquad (6.3)$$

The random, independent increment y_i has a mean value of 0. α is a constant and $E[z_i] = E[z_{i-1}] = \mu_z$. This assures stationarity. Simple calculations show that $\text{var}[z_i] = \sigma_z^2 = \text{var}[y_i]/(1 - \alpha)^2$. The correlation coefficient ρ_k relating the present value and one k measurements earlier is given by

$$\rho_k = \frac{E[(z_i - \mu_z)(z_{i-k} - \mu_z)]}{\sigma_z^2} \qquad (6.4)$$

This correlation coefficient is also called the serial correlation coefficient. It is discussed more fully in Section 9. If z_i is expressed in terms of z_{i-k} and the k-1 independent increments $y_{i-1}, \ldots, y_{i-k+1}$, it is also a simple matter to show that

$$\rho_k = \alpha^k \qquad (6.5)$$

Thus an autoregressive Markov process of intervals exhibits a non-zero correlation coefficient between intervals that are not immediate neighbors. The correlation will decrease in absolute value as the separation increases and can be either positive or negative according to the sign of α. Although we have used the autoregressive process to illustrate a Markov process, it should not be construed that the autoregresive process can always provide an adequate description of spike-generating processes. Some consideration will show that if the random increments to interval duration are independent and sufficiently negative, then the model would admit the possibility of negative interval durations, a physically unrealizable situation. In the Markov model here, negative interval durations cannot occur as long as $y_{min} \geq - \mu_z(1 - \alpha)/\alpha$. This indicates that Markov models for spike activity have to be examined with care.

Estimates of the serial covariances or correlation coefficients, the correlations between intervals in an observed sequence, can be of great value in describing the nature of the process. If all the serial correlation coefficients starting with ρ_1 are 0, the process is said to be renewal and not Markovian. Renewal processes are discussed in the following section. In experimental situations the renewal decision would be reached if all the estimated determined serial correlation coefficients $\hat{\rho}_1$, $\hat{\rho}_2$, etc., were sufficiently small. Nakahama *et al.* (1972) have investigated the Markovian behavior of spontaneous activity in several regions of the central nervous system and found indications of as high as 4th-order dependencies.

There have also been attempts to describe spike processes in Markov-like terms. One such description is the semi-Markov process (Cox and Lewis, 1966). The simplest example of this is the two-state semi-Markov process. If the process is in state 1, at the next event it has probability α_1 of remaining in that state, and probability $1-\alpha_1$ of jumping to state 2. The corresponding probabilties if it were initially in state 2 are α_2 and $1 - \alpha_2$. States 1 and 2 might represent, respectively, one with diminished spontaneous activity and another in which it is vigorous. Semi-Markov processes have not yet been applied satisfactorily as descriptions of neuronal activity. The pseudo-Markov process described by Ekholm and Hyvärinen (1966) includes the semi-Markov process as a special case and has been found to be applicable to some neuronal spike processes. In a 2-state pseudo-Markov process the process remains in a given state until a run of K intervals has been generated. The run length K is determined by a discrete probability distribution which is determined by the state. If the initial state was state 1, it jumps to state 2 with probability $1 - \alpha_1$ or remains in state 1 with probability α_1. (When state 2 is the initial state, the corresponding probabilities are $1 - \alpha_2$ and α_2.) In either case, a new run length is selected according to the new state of the process. At the end of that run, the process is again capable of jumping to the other state or remaining in its present state. Ekholm and Hyvärinen used this model to study the spontaneous activity in rabbit brain. They labeled the two states descriptively as "resting" and "bursting" and showed that the activity of about half of the cells they studied could be reasonably described as pseudo-Markovian.

A. RENEWAL PROCESSES

Here $k = 0$ in Eq. (6.1) and the length of the present interval is independent of the lengths of any preceding interval. A renewal process is one in which the previous history of the process has no effect on its present state of activity. A unit exhibiting such activity may be thought to be behaving randomly, reflecting perhaps the combined influence of some continuous noiselike process that alters its membrane potential and in addition, the convergence of unrelated presynaptic spike trains at its many synaptic terminals. However, a unit that exhibits renewal properties may be conveying information in its average spike rate if not in its interval fluctuations. It is also possible, though unlikely, that the seeming randomness of a renewal process represents some highly structured integrative coding of the afferent information in the presynaptic spike trains.

In a renewal process, the conditional probability of z_i is

$$P[z_i | z_{i-1}, z_{i-2}, \ldots, z_{i-k}] = P[z_i] \qquad (6.6)$$

Likewise, the occurrence of an event is dependent only upon the time elapsed since the preceding one. The probability distributions for intervals can take on many forms. One useful way of categorizing renewal distributions is the gamma distribution (Parzen, 1964). Here the probability density for an interval of length z is given by

$$p(z) = \frac{\nu}{\Gamma(r)} (\nu z)^{r-1} \exp(-r\nu) \qquad (6.7)$$

ν is the average rate of events. $\Gamma(r)$ is the gamma function which

301

is defined in standard calculus texts (Courant, 1937). When r is an integer, $\Gamma(r) = (r - 1)!$ The exponential density corresponds to the case when $r = 1$. The mean and variance of the interval duration are given by

$$E[z] = 1/\nu = \mu_z; \quad \text{var}[z] = 1/\nu^2 = \mu_z^2 \quad (6.8)$$

Should the process under study appear to be of the renewal type, it is useful to try to fit a gamma distribution to it by estimating from its shape the values of ν and r. A reasonably good fit, if it can be obtained, can be helpful in suggesting a physical model to fit the process. When $r > 1$, the gamma distribution has a density function which is zero at the origin. Since the minimum interspike interval of neurons is limited by refractoriness, this suggests that the gamma distribution can be of use in describing the intervals of neuron spike processes. Kuffler et al., (1957) found that the gamma distribution could provide a good fit to the spontaneous activity of cat retinal ganglion cells. Hyvärinen (1966) investigated the spontaneous activity of the developing rabbit diencephalon and found that a small but significant number of the interval histograms appeared to have gamma distributions.

B. POISSON PROCESSES

The most thoroughly studied stationary point process is the Poisson process. It occupies a position in point process analysis equivalent to that of the Gaussian process in the study of continuous processes. This is because the Poisson process is a simple though useful simplification of many of the neural processes associated with spike generation. As a "reference" type of behavior it often yields valuable insights into the process being studied. In the Poisson process the probability of an event in any small interval of time dt is proportional to the length of that interval and is independent of the occurrence of previous events generated by the process. During the small interval dt, the probability of an event occurring is νdt where ν is the average event rate, as before. The probability of more than one event occurring in dt

is negligible. It is possible to show (e.g., Parzen, 1962) that in a given time of observation T, the probability that exactly n events will occur is

$$p(n) = \frac{(\nu T)^n \exp(-\nu T)}{n!}, \qquad n = 0,1,2, \ldots \qquad (6.9)$$

This is the Poisson distribution and it applies regardless of whether the observation interval begins with an event or not. The mean and variance of n are given by $E[n] = \text{var}[n] = \nu T$, an important property of the Poisson process. The probability density function for the intervals between successive events of the process is given (Parzen, 1962) by the exponential density

$$p(z) = \nu \exp(-\nu z) \qquad (6.10)$$

Further discussion of the properties of the Poisson process and tests associated with it appear in Sections 6.6 and 6.7.

6.4. SPIKE DATA ACQUISITION

When one examines an individual neuron isolated by a micro-electrode from its neighbors, only one type of neural event is observed, the nerve action potential or spike. Its waveform has a duration shorter than that of the shortest interval between successive waveforms. Although when several neurons are observed simultaneously by a single electrode there may be occasionally overlapping waveforms, we ignore that situation here. The spike waveform is by definition a unitary event that conveys information only by way of its time of occurrence or epoch. Any point on the spike waveform, e.g., its peak value, can be adopted as a fiduciary point for epoch measurement. In a noise-free situation, this poses no problem. There are difficulties, however, when noise is present or when the amplitude of the waveform fluctuates from one event to the next. The presence of either perturbation in the data alters the derived event time. Fig. 6.3 shows spike detection as performed by an amplitude comparator. The comparator generates an output

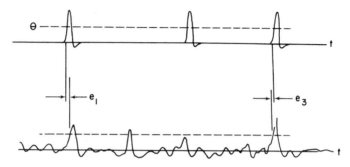

Fig. 6.3. Above, a spike train whose event times are detected when spike amplitude makes an upward crossing of threshold θ. Below, the same spike train in a noisy background. The estimated times of the first and third spikes are jittered by e_1 and e_3. The second spike is missed and a spurious spike is inserted earlier.

pulse whenever the amplitude of the spike waveform exceeds some threshold θ. Additive noise or the event-to-event amplitude fluctuation in the spike itself produces "jitter" of the estimated time relative to the true epoch. It can also suppress some event detections (the second one in the top trace) by being out of phase with the spike and it can be strong enough to be detected as a real spike (the second one in the bottom trace). As long as the waveform is short compared to the precision of interval measurement, epoch jitter is not a serious problem. It can be important when highly precise epoch estimation is required. The amplitude comparator may then prove to be unsatisfactory. An alternative device is the waveform peak detector. It is insensitive to amplitude fluctuations in the spike waveform. It does not, however, eliminate the jitter produced by background noise and may, under certain circumstances, increase it. The peak detector consists of a time differentiator followed by a threshold-crossing detector. The output of the differentiator crosses zero in the negative-going direction when the detected peak is a positive one and in the positive-going direction when the peak is negative. The threshold-crossing detector is an amplitude comparator whose threshold is set at zero. It generates a pulse at the instant its input becomes negative. Its

304

output is gated on by another amplitude comparator which detects when the spike is above the background noise. Zero crossings produced by noise will then not be able to produce an output pulse. It is also possible to perform peak detection operations on the sampled waveform if the rate of sampling is fast enough to permit a good representation of the waveform. The peak detector does not eliminate jitter or spurious events produced by background noise and may actually increase them unless care is taken. The reason is that a differentiator is a high-pass filter whose gain is proportional to frequency. It emphasizes the high frequency noise components in the input signal. If these are not to degrade the detector performance, they must be filtered from the signal prior to differentiation. The filter high frequency cutoff must be set so as to remove as much of the high frequency noise as possible without significantly reducing the frequency components in the spike waveform.

The occurrence of the timing pulse derived from epoch estimation is used to store the event times in computer memory. The passage of time is recorded by an accurate clock, usually one based upon a crystal oscillator. The measurement precision of the clock is of the order of 10 μsec or less and its accuracy is several parts per million. A clock with these properties is more than satisfactory in measuring the event times of occurrence of neural spikes. The event times can be recorded as the absolute times relative to some fixed reference time or they can be recorded as the time elapsed since the preceding event. In the latter case, there is less storage space required in the computer memory since the elapsed time contains many fewer significant bits than the absolute time. This is usually adequate unless accurate determination of periodicities in the activity is required.

Regardless of the type of event detector used, the noise may be large enough to introduce spurious events into the data or to suppress the detection of bona fide ones. The effects of these decision errors on the analysis of a point process vary in accordance with how prevalent are the errors, a matter to be discussed later in the chapter. For the present our discussions of spontaneous activity assume that the event detector provides substantially error-free estimation of the event times.

Spike data can often be analyzed by computer while being measured, provided that events do not occur too rapidly. This is certainly true for histogram analyses. When the analyses are more complex, it may be possible to perform them on the same machine within a short period of time immediately after the data have been obtained. Only when the analyses are highly complex is it necessary to defer their performance until after the completion of the experiment. The distinction between "simple" and "complex" depends primarily upon the speed and computing power of the machine in relationship to the rate at which data are acquired from the experiment.

6.5. INTERVAL DISTRIBUTION, MEAN AND VARIANCE

The event times for a spontaneous point process contain all the information there is to know about it. The interval durations between successive events, if preserved in the order in which they occur, are an equivalent representation. It is usually best to begin the study of a point process by methods which disregard the more complex temporal relationships that may be present. Then, when the simpler aspects of the process are known, one can move on to study the more detailed properties. In this procedure the interval distribution is generally the starting point. The interval distribution describes the most basic aspect of a point process, the duration of its intervals without regard to the order in which they occur. It reveals nothing at all about how successive intervals may be interrelated. But as already seen, if the process is Poisson, the interval distribution provides a complete description of the process. The estimate of the interval distributions is obtained from the interval times by sorting them into a histogram according to their durations. Suppose that in a fixed time T a sequence of N intervals was experimentally obtained from a spontaneous process. The histogram compilation dismantles this sequence but in doing so, it also destroys all the information relating to the order of interval occurrence. If the interval durations never exceed a maximum z_{max} sec, it is useful to partition the intervals into B different length bins each of whose length is $\Delta = z_{max}/B$ sec. Each measured interval is sorted into one of these bins. An interval falling into the bth bin is assigned the arbitrary duration

$$z_b = (b - 1/2)\Delta \qquad (6.11)$$

After all N intervals have been sorted, each bin contains n_b intervals such that

$$N = \sum_{b=1}^{B} n_b \qquad (6.12)$$

The histogram is a plot of bin population as a function of the bin number b and is an estimate of the interval density function. It is often useful in itself without computation of other statistics from the data. Once the interval histogram is available, it becomes possible to employ a number of tests designed to reveal some of the details of the process generating the intervals. The sample mean interval $\hat{\mu}_z$ and interval variance $\hat{\sigma}_z^2$ are useful statistics if only for estimating the average rate of the process and the magnitude of its fluctuations. Other useful tests are those designed to reveal whether the process is Poisson or, if not, to estimate the parameters of a gamma distribution that provides a good fit to the observed histogram. But because it does not preserve order information, the histogram cannot be used to test for stationarity or for the dependencies between intervals that would occur in nonrenewal processes.

The sample mean and sample variance of the interval durations are available from the interval histogram with little added computational effort. Higher order moments of the intervals can also be obtained without much difficulty. The sample mean and variance of the intervals are given by

$$\bar{z} = \frac{1}{N} \sum_{b=1}^{B} n_b z_b = \left(\bar{b} - \frac{1}{2}\right)\Delta \tag{6.13}$$

$$\overline{(z - \bar{z})}^2 = \frac{1}{N} \sum_{b=1}^{B} n_b z_b^2 - \left[\frac{1}{N} \sum_{b=1}^{B} n_b z_b\right]^2 = \left(\overline{b^2} - \bar{b}^2\right)\Delta^2 \tag{6.14}$$

The sample mean interval is also the reciprocal of the estimated average event rate, $\hat{\nu}$. ν can be estimated directly from the data by means of an event per unit time (EPUT) meter that counts the number of events in a fixed interval T sec. When νT is large, the observed number of events N in the fixed time T tends to be normally distributed with mean and variance both νT. The estimated rate N/T is therefore also normally distributed with mean ν and variance ν/T.

The sample mean duration of the N intervals when there is no quantizing error, i.e., when the bin width is very small, is given by

$$\bar{z} = \frac{1}{N} \sum_{i=1}^{N} z_i \tag{6.15}$$

and the unbiased sample variance by

$$s_z^2 = \frac{1}{N-1} \sum_{i=1}^{N} (z_i - \bar{z})^2 \tag{6.16}$$

Since $\bar{z}$ and s_z^2 are unbiased estimates, their expected values are $E[z]$ and var$[z]$ regardless of the nature of the process. However, if N is small and there is a high degree of positive correlation between successive intervals in the process or if the process is nonstationary, the estimates of interval mean and variance will tend to depart more from their expected values than is the case when the intervals are generated by a stationary renewal process. Under renewal circumstances the sample mean tends to have a normal distribution with a variance given by

$$\text{var}[\bar{z}] = (1/N) \ \text{var}[z] \qquad (6.17)$$

s_z^2, if it pertains to a process of normally distributed intervals, has a chi-squared distribution with $N - 1$ degrees of freedom. The variance of s_z^2 will therefore be

$$\text{var}\left[s_z^2\right] = [2/(N - 1)] \ \text{var}^2[z] \qquad (6.18)$$

Few other properties of sampled normal distributions lend themselves to application here, since it is not common in neurophysiology to encounter point processes which have normally distributed interval durations. One aspect that does merit consideration deals with the confidence limits for the mean interval. Assuming the interval generating process to be normal, then the ratio

$$t = \frac{\bar{z} - E[z]}{s_z / \sqrt{N}} \qquad (6.19)$$

is of interest. When z is normal, t is distributed according to what is known as the Student t distribution. It is closely related to the chi-squared distribution. Of great importance to us here is the fact that the t distribution is useful in many cases, like the present one, in which z is not distributed normally. Interspike interval analysis can therefore make use of it since interval duration is rarely normally distributed. With the estimated values $\bar{z}$ and s and the number of intervals N, one can consult the tabulated values of the t statistic to determine the confidence limits for the mean interval μ_z at any desired level α.

6.6. TESTS FOR MEAN INTERVAL AND
      RATE OF A POISSON PROCESS

Let us assume that the point process we are dealing with is Poisson. We want to estimate its mean rate and establish confidence limits for that estimate. Time is measured from an arbitrary origin to the occurrence of the Nth event at time t_N, the completion of the Nth interval. The interval mean and variance in a Poisson process are easily found from the exponential distribution of Eq. (6.10). They are

$$\mu_z = 1/\nu, \qquad \sigma_z^2 = 1/\nu^2 \qquad (6.20)$$

It is not difficult to show that the expected value of t_N is the sum of the expected values of N intervals:

$$E[t_N] = N/\nu \qquad (6.21)$$

Since the number of intervals considered is fixed at N, it is convenient to estimate the average interval duration μ_z. An unbiased estimator for μ_z is

$$\hat{\mu}_z = \bar{z} = t_N/N \qquad (6.22)$$

$\bar{z}$ is a random variable defined in terms of t_N, the time between the start of the observation and the Nth event. The mean and variance of $\bar{z}$ can be obtained by using the fact that $2\nu t_N$ has a chi-squared probability distribution with $2N$ degrees of freedom (Section 1.13). This means that $E[2\nu t_N] = 2N$ and $\text{var}[2\nu t_N] = 4N$. Then it follows that

$$E[\bar{z}] = 1/\nu = \mu_z$$

$$\text{var}[\bar{z}] = 1/N\nu^2 = \mu_z^2/N \qquad (6.23)$$

$$\text{cvar}[\bar{z}] = 1/\sqrt{N}$$

indicating that the estimator has a variance that approaches zero as N becomes large. Thus the longer the sequence, the closer $\bar{z}$ will tend toward μ_z. We therefore determine the coefficient of variation of $\bar{z}$ merely by choice of the number of intervals to measure.

The average rate of the process can also be dealt with. In this case we wish to establish confidence limits for ν. To do this we take advantage of the chi-squared distribution for $2\nu t_N$. Using N and t_N to estimate ν, we find that the high and low confidence limits ν_H and ν_L are, at the level α,

$$\nu_H = (1/2t_N) \chi^2_{2N,1-\alpha/2}$$

$$\nu_L = (1/2t_N) \chi^2_{2N,\alpha/2}$$

(6.24)

where $\chi^2_{2N,\alpha/2}$ is taken to be the value of the chi-squared random variable at the point where the cumulative distribution function has the value $\alpha/2$. $\chi^2_{2N,1-\alpha/2}$ is defined similarly. The situation can be illustrated with a diagram representing the shape of the chi-squared distribution for a typical situation. Fig. 6.4 shows

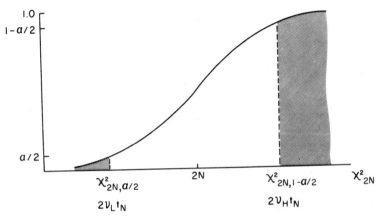

Fig. 6.4. The CDF for $\chi^2_{2N} = 2\nu t_N$. The probability that ν lies between ν_L and ν_H is $1 - \alpha$.

the chi-squared CDF for the random variable $\chi^2_{2N} = 2\nu t_N$. N complete intervals have been measured and so the variable is subscripted with $2N$. The expected value of χ^2_{2N} is $2N$ with a corresponding estimated value of N/T_N for ν. The two values $\chi^2_{2N,\alpha/2}$ and $\chi^2_{2N,1-\alpha/2}$ separate the shaded areas at left and right from the clear central region. The probability that the random variable takes on some value beyond one of the boundaries is $\alpha/2$, and the probability that it takes on some value in between is $1 - \alpha$. The corresponding values of ν at these boundaries are ν_L and ν_H. Thus, given the observation of N intervals in t_N sec, we can say

311

that the probability that the true value of ν lies between the confidence limits ν_L and ν_H is $1 - \alpha$.

The following is an illustrative example. The spontaneous activity of a neuron is observed from an arbitrary starting time to the 50th subsequent event, $N = 50$. The time duration measured is $t_N = 4.00$ sec. We then calculate

$$\hat{\nu} = \frac{50}{4.00} = 12.5 \text{ events/sec}$$

$$2N = 2 \times 50 = 100 \text{ degrees of freedom}$$

Let us choose $\alpha = 0.01$. Consulting tables of the chi-squared distributions (Abramowitz and Stegun, 1965), we find that

$$\text{prob}\{67.3 \leq \chi^2_{100} \leq 140.2\} = 1 - 0.01$$

But $\chi^2_{100} = 2\nu t_N$, so

$$\text{prob}\left\{\frac{67.3}{2 \times 4.00} \leq \nu \leq \frac{140.2}{2 \times 4.00}\right\} = 1 - 0.01$$

From this we see that

$$\nu_L = 8.41 \quad \text{and} \quad \nu_H = 17.5$$

The true value of ν has 99% probability of being between these two values. Had we been content with $\alpha = 0.10$, the corresponding confidence limits would be 9.74 and 15.5. The broad confidence limits are an indication that considerable measurement fluctuations exist in a sequence of only 50 intervals. This can also be seen by the variance of the estimate given in Eq. (6.23). With respect to $\text{cov}[\hat{\nu}]$, it is $N^{-1/2}$ which in this example amounts to .141. Note that in the preceding calculations no use is made of the shape of the interval histogram, for it has been assumed that the process is Poisson.

6.7. TESTS FOR A POISSON PROCESS

Suppose we are reasonably confident that the process is a renewal process but not certain that it is Poisson. We would like, therefore, to determine whether it can be so described. Any test we perform on the data can be expected to rely on the characterization of a Poisson process by the exponential distribution of its interval durations. We seek a test which utilizes the data in the most effective way and which is also practical to perform on a digital computer, possibly during an experiment. It sometimes occurs that these are conflicting requirements. A case in point is one involving the test of a process for a Poisson versus a gamma distribution alternative. As discussed by Cox and Lewis (1966), a test based on the interval statistic

$$- \log \bar{z} + \frac{1}{N} \sum_{i=1}^{N} \log z_i \qquad (6.25)$$

has the property of being what is called an asymptotically most powerful test of the two alternatives. That is, as N becomes large, this among all tests has the greatest probability of correctly rejecting the null (Poisson) hypothesis when the process is not Poisson. What the test does is to verify whether unity is a good estimate of the value of r in the gamma distribution of Eq. (6.7). If it is, the process is judged to be Poisson. The test has two practical drawbacks that limit its usefulness. The first is that it uses the logarithm measure of interval duration. While it is possible to extract the logarithm of an interval in real time, it can be excessively time consuming to do so. The second and more serious objection is that even before the logarithm is taken, the interval measurement has been first digitized in multiples of the bin width Δ. The duration of a small interval may be represented consequently by as little as one significant binary digit. This leads to a large relative quantization error in the measurement of small intervals and even larger errors in their logarithms. As a result, the error in the statistic can be quite severe and can drastically reduce the efficacy of the test. For this reason, the test is to be employed with great caution.

A more satisfactory test to consider is the modified mean test (Cox and Lewis, 1966). This statistic takes the form

$$S' = \frac{2}{T} \sum_{i=1}^{N} (N + 1 - i) z_{(i)} \tag{6.26}$$

Here $z_{(i)}$ represents the ith smallest interval of the N intervals measured, and T is the duration of the sequence of N intervals. After all the intervals have been measured, they are ranked in a new sequence according to increasing duration. Thus,

$$z_{(1)} \leq z_{(2)} \leq z_{(3)} \leq \cdots \leq z_{(N)}$$

If the intervals have been generated by a Poisson process and if N is reasonably large, S' will have a nearly normal distribution with mean $N/2$ and variance $N/12$. The greater the departure of S' from $N/2$, the less likely is the process to be Poisson. Because of the near normality of S' under the Poisson hypothesis, there is no difficulty in setting up confidence limits for a test at any desired level.

The computation of the S' statistic can be performed easily once a histogram of the intervals has been obtained. It requires certain minor changes necessitated by the quantization of interval length. The interval histogram has B bins of width Δ. An interval $z_{(i)}$ whose length is between $(b - 1)\Delta$ and $b\Delta$ is placed in the bth bin and assigned the length $(b - 1/2)\Delta$. The population of each bin is n_b where

$$\sum_{b=1}^{B} n_b = N \tag{6.27}$$

The total length of the sequence is taken to be

$$\hat{T} = \sum_{i=1}^{N} \hat{z}_{(i)} = \Delta \sum_{b=1}^{B} (b - 1/2) n_b \tag{6.28}$$

This assumes that we have not available an independent measure of the sequence length as obtained from a running clock. Using Eq. (6.28) we revise our equation for S' to

$$S' = 2(N + 1) - \frac{2}{\hat{T}} \sum_{i=1}^{N} iz_{(i)} \tag{6.29}$$

We now deal with the summation. In the first bin there are n_1 intervals all considered to be of equal duration $\Delta/2$. The summation of $iz_{(i)}$ over this bin is given by

$$(1 + 2 + \ldots + n_1)(\Delta/2) = (n_1/4)(n_1 + 1)\Delta \tag{6.30}$$

In the second bin the summation yields

$$[(n_1 + 1) + (n_1 + 2) + \ldots + (n_1 + n_2)]\Delta$$

$$= (3n_2/4)(2n_1 + n_2 + 1)\Delta \tag{6.31}$$

In the bth bin, when n_b is greater than zero, we have

$$[(N_{b-1} + 1) + \ldots + (N_{b-1} + n_b)](b - \frac{1}{2})\Delta$$

$$= (b - \frac{1}{2})(n_b/2)(2N_{b-1} + n_b + 1)\Delta \tag{6.32}$$

where

$$N_{b-1} = \sum_{i=1}^{b-1} n_i \tag{6.33}$$

If $n_b = 0$, then $N_b = N_{b-1}$. Thus, the summation of $iz_{(i)}$ over all bins becomes

$$\sum_{i=1}^{N} iz_{(i)} = \frac{\Delta}{2} \sum_{b=1}^{B} (b - \frac{1}{2})n_b(2N_{b-1} + n_b + 1) \tag{6.34}$$

Insertion of this into Eq. (6.29) gives, after some simplifications based upon Eq. (6.28),

$$S' = 2N + 1 - \frac{\Delta}{\hat{T}} \sum_{b=1}^{B} (b - \frac{1}{2})n_b(2N_b - n_b) \tag{6.35}$$

Note that N_b is the total number of intervals falling in or below the bth bin while n_b is the total number of intervals in the bth bin only. Both of these qualities as well as T are readily available from the histogram so that the computation of S' can be accomplished rapidly.

According to Cox and Lewis (1966) comparison of the modified mean test against one employing the statistic of Eq. (6.25) reveals that when N is large, its variance is about 1.4 times greater when the alternative distribution is of the gamma type. However, an advantage of the modified mean test is that it exhibits great effectiveness against alternatives broader than the gamma one. This fact and the comparative simplicity of the test are good reasons for its application to testing a series of events for Poisson behavior.

6.8. TEST FOR THE PARAMETERS OF A GAMMA RENEWAL PROCESS

Once the decision has been made that the process under study is a renewal process but not necessarily of the Poisson type, it may be of value to attempt to fit a gamma density to the data. Such a density, given in Eq. (6.7), can often be made to fit renewal data rather well. The problem is to estimate the two parameters of the distribution ν and r. The maximum likelihood estimate for r is given (Cox and Lewis, 1966) by solution of the equation

$$N[\log \hat{r} - \psi(\hat{r})] = N \log \bar{z} - \sum_{i=1}^{N} \log z_i \qquad (6.36)$$

The function $\psi(r)$ is called the digamma function and is available in tables (Abramowitz and Stegun, 1965) or can be computed. The solution of Eq. (6.36) requires only the experimental information obtainable from an interval histogram. There is, however, the difficulty that the solution involves logarithms of quantized intervals. As noted previously, this can be the source of computational inaccuracies when the bin widths are relatively broad.

6.9. SERIAL STATISTICS AND NONRENEWAL PROCESSES

As has been seen, interval distributions have important application to the study of renewal processes, processes in which there is no statistical dependence between any of the intervals. When the process is nonrenewal, it generates intervals that are dependent upon one another in some sequential manner. The interval distribution cannot by itself indicate this for it contains no information whatever about the order in which the intervals occurred. Therefore, in dealing with nonrenewal processes, the temporal or serial order of the intervals must be considered during the analysis.

There are several prominent ways of using the serial order for indicating the nature of interval interdependency. The first that we discuss is the serial correlation coefficient, Eq. (6.4), rewritten here in slightly different form:

$$\rho_k = \frac{E[(z_i - \mu_z)(z_{i+k} - \mu_z)]}{\sigma_z^2} \tag{6.37}$$

The correlation coefficient is an average measure of the joint behavior of pairs of intervals ordered as they occur in time. It is a measure that is normalized with respect to the variance of the intervals in the process. When ρ_k is positive, it indicates that one interval and another, k intervals later, tend to be jointly greater or less than the mean interval. Thus, if ρ_1 is positive, an interval which is longer than the mean tends to be followed immediately by another also longer than the mean; if the interval is shorter than the mean, the next interval also tends to be shorter. If ρ_2 is negative, it indicates that an interval longer than the mean tends to be followed two intervals later by another that is shorter, or vice versa. When the serial correlation coefficients are positive over a rather long range of interval separations, it is a sign that the intervals tend to be either increasing or decreasing. The serial correlation coefficient can be estimated

317

from limited sequences of N intervals by the equation

$$
\hat{\rho}_k = \frac{\sum_{i=1}^{N-k}(z_i - \bar{z}')(z_{i+k} - \bar{z}'')}{\left[\sum_{i=1}^{N-k}(z - \bar{z}')^2 \sum_{i=1}^{N-k}(z_{i+k} - \bar{z}'')^2\right]^{1/2}}
\tag{6.38}
$$

The terms $\bar{z}'$ and $\bar{z}''$ denote the estimates of the mean interval taken, respectively, from the first and last $N - k$ intervals in the sequence. The bias associated with $\hat{\rho}_k$ goes to zero as N becomes large.

To get a better understanding of the serial correlation coefficient it is helpful to consider a sequence of intervals as shown in Fig. 6.5. The intervals are numbered in their order of occurrence. The abscissa is the interval number i and the ordinate is the interval length. We may then consider the z_i as uniformly spaced sampled amplitude values of some continuous random variable z that is band limited to frequency 1/2 in terms of the interval number variable. Fig. 6.5 shows the correlogram of these intervals. The serial correlation coefficient ρ_k can be seen to be the same as the correlation function of lag k for the sampled random variable. The mean interval is the average amplitude of the samples and the variance is their mean square fluctuation about this mean. The general properties of correlation functions mentioned in Chapters 1 and 3 with respect to sampled random variables apply here equally well. But there are some special factors to take into account. The first is that we now consider the data to be noise-free. We are therefore not concerned with estimating what part of it is signal and what part is noise--for our purposes it is purely signal. But it is possible to encounter noiselike disturbances to the intervals since there can be short intervals due to spurious events and long intervals due to missed events. If the spike waveforms associated with single unit events are large compared to the interfering noise, spurious and missed events will be rare and our assumption will be a reasonable one. A second factor is that the probability distributions describing the duration of the random interval variable of a point process are, as noted before, gener-

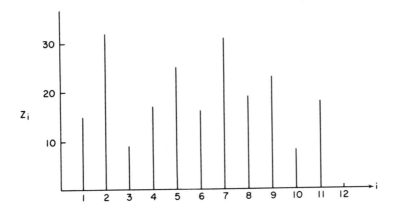

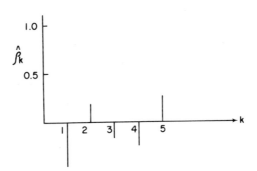

Fig. 6.5. Above, interspike interval duration z_i plotted as a function of interval number. Below, the estimated serial correlation shown for lags up to 5.

ally quite different from the Gaussian distribution commonly appropriate to fluctuating continuous signal processes. This leads to difficulty in dealing with the issue of the statistical dependency of intervals upon one another. A Gaussian process is defined completely by its first and second moments, and so lack of linear correlation implies statistical independence (Davenport and Root, 1958). This is not generally true for non-Gaussian processes. Thus there can be statistical dependence in a non-Gaussian process even though there is an absence of linear correlation. When a sequence of intervals is generated by a non-Gaussian process, even though the serial correlation coefficients may be zero for all lags, it does not necessarily follow that the intervals are statistically independent nor that the process generating them is renewal. This consideration makes the use of serial correlation coefficient tests for the renewal hypothesis somewhat inconclusive and unreliable in deciding when a process is renewal and when it is not. Nonetheless such tests are useful in giving some indication of the fitness of a renewal process description (Perkel *et al.*, 1967). Furthermore, they are presently about all the useful quantitative tests we have.

With these caveats in mind we can now discuss some of the properties of the serial correlation estimates as used in a test for a renewal process. Consider an N interval sample from the process being considered. We are interested in a test involving the low-order correlation coefficients even though we can estimate the correlation coefficients up to $\hat{\rho}_{N-1}$. The reason for confining our interest to the low-order coefficients is that the high-order ones are not of high quality inasmuch as they are computed from fewer sample products. Furthermore the estimates of the ρ_k are not independent and this fact is manifested by the nonzero covariances of the estimators themselves. This amount of covariance between the estimators of the different correlation coefficients depends upon the values of all the ρ_k of the process and it also depends upon the process itself (Cox and Lewis, 1966). It becomes small as N becomes large. Clearly, this covariance between the estimators of the correlation coefficients needs also to be kept in mind in interpreting an experimentally obtained set of correlation coefficients. For example, periodic oscillations in the sequence of the $\hat{\rho}_k$ may be due in large part to the properties of the estimators rather than those of the process. This is reminiscent of the behavior of covariance function estimates for the continuous processes dealt with in Chapter 3.

The test that we use on the low-order correlation coefficients is a simple one: If the $\hat{\rho}_k$ are different enough from zero,
independence is rejected. The acceptance region will vary with the
order of the correlation coefficient. The first serial correlation
coefficient $\hat{\rho}_1$ is the most practical one to deal with, yielding results which are easiest to interpret. Useful results for its estimate are given by Moran (1967), namely,

$$E(\hat{\rho}_1) = \frac{-1}{N-1} \quad \text{and} \quad \text{var}(\hat{\rho}_1) \leq \frac{N-2}{N(N-1)} \tag{6.39}$$

The expected value inequality is true for any interval distribution
as long as the process is renewal. The exact variance of $\hat{\rho}_1$ depends
upon the interval distribution. For a more detailed discussion, see
Lewis (1972). A specific test for the renewal hypothesis can be
based upon the behavior of $\hat{\rho}_1$ when N is large. The distribution
of $\hat{\rho}_1 (N - 1)^{1/2}$ in this case tends toward the unit normal (Cox and
Lewis, 1966) if $\rho_1 = 0$. Consequently, it is possible to test for
a renewal process by using just the first serial correlation coefficient estimate. A confidence level α can be adopted for the test.
The renewal hypothesis will then be rejected at this level if

$$|\hat{\rho}_1| > \frac{C_{\alpha/2}}{\sqrt{N - 1}} \tag{6.40}$$

$C_{\alpha/2}$ is the threshold which a normally distributed random variable
(0, 1) will exceed in $\alpha/2$ of the trials. Notice again that this
test is based only upon the first serial correlation coefficient.
For a more assured acceptance of the renewal hypothesis, higher
order correlation coefficients should be inspected as well. When
the number of intervals N is large and the process is renewal,
$\hat{\rho}_k$ also tends to be normally distributed with mean 0 and variance
of the order of $1/(N - k)$. But when N is not very large, the estimates of the different correlation coefficients suffer from possible
correlation, as has already been noted. These correlation effects
make the interpretation of the estimates of a sequence of estimated
correlation coefficients difficult, and it is probably best to

restrict one's attention to $\hat{\rho}_1$. Another important consideration is that the tendency toward the normal distribution with increasing N can be quite slow and dependent upon the interval distribution. Even when N is of the order of several hundred or perhaps more, the normal approximation may be unsatisfactory. Particular effects involving $\hat{\rho}_1$ are discussed by Lewis (1972).

One way to circumvent the difficulties associated with the distribution of $\hat{\rho}_k$ is to employ (Cox and Lewis, 1966; Perkel *et al.*, 1967) a test based upon estimated correlation coefficients obtained from a random permutation or shuffling of the intervals in the sequence. The shuffling procedure makes the test independent of the interval distribution. More will be said of shuffling tests later in the section. Some further simplification can be obtained by dealing with the sample product moment instead of the correlation coefficient. The sample product moment is defined by

$$r_k = \sum_{i=1}^{N-k} z_{i+k} \, z_i \qquad (6.41)$$

It is computationally easier to deal with than the estimated serial correlation coefficient of Eq. (6.38) and yields results which are equivalent to those obtained with that statistic. This includes the fact that there is correlation between the estimates of sample product moments for different orders of lag.

The sample product moment statistic can be employed in a special way that results from replacing the values of the z_i by their ranks $z_{(i)}$ in a histogram of the interval data. (See Section 6.7.) This exchange of rank order for actual size is made for all the intervals. We then obtain the rank product moment statistic (Cox and Lewis, 1966)

$$R_k = \sum_{i=1}^{N-k} z_{(i+k)} \, z_{(i)} \qquad (6.42)$$

The advantage of this statistic is that its distribution tends to the normal as N becomes large. For N of the order of 200 or more, a frequent situation in the study of spontaneous neuronal activity, the mean and variance of R_1 are approximately given by

$$E[R_1] \simeq \frac{1}{4}N^3 \quad \text{and} \quad \text{var}[R_1] \simeq \frac{N^5}{144} + \frac{N^4}{45} \qquad (6.43)$$

When the process is renewal, the approach to the normal is independent of the particular distribution of the intervals. The near normality of R_1 makes it easy to test for the validity of the null renewal process hypothesis. But, once again, this decision is based upon the properties of neighboring intervals of the sequence.

A difficulty in obtaining the R_1 statistic is that some intervals may be tied in their rank positions when Δ is relatively large compared to the spread of interval durations. Consider an interval histogram of interspike intervals. When the intervals are sorted into bins, all those that fall within the same bin will effectively be tied in rank for there is no further way to differentiate between them in length. To get around this, we can assign an "average rank" to each interval in the bth bin. It is

$$z_{(i)} = \sum_{j=1}^{b-1} n_j + \frac{n_b}{2} \qquad (6.44)$$

where n_j is the number of intervals in the jth bin. The exact effect of the averaging rule is not known but it will clearly become small as the bin size decreases.

An interesting variant of the order statistic for sample products is the statistic based upon the use of the "exponential scores" of the ranked intervals (Cox and Lewis, 1966). The exponential score of the nth smallest interval of N intervals is defined as

$$e(n;N) = \sum_{i=1}^{n} \frac{1}{N - i + 1} \qquad (6.45)$$

It is the expected value of the nth smallest of N intervals which are independent and arise from a Poisson distribution of interval duration. For example, if there are 10 intervals in a sequence,

the smallest ($n = 1$) has the score $e(1;10) = 0.1$; the second smallest has score $e(2;10) = 0.211$; etc. Using the exponential scores
of the ranked intervals, the previous test for a renewal process
is modified to a test of score products:

$$R'_1 = \sum_{i=1}^{N} e(n_i;N) \; e(n_{i+1};N) \tag{6.46}$$

Both the rank statistic and the exponentially scored ranked
statistic converge very slowly to a normal distribution as N becomes large. So does the distribution for the ordinary serial
correlation coefficient. Because of differences in the skew of
the distributions, the rank test tends to emphasize correlations
between small intervals whereas the exponential score test tends
to emphasize correlations between large intervals. Beneficially,
both tests tend to minimize the effect of the intervals that are
produced when events are falsely dismissed. The reason is that
the aberrantly long intervals are handled according to their rank
rather than their actual duration. In this way the ranking procedure for interval duration is similar to the median response discussed in Chapter 4. Just how the ranking procedure is affected
by spurious events which tend to produce shorter intervals than
the process ordinarily generated is not clear except that these
spurious events, being independent of the process, would predispose
any renewal process tests to decide in favor of the null hypothesis.
Further details on the rank test and the exponential score test can
be found in Cox and Lewis (1966) and Lewis (1972).

6.10. INTERVAL SHUFFLING AS A TEST
      FOR RENEWAL PROCESSES

A procedure which has been frequently employed for testing
for a renewal process is one which randomly "shuffles," i.e., re-
arranges or permutes the order of the intervals in an observed
sequence. This test utilizes a computer to perform the shuffling
of the intervals. Once adequately shuffled, the resulting sequence

of intervals can be considered to represent the output of a renewal process. The sample product moments or serial correlation coefficients of this renewal process are then determined. The shuffling procedure is repeated on the same data a large number of times in order to build up an empirical distribution of the resulting r_k or $\hat{\rho}_k$, all presumably from renewal processes. The values obtained from the unshuffled sequence can then be tested against these empirical distributions to see whether they also are likely to have arisen from a renewal process. The renewal hypothesis is rejected if the unshuffled r_k or $\hat{\rho}_k$ fall too far out on the tails of the distributions.

The shuffling test depends upon the ability of a computer shuffling algorithms to produce a satisfactory realization of a renewal process sequence from the original sequence. The tests performed upon the shuffled and original sequences are the same serial correlation coefficient tests described in the preceding paragraphs. With well-designed algorithms, shuffling and rank order tests appear comparable in efficiency although it may be that the latter are preferable in terms of requiring less computer time. Also, as more becomes known about the properties of the rank order tests for moderately large N, they may be found to be more reliable than the shuffling tests. Shuffling is also discussed in Sec. 6.11.

6.11. THE EXPECTATION DENSITY AND
      COVARIANCE FUNCTION OF POINT PROCESSES

The interval serial correlation and periodogram aspects of a point process yield only a limited view of the dynamics of the process. A variety of alternate statistical methods is necessary if a better understanding of the mechanisms controlling the processes is to be obtained. One such method is the expectation density (Huggins, 1957; Poggio and Viernstein, 1964). It has also been called the intensity function (Cox and Lewis, 1966), the renewal density (Perkel et al., 1967), and the autocorrelation (Gerstein and Kiang, 1960). We prefer the expectation density name since it is suggestive of the way in which the function is defined. The expectation density deals with the times of the events rather than the intervals between them. But, as with the interval approach, it deals only with the second-order statistics of the process, albeit in a somewhat different way. Still, it has certain advantages which make it of considerable value. One of them is that time appears directly rather than being concealed in the interval number. This facilitates interaction studies of simultaneously occurring processes, both point and continuous. Expectation density and correlogram analysis are in many ways complementary to each other, each indicating aspects of the process that cannot be seen with the other. However, their limitation to second-order statistics must always be kept in mind.

The expectation density arises when one considers the sequence of events to be a continuous process consisting of very brief pulses of the same shape and polarity. These represent the occurrence of events. This in fact is close to what we see when viewing the discharges of a single neuron on an oscilloscope whose sweep time is much longer than the duration of an individual spike. Actually, the waveform may vary from spike to spike but, according to current neurophysiological concepts, waveform is of no significance in terms of a neuron's ability to convey information. Therefore, we ignore it and idealize each spike event into the short pulse that is a Dirac delta function. Having done this we can consider the autocovariance function (acvf) of the sequence of events $s(t)$ using the techniques of Chapters 1 and 3:

$$c_{ss}(\tau) = \lim_{T \to \infty} \frac{1}{T} \int_0^T [s(t) - \mu_s][s(t + \tau) - \mu_s] \, dt \qquad (6.47)$$

μ_s, the average value of $s(t)$, is equal to the average rate of events ν. Let us consider some of the properties of $\hat{c}_{ss}(\tau)$, the finite time estimate of $c_{ss}(\tau)$ when N events occur during the observation time T. For a time lag of 0, $\hat{c}_{ss}(0)$ has the value $(N/T)\delta(0) - (N/T)^2$. The delta function at $\tau = 0$ results from the complete overlap of all the spikes in the original sequence with those in its 0-shifted replica. $(N/T)\delta(0)$ is thus the total power in the spike sequence, while $(N/T)^2$ is the power associated with only the average value of the spike sequence. N/T is the estimate $\bar{\nu}$ of the average rate of events. At a nonzero time lag, τ_i, $\hat{c}_{ss}(\tau_i)$ takes on the value $n(\tau_i)\delta(\tau - \tau_i)/T - (N/T)^2$. $n(\tau_i)$ is the number of times in the observation time T that an event in sequence $s(t)$ coincides with an event in $s(t + \tau_i)$. If we go to the limit, we find that for an aperiodic process, $c_{ss}(\tau)$ is given by a delta function $\nu\delta(\tau)$ plus a continuous component ranging over all other values of τ. This will be developed in the following discussion. Figure 6.6 illustrates a T sec segment of a spike train and, below

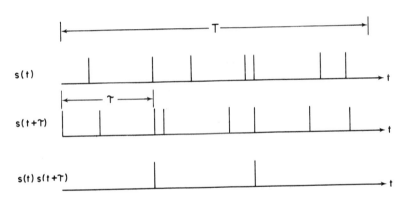

Fig. 6.6. A T sec sequence of events s(t) and its time shifted version. (A positive value of τ produces a shift to the right.) The bottom trace is the product of the upper two and indicates two temporal coincidences.

it, its time shifted version. There are two instances shown in which there is coincidence between spikes in the two trains. $\hat{c}_{ss}(\tau)$ for the delay chosen thus has the value 2. If there were N events in the observed sequence, the total number of coincidences possible for all the values of τ ranging from 0 to T is $N(N + 1)/2$. $\hat{c}_{ss}(\tau)$ when plotted has the appearance of a collection of delta functions of different strengths tending to cluster at different regions along the τ axis. This is especially evident when $s(t)$

arises from a random process. The density of the cluster around a particular value of τ is a measure of the preference for events to be separated from each other (ignoring intervening events) by that time delay. The estimated autocovariance function for the spike sequence of Fig. 6.6 is shown in Fig. 6.7. A more useful way to

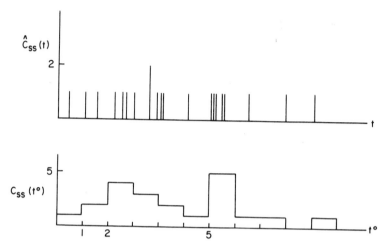

Fig. 6.7. Above, the acvf estimate $\hat{c}_{ss}(\tau)$ indicating the lengths of all intervening intervals within a T sec data segment. Below, a histogram version of the same data with time quantized into bins of width Δ = 1.

present this data is to subdivide the τ axis into bins Δ sec wide, count the number of coincidences or delta functions in each, and plot that number as a function of τ°, the delay as measured by the number of the bin. The ordinate value at τ° alternatively represents the number of times that an event in $s(t)$ followed some preceding event by a delay of $(\tau° - 1)\Delta < \tau \le \tau°\Delta$. The gain in the effectiveness of the presentation is clear.

There is a more satisfactory way of dealing with the acvf concept for a point process. To develop it, let us return to the original sequence of events and consider the probability that if an event occurred at time t, another will occur within the indicated delay increment. This probability is given by

$$m(\tau)d\tau = \text{prob}\{\text{event in } (t + \tau, t + \tau + d\tau) \mid \text{event at } t\}$$

(6.48)

The quantity $m(\tau)$ is called the expectation density of the point process. $m(\tau)$ is a probability function for the occurrence of another event τ sec after an earlier event. There may have been any number of events or none at all occurring between t and $t + \tau$. Thus, $m(\tau)$ pertains to the probability that any two events in the sequence are separated by τ sec. Note that as τ becomes large

$$\lim_{\tau \to \infty} m(\tau) = \nu \qquad (6.49)$$

the expected rate of events. For large τ, the probability of an event in the small interval $d\tau$ starting at τ is just $d\tau$ times the average rate of events. The rate at which this limit is approached depends upon the process involved. For a Poisson process it is immediate since $m(\tau) = \nu$ for all τ. $m(\tau)$ is estimated from a T sec segment of a spike sequence. This segment will have about $N = \nu T$ events in it. The total number of τ sec lagged coincidences in T is $n(\tau)$ and is given by $\nu T \hat{m}(\tau)$, where $\hat{m}(\tau)$ is the T sec estimate of $m(\tau)$. Division by T as in Eq. (6.47) shows that $\nu \hat{m}(\tau) = n(\tau)/T$, the amplitude of the delta function contribution to $\hat{c}_{ss}(\tau)$ at time τ. Attention should be drawn to the fact that $m(\tau)$ is not a true probability density function in the sense that it is not the derivative of a CDF whose value is 1 at $\tau = \infty$ and 0 at $\tau = 0$. Consideration of the fact that $m(\tau)$ has the limiting value of ν will also make this clear.

The expectation density can also be derived from the interval densities of the process. It is instructive to see how this is done. Let the interval between an event and its immediate successor be referred to as a first-order interval; the interval between an event and the second one following it, as a second-order interval; and the interval between an event and the nth one following it, as an nth order interval. The probability density functions for each of these types of intervals are, respectively, $m_1(\tau)$,

$m_2(\tau)$, and $m_n(\tau)$. Since an event occurring τ sec after an earlier one must terminate one of these types of intervals, the sum of these probability densities must yield the expectation density,

$$m(\tau) = \sum_{n=1}^{\infty} m_n(\tau) \tag{6.50}$$

The estimated expectation density in Fig. 6.7 was constructed as a histogram between an event and any of its successors. It can now be seen to have the alternative interpretation as a summation of the experimentally obtained estimates of the interval density functions $m_1(\tau)$, $m_2(\tau)$, etc. Just how many of these density function estimates we need to deal with is determined by the range of τ over which we wish to estimate the expectation density. As an illustration, consider a process in which after an event occurs there is zero probability of another event for the next 1/2 sec. Then, somewhere within the next 1/2 sec another event is sure to occur. The process is a renewal one so that the next interval does not depend upon the preceding one. Returning to the expectation density as given in Eq. (6.50), we may now refer to Fig. 6.8. It

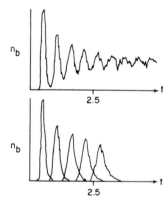

Fig. 6.8. Composition of the estimated expectation density from the estimates of the interval densities. The process is one which simulates a noisy pacemaker with mean interspike interval of 0.47 sec. n_b is the number of occurrences per bin. Above, the estimated expectation density; below, a superimposition of the first five interval densities. [Adapted from Perkel, et al. (1967)]

shows how the estimated expectation density is composed by summation of the first and higher order interval density estimates. The first-order intervals range from 0.4 to 0.9 sec, the second-order intervals from about 0.8 to 1.7 sec, the third-order intervals from about 1.3 to 2.7 sec, and so on for the higher order intervals. This means that at the progressively larger values of τ, $m(\tau)$ is contributed to by more and more of the interval density functions. It has already been pointed out that as τ becomes large, $m(\tau)$ approaches the limiting value ν. Figure 6.8 shows that the approach to this constant value can be slow. We also note here that although we may estimate the expectation density from the interval densities, we cannot do the opposite.

The exact relationship between $m(\tau)$ and $c_{ss}(\tau)$ can be obtained by considering events to be generated by a process derived from the original sequence of events, the counting process $N(t)$ (Parzen, 1962). This is a process whose initial value is 0 and which receives a unit increment whenever an event occurs. It is a function appearing as a sequence of unit amplitude steps occurring at the event times. Closely associated with the counting process is the differential counting process $\Delta N(t)$. It represents the rate of change of the counting process and so appears as a sequence of delta function spikes at the event times. These functions are mathematically tractable and turn out to be quite useful in understanding the relationship between the expectation density, the covariance function, and the spectrum of a point process. More will be said of this in Section 6.12. In effect, $\Delta N(t)$ corresponds to the original sequence of neural spikes except that their shape has been idealized into delta functions. When the point process is stationary, it is possible to show (Lewis, 1970) that the autocovariance function of $\Delta N(t)$ is given by

$$c_{ss}(\tau) = \nu\delta(\tau) + \nu[m(\tau) - \nu] \tag{6.51}$$

This is the result we had anticipated earlier in the section and consequently we have used the same symbol to represent the acvf.

It is evident that $c_{ss}(\tau)$ and the expectation density are proportional and can be obtained from each other. Note also that $c_{ss}(0)$ = $\nu\delta(0)$ and $c_{ss}(\infty) = 0$. Although the relationship between $c_{ss}(\tau)$ and $m(\tau)$ has been derived only for positive τ, it can be extended to negative τ by recognizing that the expectation density $m(\tau)$ is symmetrical about 0. Therefore, $c_{ss}(\tau)$ will be symmetrical about 0 also. This symmetry is useful when the spectrum of a point process is considered. In subsequent discussions, when referring to the acvf of a point process we shall mean the acvf of its differential counting process representation.

The standard approach used in estimating the expectation density chooses each event in the spike sequence in its turn as a time origin. The times from the fiducial spike to subsequent spikes are measured and used to construct a histogram of interval durations. Since the histogram is determined only up to some maximum time duration $B\Delta$, only intervals shorter than this need to be measured. Those intervals longer than $B\Delta$ are placed in the last bin. When all the events in the sequence have served as reference spikes, the expectation density histogram is complete. A useful technique for compiling an expectation density histogram in real time has been described by Arnett and Ellert (1976). It uses a buffer memory (look-back registers) capable of storing past events occurring within the $B\Delta$ time span prior to a current event. All intervals between these earlier events and the current one are measured. This is in contrast to a less effective but popular method which selects events that are $B\Delta$ or more apart to be the leading events in interval measurements. Because this method measures only those intervals, it can lead to a biased estimate of the expectation density. It should also be evident that the procedure for computing $\hat{m}(\tau)$ from the interval density estimates guarantees that $\hat{m}(\tau)$ contains all the shorter intervals that are in the record. Only the longer intervals are disregarded, partially or totally. The bias against the longer intervals depends upon how many interval densities we used to obtain $\hat{m}(\tau)$. A dis-

cussion of the effect of the bias on the expectation density estimate is given by Cox and Lewis (1966). And, as with the acvf of
continuous process discussed in Chapter 3, it is worth noting that
the mean square error in the acvf estimate is larger when the unbiased instead of biased estimate is used. As a result, the unbiased estimate is usually ignored in estimating the acvf. Another
point of interest is that the higher order interval density estimates are formed from fewer samples. They therefore tend to have
higher variance. When the number of events in the T sec sample is
large and only several interval distributions are estimated, this
will be of minor concern as will the bias against longer intervals.

Suppose now that the process under study is renewal. Then
the higher order interval densities have the property of being con-
volutions of the lower ones. Thus $m_2(\tau) = m_1(\tau) * m_1(\tau)$;
$m_3(\tau) = m_2(\tau) * m_1(\tau) = m_1(\tau) * m_1(\tau) * m_1(\tau)$; etc. This is so
because (a) in a renewal process successive intervals are independ-
ent, and (b) the probability density for the sum of two independent
random variables is the convolution of their individual densities.
In the case of a renewal process these individual densities are
identical; thus the relations given above. Departures of the higher
order interval densities from the convolution property can serve as
an indication of a renewal process. This type of test is not as
effective, however, as those based upon serial correlation coefficients or the spectrum of intervals or upon the randomizing or
shuffling of the temporal order of the intervals. In the latter
type of test one compares the expectation density of the shuffled
sequence with that obtained from the original sequence. Adequate
shuffling should separate possibly dependent intervals that were
close in time and result in a sequence with renewal properties.
Therefore significant differences in shape between the shuffled and
unshuffled expectation densities would indicate that the process is
not renewal. Measures of differences in the shapes of the functions could be obtained by a chi-squared test. But it must be kept
in mind that the shuffled sequence itself must be considered with

care for it is no more than a particular attempt to randomize the sequence of intervals so as to yield a new sequence with renewal properties. A shuffle may or may not be successful and one has to
guard against the latter possibility by taking the effects of different shuffles into account. When the process being studied has a
tendency toward being periodic, as with near-periodic pacemaker
types of cell discharges, it may be difficult to decide from the
shuffled and unshuffled expectation densities that the process is
renewal. Perkel *et al.* (1967) have pointed out that shuffling can
sharpen or flatten the peaks of the expectation density according
to whether the process exhibits positive or negative serial correlation between successive intervals. Their example showing how
shuffling sharpens peaks in the expectation density is provided
in Fig. 6.9. The data are from a semi-Markov process in which long

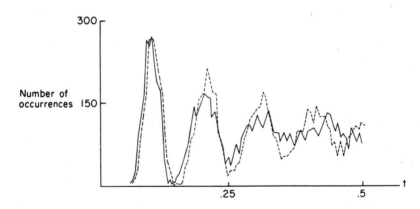

*Fig. 6.9. Expectation densities of a semi-Markov process
before (solid line) and after (dash line) shuffling of intervals.
Note the sharpening of peaks.   [Adapted from Perkel, et al. (1967).]*

intervals tend to follow long, and short intervals tend to follow
short. The expectation density for the unshuffled data is shown
in (a), and for the shuffled data in (b).

    If the departure of a process from renewal is not pronounced
or if there are other factors at play, such as nonstationary trends,
the difference between the expectation density and its shuffled

version may not be marked enough to confidently affirm or deny the
renewal process hypothesis. Nonetheless, the expectation density
can often give a useful picture of the behavior of the process.
Serial correlograms, on the other hand, appear to be more useful
in deciding between renewal and nonrenewal alternatives. The serial
correlation coefficients are easy to estimate and, except for ρ_0,
all of them are zero when the process is a renewal one. For a posi-
tively correlated Markov process, the serial correlation coefficients are all positive, decaying to zero with increasing interval
lags; for a negative correlated Markov process, they alternate between negative and positive values within a decaying envelope.
Thus, the serial correlation coefficients can give a rather clear
picture of the process in such instances. Taken overall, this indicates that in many situations it may be desirable to analyze a
point process using both expectation densities and serial correlograms.

6.12. SPECTRAL ANALYSIS OF SPIKE SEQUENCES

A. *RELATIONSHIP TO THE EXPECTATION DENSITY*

Now that we have introduced the expectation density and the
autocovariance function for a sequence of spike events, we can move
to another way of analyzing the sequence, its spectral description.
This is closely related to the acvf by way of the Fourier transform,
just as it was for continuous processes. There are two types of
spectral descriptions that can be given of a point process, the
first arising from the Fourier transform of the expectation density,
the second from the Fourier transform of the serial correlogram of
intervals. Of the two, the one based upon the expectation density
seems more useful especially when the dynamics of the process are
to be compared with the concurrent activity of other processes,
point or continuous. This is the spectrum we consider first. Spectral analysis based upon serial correlograms is discussed afterwards.

The spectrum of a point process is defined as the Fourier transform $C_{ss}(f)$ of $c_{ss}(\tau)$, the autocovariance function of the differential counting process representing the spike train.

$$C_{ss}(f) = \nu \left\{ 1 + \int_{-\infty}^{\infty} [m(\tau) - \nu] \exp(-j2\pi f\tau)\ d\tau \right\} \qquad (6.52)$$

Note that since the acvf has a delta function in it at $\tau = 0$, something not encountered in the acvf of continuous processes, there will be a constant term in $C_{ss}(f)$. Note also that the spectrum is proportional to the average rate of events, so it is sometimes useful to normalize with respect to this rate. And as before, the symmetry of $c_{ss}(\tau)$ about zero assures that the spectrum is symmetrical about zero frequency so that we need to consider $C_{ss}(f)$ only at positive frequencies. The normalization is given by

$$C'_{ss}(f) = \frac{C_{ss}(f)}{\nu}$$

$$= 1 + \frac{2}{\nu} \int_{0}^{\infty} [m(\tau) - \nu] \cos 2\pi f\tau\ d\tau, \quad f > 0 \qquad (6.53)$$

It is useful when a single isolated process is considered. It may not be of much value when interactions between processes are of interest because the average rate of one process can be affected by the other.

In an experimental situation we must deal with the estimate of the expectation density $\hat{m}(\tau)$. This is obtained, as previously noted, by measuring all the intervals between the N spikes in the sequence observed. Each interval of length τ is represented as a delta function located along the τ axis. Thus, the interval between the ith spike and the $(i + k)$th spike is represented as $\delta(t_{i+k} - t_i - \tau)$. Furthermore, although $m(\tau)$ has been defined in terms of intervals starting with an earlier event and ending with a later one, it also applies to intervals measured in the opposite time direction. For a given value of τ, we have $m(\tau) = m(-\tau)$.

Then $\hat{m}(\tau)$ can be written as

$$\hat{m}(\tau) = \frac{1}{N} \sum_{i=1}^{N-1} \sum_{k=1}^{N-i} \delta(t_{i+k} - t_i - |\tau|) \tag{6.54}$$

Division by N expresses the apportionment of the $N(N - 1)/2$ intervals equally among the N events in the data. This gives $\hat{m}(\tau)$ the desired form of a probability; but some further consideration of the equation indicates that it yields a biased estimate of $m(\tau)$. The reason is much the same as that which causes the estimated acvf of a continuous function to be the biased one shown in Eq. (3.99). That is, we are dealing with N events in a T sec segment of the process. Consequently, as we move to the later occurring events, they will be the leading events in progressively fewer intervals in the histogram of intervals. In particular, an event occurring u sec after the start of the specimen cannot be the starting event in any interval that is longer than $T - u$. Although it is possible to employ an unbiased estimator for $m(\tau)$ (Cox and Lewis, 1966), it is usually not advantageous to do so because, as with the unbiased estimator for the acvf of a continuous process, it leads to large estimate variances at large values of τ.

By using the fact that $m(\tau)$ is symmetrical about 0, the Fourier transform of $\hat{m}(\tau)$ is found to be

$$\hat{M}(f) = \int_{-\infty}^{\infty} \hat{m}(\tau) \exp(-j2\pi f\tau) \, d\tau$$

$$= \frac{1}{N} \left\{ \sum_{i=1}^{N-1} \sum_{k=1}^{N-i} \exp[-j2\pi f(t_{i+k} - t_i)] \right.$$

$$\left. + \sum_{i=1}^{N-1} \sum_{k=1}^{N-i} \exp[j2\pi f(t_{i+k} - t_i)] \right\}$$

$$= \frac{2}{N} \sum_{i=1}^{N-1} \sum_{k=1}^{N-i} \cos[2\pi f(t_{i+k} - t_i)] \tag{6.55}$$

$\hat{M}(f)$ can now be compared with the periodogram of the same T sec sequence of spikes. This is done by first taking the Fourier transform of the original sequence of delta function spikes $s(t)$. The periodogram of a T sec segment of a continuous (unsampled) process is given by $P_{ss}(f) = |S(f)|^2/T$. It is a measure of the spectral distribution of power, not energy. Because the process here consists of spikes that can occur at any time, not just at uniformly spaced sample times, the periodogram is not band limited. We shall deal with this matter later. When there are N delta function spikes in the T sec segment,

$$P_{ss}(f) = \frac{1}{T}\left| \sum_{i=1}^{N} \exp(-j2\pi ft_i) \right|^2 \tag{6.56}$$

Here power is equivalent to spike rate and energy to the total number of spikes. $P_{ss}(f)$, after some algebraic simplification and comparison of terms with those in Eq. (6.55), is found to be given by

$$P_{ss}(f) = \hat{\nu}[1 + \hat{M}(f)] \tag{6.57}$$

Observe that this estimate of the spectrum essentially differs from $C_{ss}(f)$ in Eq. (6.52) only by lacking the term

$$-\int_{-\infty}^{\infty} \nu \exp(-j2\pi f\tau)\ d\tau = -\nu\delta(f) \tag{6.58}$$

The reason for the discrepancy is that $P_{ss}(f)$, having been obtained directly from the sequence of spikes, contains the dc effects of the average spike rate ν. $C_{ss}(f)$ does not contain these effects for it has been obtained from the covariance function which specifically removes the effects of the average value. The contribution of the average spike rate to the spectrum is just $\nu^2\delta(f)$, a dc bias component represented by a delta function at $f = 0$. $P_{ss}(0)$ contains the dc bias which has an average value of

$$E[P_{ss}(0)] = \nu\{1 + E[\hat{M}(0)]\} = \nu[1 + (\nu T - 1)] \tag{6.59}$$

This was obtained from Eq. (6.55) by using the fact that there are $N(N - 1)/2$ terms in the double summation there. The bias in the periodogram is given by

$$E[P_{ss}(0)] - C_{ss}(0) = \nu(\nu T - 1) - \int_{-\infty}^{\infty} [m(\tau) - \nu] \, d\tau \simeq \nu^2 T \qquad (6.60)$$

This is the amplitude of the delta function at $f = 0$. When a T sec sample of data is used for estimation of the spectrum, the dc component at 0 is smeared into a spectral peak given by $(\hat{\nu})^2 T [\sin 2\pi f T / \pi f T]^2$. This is the leakage effect discussed previously in Chapter 3. To remove or minimize leakage near $f = 0$, the estimated average rate $\hat{\nu}$ should be subtracted from $\hat{m}(\tau)$ before its Fourier transform is taken, as in Eq. (6.55). If the spectrum is estimated directly from the spike record, there will be no leakage at harmonics of the fundamental frequency $1/T$. Quantizing time, to be discussed later, will also eliminate aliasing effects. In either case, the removal of the average value, though imperfect, will greatly reduce the leakage.

The major difficulty with the periodogram, as pointed out in Chapter 3, is that it is not a consistent estimator of the spectrum. The variance of the periodogram at frequency f does not go to 0 as the length of the observed sequence of intervals increases. For a Poisson process of average rate ν, the mean of the periodogram at any frequency different from 0 is

$$E[P_{ss}(f)] = \nu \qquad (6.61)$$

The variance of the periodogram at a frequency that is an integer multiple of $1/T$ can be shown to be (Lewis, 1970)

$$\text{var}[P_{ss}(f)] = \nu^2 [1 + (1/\nu T)] \simeq \nu^2 [1 + 1/N] \qquad (6.62)$$

From this we have

$$\text{cvar}[P_{ss}(f)] \simeq (1 + 1/N)^{1/2} \qquad (6.63)$$

Since the same experimental data are used to estimate the spectrum at all frequencies, there is, as might be expected, covariance between these spectral estimates. When f_1 and f_2 are multiples of $1/T$,

$$\text{cov}[P_{ss}(f_1), \, P_{ss}(f_2)] = \nu/T \simeq \nu^2/N \tag{6.64}$$

This shows that the covariance is nonzero and independent of the frequency separation, but becomes small as N, the number of intervals measured, becomes large.

Since the Poisson process plays much the same role in the study of point processes that the Gaussian white noise process does in the study of continuous processes, it is useful to contrast these results for the Poisson point process with those previously obtained for the Gaussian continuous process. As shown in Chapter 3 for the latter process the coefficient of variation of the periodogram at frequency f is unity regardless of the duration of the sample. In this regard the periodograms of continuous and point processes are similar when N is large. For the continuous process, the covariance between spectral estimates at frequencies that are multiples of $1/T$ is always 0. This latter property contrasts somewhat with that for the Poisson point process where the covariance becomes small only when the number of intervals is large. Further, as noted above, the 0 frequency component $P_{ss}(0)$ of a point process periodogram contains a bias term at $f = 0$. And finally, for a large class of point processes the spectrum estimate $P_{ss}(f)$ has an expected value that only approaches $C_{ss}(f)$ as a limit as T becomes large. Thus there are major differences between the spectral of point and continuous processes and special consideration has to be given them if useful spectral estimates are to be obtained.

B. *SMOOTHED ESTIMATES OF POINT PROCESS SPECTRA*

To obtain a consistent spectral estimate, the periodogram of a point process needs to be smoothed. This is the same situation that prevails in estimating the spectrum of a continuous process.

Spectral smoothing can be done directly upon the periodogram estimate or by first applying a lag window to the estimated acvf. Since
the spectrum and the acvf are related by the Fourier transformation,
the two approaches yield equivalent results. This has been shown
previously in Chapter 3. The criteria for successful smoothing of
a point process spectrum have several factors additional to those
involved in smoothing a continuous process. These include taking
into account both the bias term at 0 frequency and the number of
intervals making up the data sample. The latter bears directly
upon the statistical degrees of freedom of the estimate and its
variance. Also, it must be pointed out that although the smoothing
procedure is indifferent to the nature of the process generating
the data, the goodness of the estimate is not.

The direct approach to spectral smoothing deals with the
periodogram by applying a spectral window to it. The amplitudes
of the periodogram frequency components within the window are
weighted and averaged. This average is the smoothed spectral
estimate at the frequency that the window is centered upon. As
discussed previously in Chapter 3, the width of the window may be
varied to adjust the spectral resolution and the variance of the
estimate. An increase in the window width means an undesirable
decrease in spectral resolution but brings with it a desirable
reduction in the variance of the smoothed estimate. Consequently,
some compromise in smoothing filter bandwidth has to be made. The
compromise will depend upon what aspect of the process is of most
importance to the observer. A more detailed discussion of smoothing as it applies to point processes is given by Lewis *et al.*
(1969).

The second approach to smoothing the spectrum starts with the
estimated acvf obtained from the expectation density. The estimated acvf is multiplied by $w(\tau)$, the weighting function of a lag
window and the Fourier transform of the resulting product is taken.
This is the smoothed spectral estimate. Note that there is a constant or frequency independent contribution to the smoothed spec-

trum [see Eqs. (6.52) and (6.57)] which arises from the average rate of events and not the shape of the expectation density or acvf. This constant term shows up regardless of whether the smoothed spectrum is derived directly from the periodogram or from the expectation density.

To the weighting function $w(\tau)$ of the lag window there corresponds a spectral filter $W(f)$ which, if convolved with the periodogram $P_{ss}(f)$, would yield the identical smoothed spectrum. That this should be so follows from the fact that the periodogram (ignoring the dc term) is the Fourier transform of the estimated expectation density $\hat{m}(\tau)$.

A useful method of spectral smoothing is the Bartlett method which partitions the data sample of T sec into K segments of L sec each. Each segment can have its spectrum estimated directly or by way of the estimated acvf. If these raw spectral estimates are then averaged together, the result is a smoothed spectrum. The spectral window for this type of smoothing has the shape

$$W(f) = L[(\sin \pi fL)/\pi fL]^2 \qquad (6.65a)$$

The corresponding lag window is

$$w(\tau) = \begin{cases} 1 - (|\tau|/L), & |\tau| \leq L \\ 0, & |\tau| > L \end{cases} \qquad (6.65b)$$

It was shown that since successive estimates of the spectrum are averaged to obtain the smoothed estimate, the variance of the estimate at each frequency will be inversely proportional to the number of data segments. However, if the total time of observation T is constant, the spectral resolution will decrease with the number of data segments since the width of the spectral window is proportional to $1/L = K/T$. Another important factor to be considered is that the length of the individual segments needs to be long enough to insure that there is small covariance between periodogram estimates at different frequencies. The advantage of Bartlett-type smoothing is that it also permits one to examine the process for stationarity, to see whether there are trendlike changes from segment to segment.

Spectral smoothing by whichever of the methods selected yields a consistent spectral estimate, one whose variance decreases as the number of intervals in the spike train increases. Having such an estimate available, it is now useful to inquire as to how effective smoothing is in terms of (a) the resolution of peaks and valleys within the spectrum, and (b) the confidence limits of the spectral density estimate at a particular frequency.

6.13. GENERAL CONSIDERATIONS IN SPECTRAL SMOOTHING

It has already been pointed out that the smoothed spectral estimate can be arrived at by starting with either the periodogram or the estimated expectation density. With continuous processes, the former is to be preferred since the fast Fourier transform can bring about substantial savings in computation time. It would be useful to be able to apply this method to point processes. In point processes, however, events can occur at any point in time and so the FFT seems at first glance to be inappropriate since it requires a T-discrete representation of band-limited data. But this can be obtained if we are willing to quantize our measurement of event times into Δ sec increments such that an event occurring at time $(t° - 1)\Delta < t \leq t°\Delta$ is assigned to the time bin $t°$. When this is done and the event considered to be a sample of unit amplitude rather than a delta function, the point process has the appearance of a sampled continuous process whose amplitude is either zero or unity. The results for covariance functions and power spectra of a band-limited process can then be applied to describe the sequence. An alternative approach has been employed by French and Holden (1971). It consists of digitally filtering the spike data with a low-pass rectangular filter whose cutoff frequency F is the highest frequency of interest. The filter impulse response is $(\sin 2\pi Ft)/2\pi Ft$. The filtered output is then sampled at the

Nyquist rate $2F$. The resulting sampled output is in no way different from that obtained from any continuous band limited process.

Since in any computational analysis of a point process time must always be quantized, the real question is: How much information about the process is lost as the quantizing interval is made larger? There are several aspects to the answer. First, Δ should be kept small enough to insure that events occurring at the highest possible rate will always have at least one empty bin between them. This eliminates the aliasing problem. Thus, the maximum value Δ should have for studying a single isolated neuron is 1/2 the absolute refractory time for the neuron. (When more than one neuron is observed simultaneously, we must also admit the necessity of calling their discharges simultaneous when they fall into the same time bin.) A more difficult question is how small Δ should be to make it possible to detect fluctuations in interval duration. This problem occurs primarily in the analysis of pacemakerlike units which have a high degree of regularity in interval duration. Obviously, the smaller Δ is, the greater will be the ability to detect fluctuations in interval duration. To see what the factors are that affect the analysis of such activity, we consider a simple model of pacemaker activity. This is a unit whose spike generation is a renewal process in which the interval z between successive spikes fluctuates or jitters. Let the fluctuating interval duration be described by a normal random variable (μ, σ). The expectation density for such a process is shown in Fig. 6.10. It is possible to show, using methods described by Huggins (1957), that this process has an expectation density given by

$$m(\tau) = \sum_{k=1}^{\infty} \frac{1}{\sigma\sqrt{2\pi k}} \exp\left[\frac{-(\tau - k\mu)^2}{2k\sigma^2}\right], \quad |\tau| > 0 \qquad (6.66)$$

As τ becomes large, $m(\tau)$ approaches $1/\mu = \nu$ as a limit. The Fourier transform of $m(\tau)$ is

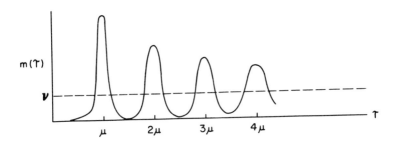

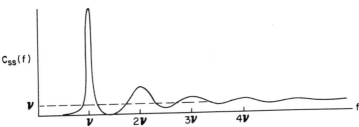

Fig. 6.10. Above, the expectation density $m(\tau)$ of a jittered renewal process whose intervals have a normal distribution. The average interval duration is μ sec. In this case there is a 10% interval fluctuation, i.e., the coefficient of variation $\sigma/\mu = .1$. Below, the power spectrum $C_{xx}(f)$ of the process. It is given by the equation $C_{xx}(f) = \nu[1 + M(f)] - \nu^2\delta(f)$. The 0 frequency term $\nu^2\delta(f)$ is not shown. The limiting value for $C_{xx}(f)$ as f becomes large is $\nu = 1/\mu$. Note that this is the same as for the expectation density.

$$M(f) = \frac{2G(f)[\cos 2\pi f\mu - G(f)]}{1 + G^2(f) - 2G(f) \cos 2\pi f\mu} \tag{6.67}$$

where $G(f)$ is the Gaussian function $\exp(-2\pi^2\sigma^2 f^2)$. The spectrum of the process can be obtained by substituting Eq. (6.67) into Eq. (6.52). The spectrum consists of a series of gradually diminishing and broadening peaks spaced at the harmonic frequencies ν, 2ν, ... The amplitude of the peak at the kth harmonic is given by

$$C_{ss}(k\nu) = \nu \frac{1 + G(k\nu)}{1 - G(k\nu)} \tag{6.68}$$

At high frequencies the spectrum becomes flat and equal to ν. The rate at which the peaks smooth out to the average is determined by the coefficient of variation of the intervals; the smaller it is, the slower the decay. This can be seen by evaluation of Eq. (6.68) when $f = k\nu$. For cvar[z] = 0.01, the peak at the 25th harmonic is still twice the average value of the spectrum. When cvar[z] = 0.1, the peak diminishes to 1.4 times the average value at the third harmonic. This is for the point process before it has been time quantized during the measurement of its intervals. What the quantization does is to suppress the higher frequency peaks. If we wish to make spectral measurements up to the Kth harmonic, we must choose $\Delta = \mu/2K$. Thus, if the process has a mean interval of 0.1 sec and we wish to distinguish the 25th harmonic, then $\Delta = 2$ msec. Once the time bin width has been selected, the ability to detect interval fluctuations will be determined by the average rate of the process. Fluctuations in high rate processes will be less detectable than those in slower ones. A limiting situation might be the desire to detect the presence of a 10% interval fluctuation in a process whose average interval duration is 10 msec. If we confine ourselves to a spectrum limited to the third harmonic of this process ($K = 3$), we have $\Delta = 1.67$ msec.

Besides the jittered process having peaks in the spectrum at the harmonic frequencies $k\nu$, the width of these peaks is also characteristic of the process. When the coefficient of interval variation is small, the width of these peaks between half amplitude points is, for small values of k, approximately $2\pi k^2 (\sigma/\mu)^2 \nu$.

That is, peak width is proportional to the square of the cvar[z]. This holds for jittered renewal processes in general. The ratio of peak width to peak separation is $2\pi k^2 (\sigma/\mu)^2$. For a process in which cvar[z] = 0.01, the width of the first peak is 6.2×10^{-3} Hz when $\mu = 100$ msec. When cvar[z] = 0.1 and $\mu = 10$ msec, the width of the first peak at 100 Hz is about 6 Hz. This means that in order to determine that this peak has breadth and is not a pure frequency component, a sufficiently long data record must be obtained, one that is consistent with the spectral resolution and variance considerations. Note also that if the spectrum is to be obtained by Fourier transformation of the expectation density, that density should be estimated out to sufficiently large values of τ so as to hold spectral leakage within the bounds required for determination of peak width. In the example of the 100/sec sequence with 10% jitter, an expectation density extending out to about 1 sec would be desirable. See Chapter 3.

6.14. THE SPECTRUM OF INTERVALS AND ITS RELATIONSHIP TO THE SERIAL CORRELOGRAM

There is an alternative spectral representation for point processes that is of importance. It is one that arises from considering the point process in terms of the intervals z_k between its successive events. The interval lengths are treated as though they were samples of a continuous band-limited process, always positive, whose independent variable is not time but the index k which refers to the position of the interval in the sequence of N intervals. The z_k are spaced one unit apart ($\Delta = 1$) along this axis. The discrete Fourier transform of an N interval specimen of this process of intervals is

$$Z_N(n) = \sum_{k=0}^{N-1} z_k \exp \frac{-j2\pi nk}{N}, \quad \frac{-N}{2} \leq n < \frac{N}{2} \qquad (6.69)$$

The index n is a harmonic of the fundamental frequency $1/N$ and can range up to the band-limiting frequency $1/2$. The average interval duration $\bar{z}$ is given by $Z_N(0)$. The sample spectrum or periodogram of the sequence $P_{zz}(n)$ is defined as

$$P_{zz}(n) = (1/N) \left| Z_N(n) \right|^2 \qquad (6.70)$$

This is the same as the definition of a continuous process. The average length of the intervals can be subtracted from the individual intervals before taking the DFT so as to make $Z_N(0) = 0$.

The major feature of the spectrum of the intervals is that it indicates the presence of periodicities in the duration of the intervals. It does this in terms not of time but of the ordinal separation of the intervals. Thus, if intervals in a nonrenewal process had a tendency to diminish and then lengthen in a cycle that was 10 intervals in duration, there would be a peak in the spectrum at a frequency of 1/10. This periodicity, however, tells us nothing of the event rate of the process. $P_{zz}(n)$ can also be seen to be the estimate of the spectrum of the serial covariances $c_{zz}(k)$ of the intervals where

$$c_{zz}(k) = E[(z_{m+k} - \mu_z)(z_m - \mu_z)] \tag{6.71}$$

The frequency of the interval fluctuation in real time can be estimated by $1/10\bar{z}$. The dimension of $P_{zz}(n)$ is (sec)(interval)^2. The integral of the spectrum over a range of frequencies gives the amount of interval fluctuation that is contributed by frequencies in that region. The total fluctuation in interval duration, the interval variance, is related to the spectrum by

$$\int_{-1/2}^{1/2} P_{zz}(f)\ df = \text{var}[z] \tag{6.72}$$

The mean interval has been removed so that $P_{zz}(0) = 0$. Similar statements can be made for the spectrum of serial correlation coefficients. A spectrum of intervals without peaks indicates, of course, a lack of periodicities in the interval generation process. Several tests for the flatness of the sample spectrum of intervals have been proposed (Cox and Lewis, 1966, and Lewis, 1972). Thus far they appear not to have been applied to neurophysiological spike data.

If one is interested in determining the relationship between individual point processes or between a point process and a concurrent continuous process, the spectrum obtained from serial correlograms presents a major difficulty: Time is not related simply to the frequency of its spectral representation. This makes it difficult to define a meaningful serial cross covariance function linking either the intervals of two point processes or the intervals of one point process with the amplitude of a continuous process. It seems, therefore, that the applicability of serial correlograms and their spectra is restricted to point processes in isolation. Here, they can reveal aspects of a point process that are not accessible to the expectation density and its spectrum. The reason for this can be understood by comparing the approaches used in arriving at the expectation density and the serial correlogram. For the expectation density, the point process is considered from the point of view of the counting process $N(t)$, the number of events which have occurred since the start of observation. $N(t)$ jumps by one unit at each event time. From $N(t)$ we derive the differential counting process $\Delta N(t)$ and then the expectation density. When it comes to the serial correlogram, the process is considered as a sequence of the intervals z_k between the kth event at t_k and the preceding event at t_{k-1}. The time from the start of observation (the event at $t = 0$) to the Kth event is

$$T_K = \sum_{k=1}^{K} z_k \tag{6.73}$$

Now at t_k the counting process assumes the value $N(t_k)$ and remains at this value until t_{k+1}. Therefore at those times prior to T, $N(t)$ will be less than $N(T_K) = K$. We can express this statement in the probabilistic relation

$$\text{prob}\{N(t) < K\} = \text{prob}\{T_K > t\} \tag{6.74}$$

This is the fundamental probability relation between the counting and interval representations of the point process. If we know one of these distributions, we also know the other. But in practice we are limited to far less: knowledge of the second-order properties of the counting process, the expectation density; or the second-order properties of the intervals, the serial correlogram. Neither one is adequate to obtain the other nor do they lead to the probability distribution of Eq. (6.74). Therefore, each has some information about the point process that the other does not. This is also true of their spectra. Consequently, there is value in considering a point process both as a counting process and as a sequence of intervals. Of the two, however, the counting process is more closely tied to time and therefore to other possibly related continuous and point processes.

While one can assume that spontaneous neuronal activity represents a response to an as yet unidentified and uncontrolled stimulus, it is more likely that it represents some ongoing neural state that is independent of external stimuli. It is not known whether spontaneous activity in itself conveys information from neuron to neuron. In a sense it may be closely analogous to the noise inherent in electronic communication systems. The properties of spontaneous activity can reveal to what extent it is a manifestation of (a) the physiological properties of the individual neuron, and (b) the connective properties of the neuronal network that the neuron forms a part of. But if we are to understand how the nervous system processes information, we must go beyond spontaneous activity and examine how neurons respond to external stimuli. It is within the stimulus-response relationships, obtained under a wide variety of stimulus parameters, that the key to information processing properties of the nervous system lies. The response of a neuron to a stimulus is determined in part by its synaptic relationships with other neurons and in part by its own cellular mechanisms. To some extent the latter are stochastic in nature so that the overall responsiveness of a neuron to an invariant stimulus is itself never invariant. This fluctuation of a neuron's activity in even the most well-controlled preparation is well established. It means that the description and interpretations of stimulus-response relationships must be made on a statistical basis that is closely connected to the properties of random processes. The study of stimulus-response relationships at the neuronal level begins most appropriately with the response of the isolated single neuron. Isolation here means that the experimenter considers the activity of only one neuron at a time, deliberately ignoring the activity of any other unit also being observed at the same time whether by the same microelectrode or another.

6.15. DRIVEN SINGLE UNIT ACTIVITY

A variety of useful experimental procedures and data processing techniques have been developed that permit some rather detailed analysis of the relationships between the stimulus and the responses of a single unit. To a large extent these have resulted from the use of the real-time computer for it gives the experimenter the ability to determine during the experiment whether the stimulus and the response are related and to ascertain which stimulus parameters are important in evoking a response. While the ultimate goal of these kinds of experiments is an understanding of the responsive behavior of groups of interacting neurons, most work thus far has been limited to studying the stimulus-response relationships of the single neuron. Many fundamental discoveries of nervous system behavior have been made in this area and a considerable amount of insight has been gained into the richness in the response of a single unit under a wide variety of experimental conditions. Although attention is now gradually shifting to the responsive behavior of groups of neurons, the techniques of analyzing the responses of a single unit are of fundamental importance for they can often be extended into techniques of analyzing the responses of several interacting neurons. At present these extensions are still rather incompletely developed and much work remains to be done on them.

A burst stimulus is one which is delivered to the preparation for only a brief period of time. Often the burst is repeated in a sequence which may or may not be periodic. For our purposes the particular modality of the stimulus is unimportant. It can be sensory, electrical or other. The properties of the stimulus that are important to us are its temporal and/or spectral representation:

351

(1) The duration of an individual burst;

(2) The nature of the sequence it forms a part of;

(3) The temporal variation of the stimulus parameters within the burst and within the sequence.

All of these are usually easily controlled by the experimenter. For example, intensity may be varied during each stimulus or it may be constant in a given stimulus but be altered for each stimulus in some predetermined way. Other stimulus parameters which may be varied are frequency (as in auditory stimulation) and physical location (as in tactile stimulation). One may also wish to deal with multiple stimuli delivered in the same or different stimulus modalities. The considerations that arise in such situations represent extensions of what can be said about the individual stimulus and we shall not deal with them. For an indication of what is involved in analyzing responses to multiple stimuli, see McCann (1974). The duration of the stimulus can range from the delta function to the continuous. In the latter case response analysis techniques are the same as in spontaneous activity except for the necessity of relating the response properties to the other, nontemporal parameters of the stimulus. When the stimulus is delivered in brief bursts, important new factors enter. These concern the relationships of the response to both (a) stimulus onset and termination, and (b) the temporal position of the burst stimulus within its own sequence. Just how significant these factors are can be appreciated by recognizing that a responsive unit, even if its spontaneous activity were stationary, becomes nonstationary for some period of time following the delivery of the stimulus. This nonstationarity in the response is prevalent in situations in which neural activity is influenced by habituation, adaptation, and accommodation. Consequently, many of the statistical tests for the spontaneously active process or the continuously stimulated one are inappropriate to use with burst stimuli. Other tests need to be employed which can deal with the prominent issue of describing the nature of the nonstationarities in unit activity.

Here the available statistical apparatus remains meager and cumbersome.

It is usually true of unit responsiveness that the effects of a stimulus gradually diminish with the passage of time, although the time course of diminution may differ according to the parameters of the stimulus. Adaptation and habituation effects may occur in the same experiment and can vary considerably in different parts of the nervous system and with the state of the animal. Separation of these effects from one another can be difficult. The slow changes brought about in a point process by habituation may be particularly troublesome because the number of neuronal spikes associated with any single stimulus may be small and the resulting response variability rather large. Such variability makes the discernment of slow changes in the process difficult to ascertain reliably. The situation is somewhat worse than with ongoing response processes since the latter often contain many more spikes and permit the use of more reliable statistical measures for detecting response changes.

The natural way of measuring the relationships between stimulus and response is to refer the spike event times in the response to the onset time of the stimulus. There are also occasions when response phenomena are more associated with the termination or offset of the stimulus and it is advantageous in those cases to refer response properties to the time of termination. When the burst stimulus is sufficiently brief to be characterized as an impulse, both onset and termination obviously occur simultaneously, resulting in some measurement simplification. Often the stimuli are temporally complex as when a stimulus parameter is graded during onset and offset or perhaps changes during the course of its delivery. In these circumstances, it is necessary to preserve the temporal features of the stimulus so that the more detailed relationships between stimulus and response can be established. Still, the most important information in a stimulus is its initial onset time or epoch. The times of other stimulus variations can be related to it.

Any neuron that can be driven by a stimulus exhibits a threshold effect: lack of response below a given stimulus intensity level, presence of a response above. The boundary intensity is the neuron's threshold, the lowest stimulus intensity which gives rise to a response that is measurably different from what is seen in the absence of a stimulus. An auditory click, for example, will evoke no response from a neuron in the auditory system if its intensity (sound pressure level) is too low. As intensity increases, a point will be reached at which the neuron's discharge activity indicates that it is being driven by the click: The pattern of spike activity departs from random and begins to show some form of "time locking" to the stimulus. As stimulus intensity increases above threshold, there is a more or less gradual transition in the strength of this locking of the neuron's response. The threshold stimulus intensity is that at which the neuron's response becomes distinguishable from its random spontaneous activity at some preassigned level of confidence. The criterion employed by the experimenter to test for this threshold may or may not correspond to that employed by the nervous system in establishing its own detection threshold. One important aspect of single unit threshold determination is to see how well it can be correlated with the behavioral threshold measures exhibited by the intact, conditioned animal of the same species, perhaps the one being recorded from.

The threshold measurement situation we consider here is one in which the observed neuron is discharging spontaneously. Observation of its discharge over a reasonably long period of time permits calculation of interval histograms, serial correlation coefficients or any other of the measures we have already discussed. In addition, when a sequence of stimuli is applied, peristimulus time histograms (to be discussed shortly) can be used to obtain a cross comparison of unit activity prior to stimulus delivery with that occurring after stimulus delivery. Any one of these unit activity measures can be examined to see whether it shows a significant alteration that is related to the presence of the stimulus. If so, the stimulus level is suprathreshold. It can be seen from this that a threshold level is best determined by examining the average response to a stimulus delivered a large number of times. If we look at the neural activity following just one of these near-threshold stimuli, it may be quite difficult to determine whether it represents a response to the stimulus (detection) or not. This is because the unit itself is operating upon weak signals in this situation, a few signal-conveying EPSPs immersed in the spontaneous EPSPs generated by other presynaptic cells and the intracellular noise of the neuron itself. The unit has to decide whether or not a stimulus has occurred. The probability of either decision is about equal. The detection principles describing the unit's response are quite similar to those involved in the behavioral responses animals make to sensory stimuli and in the psychophysical decisions humans make during signal detection tasks. Green and Swets (1966) have discussed threshold detection problems of this latter sort while Werner (1974) has related such psychophysical problems to single unit activity. We shall not pursue the matter.

When the observed neuron is not spontaneously active, any spike activity after stimulus delivery is an indication that the neuron has detected the presence of the stimulus. Usually as the stimulus intensity is increased, the proportion of stimuli to which the neuron responds increases until at intensities well above threshold, each stimulus is followed by a response of one or more spike discharges, with the initial one perhaps of varying latency. Under these conditions it is useful to refer to threshold as that intensity level which evokes a response to P% of the stimuli. P values between 10 and 50 are common criteria levels. Other facets of the response properties such as spike latencies (Kiang, 1965) and the number of spikes elicited by an individual stimulus (Mountcastle *et al.*, 1957) also can be considered.

Closely related to the problem of threshold response determination is the problem of determining how a neuron's response varies with some particular stimulus parameter. In these situations the neuron is already known to be responsive in some way to the stimulus. What we are concerned with is determining the extent to which the stimulus parameter must be changed before the neuron response is altered significantly. It may be seen that this approach is closely related to that of determining a detection threshold in the spontaneously active neruon. The problem now is to detect an alteration of unit activity that is correlated with the change in the stimulus. The alteration is not just a change from spontaneity but a change in such response properties as latency and number of spikes per response. If spontaneous activity is also present, it will tend to obscure what might otherwise be an easily detectable change. In the next section we consider the analysis of driven single unit activity from this point of view.

The stimulus onset times themselves can be considered to be events of another point process, commonly one which is repetitive and periodic. Increasingly, however, effort is being made to randomize stimulus delivery since this leads to certain advantages in response analyses that are not encountered with periodic stimulus delivery. Stimulus randomization minimizes the occurrence of anticipatory effects in awake animals. It also aids in frequency response analysis of neuronal activity even when behavioral factors are not relevant. This holds also for stimuli that are continuous rather than point processes (French, et al., 1972). Randomization of stimulus parameters, intensity, for example, tends to reduce the effects of temporal trends and other factors not related to the stimulus. Our interest here is only in randomization of stimulus delivery times. For this reason we consider the stimulus sequence as a point process representing the stimulus onset times. Response analysis can then be said to be an investigation of how one point process is related to another. This same point of view will be used in the next chapter when we discuss multiple unit activity.

6.16. PERISTIMULUS TIME HISTOGRAM ANALYSIS OF DRIVEN ACTIVITY

The spike activity evoked by a burst stimulus fits the description of a random evolutionary process. One of the most useful ways to analyze this driven activity is by means of histograms of the times from stimulus onset to any subsequent response. It is also useful to include within the histogram a measure of the unit's prestimulus activity. This serves as a baseline indicator of how the stimulus has altered the unit's activity. Such a histogram is easily constructed since the experimenter knows exactly when a stimulus is to occur. He merely makes the initial bin of the histogram correspond to a given time prior to the delivery of a stimulus. The duration of the histogram then covers the desired range of pre- and poststimulus time. For this reason the histogram is referred to as a peristimulus time histogram (PSTH).

The PSTH is an estimate of the cross expectation density $m_s(\tau)$, relating response events to stimulus onset. $m_s(\tau)$ is defined by

$$m_s(\tau)d\tau = \text{prob}\{\text{a response event occurs between } \tau$$
$$\text{and } \tau + d\tau | \text{stimulus onset at } \tau = 0\} \quad (6.75)$$

It can be seen to be an extension to two point processes of the expectation density of an isolated point process. A basic property of the cross expectation density is that for large values of τ, $m_s(\tau)$ approaches ν, the average rate of events when there is no stimulus. That is,

$$\lim_{\tau \to \infty} m_s(\tau) = \nu \quad (6.76)$$

This is similar to Eq. (6.50) since, as the time from the last stimulus increases, the process reverts to its spontaneous behavior. It may be that rather long periods of time are required before the limit is reached. When the stimulus-driven unit is not spontaneously active, the limiting value of $m_s(\tau)$ is, of course, 0. We must also be aware that the very act of stimulation may have altered the discharge process of the neuron so that there is a long-lasting, perhaps permanent alteration in its spontaneous acti- vity. This might occur, for example, during some form of learning situation. Equation (6.76) is to be interpreted, therefore, with restrictions such as this in mind.

Returning to the PSTH, we see that if, after N_s stimuli have been delivered, the $\tau°$ bin of the histogram has accumulated $n_{\tau°}$ responses, we arrive at an estimate of the cross expectation den- sity:

$$\hat{m}_s(\tau°\Delta) = n_{\tau°}/N_s\Delta \tag{6.77}$$

The cross expectation density leads also to the cross covariance function between the processes and thence to cross spectral de- scriptions of them. Both are considered in more detail in the next chapter.

6.17. TESTS FOR RESPONSE DEPENDENCY ON THE STIMULUS

Perhaps the simplest test for dependency of spike activity upon the stimulus is one which compares the average rate of spike activity occurring before and after a stimulus. In this procedure one compares the total number of spikes N_b that have occurred in some arbitrary T_b sec epoch before each of the N_s stimuli with the number of spikes N_a that have occurred in the T_a sec after. If the spike-generating process is reasonably close to either Poisson, Gaussian, or gamma, the difference between the two spike counts is amenable to a t-test (Burešová *et al.*, 1964). When the stimulus has no effect upon the unit activity, the estimates of before and after spike activity will originate from the same spike-generating process and should not differ significantly from one another. The null hypothesis, therefore, is that the spike-generating process

is stationary, unaffected by the stimulus and near enough to
Poisson to be suitable for the use of t-test statistics. When N_b
and N_a are large and $T_a = T_b$, the t-test takes the form

$$ t = \frac{N_a - N_b}{\sqrt{N_a + N_b}} \qquad (6.78) $$

The denominator is the estimated composite standard deviation for
the spike activity in the before and after epochs. The statistic
has the t distribution with $2(N_s - 1)$ degrees of freedom so that
the null hypothesis can be easily tested at any desired confidence
level with a two-tailed examination of t. When the Poisson assumption is not a good one, the composite standard deviation can be
estimated by methods described in Cox and Lewis (1966). These
tests deal with differences in average rates of occurrences, however, and are not particularly suited for determining whether the
process itself has changed. PST histograms should detect this.

This test of the ability of a stimulus to alter spike activity
is not a very strong one. For one thing, it disregards where the
spikes occur in the poststimulus epoch. Suppose, for example, that
for a brief time after stimulus delivery there is increased spike
activity followed by a transitory reduction in activity. This
alteration of the pattern of spike discharges could easily go undetected by a comparison of gross activity in the pre- and poststimulus epochs. The test has also been noted to be dependent to
some extent upon the suitability of the t-test to the process that
describes the spike activity. The less appropriate the t-test is
to the spontaneous or driven activity, the less is the assurance
that the test is a valid one. To get around such problems, nonparametric tests of spike activity can be used with advantage.
One example of these is the sign test (Bradley, 1968) which compares the number of pre- and poststimulus spikes on a trial-by-
trial basis. The judgment of stimulus effect upon the response
depends upon how frequently the number of prestimulus spikes exceeded poststimulus spikes or vice versa. The validity of the

test does not depend upon assumptions of the properties of the process. Trial-by-trial examinations also permit one to examine the response of the unit for the temporal trends that might be encountered in habituation or adaptation. Some of these aspects of unit activity are discussed in a later section.

More sensitive tests of unit dependency upon the stimulus can be based upon the poststimulus region of the PSTH. Under the null hypothesis that the neuron is unresponsive to the stimulus, $\hat{m}_s(\tau)$ will tend to a straight horizontal line indicating that a nerve spike is as equally likely to fall into any positive time bin of the PSTH. The mean height of the PSTH in this region is an estimate of the average unit activity following the stimulus onset. Departure of the PSTH from this average can be measured by its squared deviation from the line. If the number of bins in the poststimulus region is B_a and if N_a events occur there, the average bin population will be N_a/B_a. The actual number of intervals that fall into the τ°th bin is $n_{\tau°}$. The chi-squared statistic is an appropriate test for the departure of the experimental histogram from the straight line when N is large (Cramér, 1946). It is

$$y = \frac{B_a}{N_a} \sum_{\tau°=1}^{B_a} \left(m_{\tau°} - \frac{N_a}{B_a} \right)^2 = \frac{B_a}{N_a} \sum_{\tau°=1}^{B_a} n_{\tau°}^2 - N_a \qquad (6.79)$$

For large N_a, y has approximately the chi-squared distribution with B_{a-1} degrees of freedom as long as $N_a/B_a > 10$. Bins may have to be pooled to achieve this. Departure of the expectation density from a constant value can be tested at the desired level. If the experimental value exceeds this criterion, the null hypothesis that the neuron's response is not affected by the stimulus is rejected.

An alternative test deals with the histogram of the latency to the first event following stimulus delivery, $m_{s1}(\tau°)$. This is an estimate of the probability of time between stimulus onset and the first occurring response. Again, the null hypothesis is that the neuron is not affected by the stimulus. We assume that prior to application of a stimulus, the spontaneous activity of the neuron has been observed for a period of time sufficient to obtain a good estimate of its interspike interval distribution. With this distribution we can construct the estimated waiting time (or forward recurrence time) distribution (Cox and Lewis, 1966). This is the distribution for the length of time between an arbitrary event independent of the process and the next event within the process. If the stimulus has no effect on the unit's response, the onset time of any of the stimuli can be considered an arbitrary event. The waiting time distribution $r(\tau)$ for the spontaneous activity process is given by

$$r(\tau) = \nu R(\tau) \qquad (6.80)$$

where $R(\tau) = 1 - F(\tau)$ is the probability that an interval in the spontaneous activity process exceeds τ. $R(\tau)$ is also called the survivor function of the process. The waiting time distribution can be estimated from the histogram of spontaneous activity and can then be compared with the latency histograms obtained during the times of actual stimulation. The simplest way of doing this is by means of the same chi-squared goodness-of-fit test already discussed. The estimate of the histogram of the waiting time distribution is given by

$$r_{\tau^\circ}\Delta = \hat{\nu}\Delta \sum_{k=\tau^\circ+1}^{B} n_k \qquad (6.81)$$

B_a is chosen so that there are few intervals longer than $B_a\Delta$. These few are assigned the maximum length in the histogram in the estimation of r_{τ°. The chi-squared test then becomes

$$y = \frac{1}{N_a\Delta} \sum_{\tau^\circ=1}^{B_a} \frac{\left(n_{\tau^\circ} - N_a r_{\tau^\circ}\Delta\right)^2}{r_{\tau^\circ}} \qquad (6.82)$$

where N_a is the total number of poststimulus intervals obtained. For best results, $N_a/r_{\tau^\circ}\Delta > 10$ for all τ°; if not, bins should be pooled. Since the null hypothesis is that the latency histogram

361

is the same as the waiting time distribution and since Eq. (6.82) has the same form as Eq. (6.79), it is tested for in the same manner.

These two tests deal with experimental information in somewhat different ways and so they are not entirely equivalent. The peristimulus time histogram has used all the stimulus-response intervals that were shorter than $B_a \Delta$, whereas the waiting time histogram has used only the intervals between each stimulus and the first subsequent neuronal spike. It is difficult to say which is superior as a detector of stimulus-driven activity and better to consider them as complementing each other. Agreement of both test results provides more convincing results than either one would by itself. Should the results disagree, however, additional tests would be desired. Possible candidates would be tests involving the comparison of the spontaneous activity waiting times to the second and later events with latencies to the corresponding events following a stimulus. The test procedures would be the same as for the first-order tests.

6.18. RESPONSE TRENDS

The analysis of unit activity discussed here has assumed that a unit's responses to repetitive stimuli are ascribable to a process that does not vary from stimulus to stimulus. This means that the random differences that occur from response to response would not appear any different if we shuffled or randomized the stimulus order. In many situations because of evolutionary changes due to habituation, adaptation or learning, this is only an approximation to real unit activity, an approximation which can become more valid as the time between successive stimuli increases. But to ignore the phenomena of responsiveness changing with either time or stimulus order is unduly confining, for it removes from our consideration some of the most interesting properties of the nervous system. Though the added difficulties introduced into response analysis when such variations are encountered are substantial and much remains to be learned about how to deal with them, there are data processing techniques which merit consideration. Here we are interested in seeing whether temporal response trends can be detected by the change in the latencies of the responses to the stimuli as the stimulating process continues.

Let us consider examining the responses to a sequence of stimuli to see whether there is a trend in the latency time to the occurrence of the first spike after each stimulus. To do this we consider only the intervals between a stimulus onset and the first following spike and construct from them a new sequence of first response times. For N stimuli, the sequence will be N intervals long. If there is no response to a particular stimulus, the corresponding interval is the stimulus period. We wish to determine whether these fluctuating interval durations exhibit some increasing or decreasing trend during the duration of the stimulus process. For simplicity we begin with a situation in which the data appear to be reasonably fit by a time-dependent Poisson process (Cox and Lewis, 1966) whose rate is defined as $\nu(t) = \exp(\alpha + \beta t)$. The probability density for an interval that begins with the kth event at t_k is

$$\nu(t_{k+1}) \, \exp\left\{ -\int_{t_k}^{t_{k+1}} \nu(\mu) \, d\mu \right\} \qquad (6.83)$$

The exponential definition is preferred to a linear $\nu(t) = \alpha + \beta t$ because in the former the possibility of negative spike rates is precluded. β is a measure of how rapidly the process is changing with time. When $\beta = 0$, the process is trendless and the average rate of spikes is $\exp \alpha$. Positive β means that the average rate increases with time, while negative β means the average rate decreases with time.

An estimate of β is obtained from measurements of the N latencies measured from the onset of the sequence. A convenient way of estimating is by means of the likelihood function for the times of event occurrences (Cox and Lewis, 1966). When $|\beta t|$ is 0.1 or less, corresponding to a 10% or smaller change in $\nu(t)$ during the course of the observation, a Taylor's series expansion of the likelihood function shows that the maximum likelihood estimate for $\hat{\beta}$ is given by

$$\hat{\beta} \approx \frac{2}{t_N} - \left[\frac{N}{\sum_{k=1}^{N} t_k} \right] \tag{6.84}$$

The t_k are the event times while T_N is the time of occurrence of the Nth event and the duration of the entire sequence.

Although the estimated value $\hat{\beta}$ is of some interest in assessing the magnitude of a trend, what is usually of greater interest is the validity of the null hypothesis that there is no trend, that is, $\beta = 0$. In the trendless circumstance, it can be shown that the first $N - 1$ values of t_k are independent random variables uniformly distributed over the time interval from 0 to t_N. The distribution of their sum as N becomes large tends to the normal with mean $(N - 1)t_N/2$ and variance $(N - 1)t_N^2/12$. Thus, to see if the null hypothesis is to be accepted, we test the standardized random variable u which is approximately normal $(0, 1)$:

$$u = \frac{\frac{1}{N-1} \sum_{k=1}^{N-1} t_k - \frac{t_N}{2}}{t_N [1/12(N - 1)]^{1/2}} \tag{6.85}$$

We can fix the confidence limits within which to accept the null hypothesis by choice of the confidence level. If the null hypothesis is rejected, we can assign to β the value estimated in Eq. (6.84) provided that $|\beta T|$ is small.

The summation of the event times employed in Eqs. (6.84) and (6.85) is easily performed during an experiment. Therefore, testing for this type of trend can be done at the conclusion of an experimental trial or at any time later if the latencies are stored. One might, if desired, also compute the confidence limits for β (Cox and Lewis, 1966). Note finally that insofar as the process has Poisson characteristics, the test can be applied to interspike intervals arising either from spontaneous activity or from continuous stimulation.

The method of analyzing trend just described assumes a Poisson process varying slowly in one direction. The test efficiency deteriorates when this assumption is not valid, a not uncommon situation especially during stimulation. A Poisson process may not be a good description of the activity. For one thing, there is almost always some minimum latency between stimulus and response, and especially between successive responses. Trend-testing techniques that are not dependent upon the Poisson assumption can therefore be valuable. Cox and Lewis (1966) describe one such method which utilizes the "exponential scores" of the intervals. The exponential score of an interval is based upon its ranking by duration in the sequence. Although the score value assumes that the intervals are independently and exponentially distributed, it also turns out to be effective when the latter situation is not true. If the N intervals being considered are normalized so that their mean length is unity, the score or expected value of the rth smallest of them is (see Eq. (6.45):

$$e(r;N) = \sum_{i=1}^{r} \frac{1}{N - i + 1}, \qquad r = 1,2, \ldots, N \qquad (6.86)$$

The trend test examines the regression of interval score on its serial number in the sequence. It compares the value obtained with the value to be expected under the null hypothesis of no trend. This procedure seems reasonable when one is trying to ascertain a dependency of interval duration upon its position within its own sequence. The exponential score test seems to have good ability to detect trends in general renewal processes. For further details, see the reference cited.

Another aspect of trend analysis is the isolation of its effects from those produced by other sources of interval fluctuation. Sometimes these other sources may be deemed to be the more

physiologically interesting ones while the trend itself is considered to be in large part due to imperfect experimental conditions.
Because trend is inherently a slow or low frequency phenomenon, it
is amenable to removal by high frequency filtering techniques that
can be employed in a variety of ways. Firth (1966), while studying
the highly regular activity of crayfish stretch receptors, used a
filtering method based upon the fluctuations of higher order differences between interval durations. These are defined in the following way. $_1\Delta_k$ is the difference between the kth and the $(k + 1)$th
interval duration; $_2\Delta_k$ is the difference between $_1\Delta_{k-1}$ and $_1\Delta_k$.
The higher order differences are defined similarly. Differencing
is the discrete counterpart of the derivative operation on continuous data. Both perform high-pass filtering and remove low frequency
components from the data, though at the expense of emphasizing the
the high frequency components. The transfer function properties of
the differencing filters may be worked out according to the methods
introduced in Chapter 2. The higher the order of the difference,
the more strongly are the high frequency components weighted, with
the weighting increasing with frequency. This is acceptable in interval fluctuation analysis since, as we have seen, a sequence of
intervals may be considered to represent a process band limited to
$F = 1/2$. Firth's technique applies to the serial correlogram view
of a point process but other high-pass filtering techniques can be
devised for use with the expectation density approach. Spectral
analysis will itself tend to show the contribution of low frequency
trend components to interval variability.

Our discussion has covered only a limited aspect of temporal
changes in unit activity. Because one of the greatest challenges
the CNS offers us is to understand its plasticity, we need to develop a broad variety of tests for describing temporal change so
that we can examine what happens to unit activity during phenomena
such as learning, habituation, and adaptation. Finally, it is also
worth remarking that point processes have been used to describe
aspects of temporal change in CNS function other than those of

single unit activity. An interesting treatment of one of them, operant responses, is given by Weiss (1970).

6.19. DATA DISPLAYS

The meagerness of the available statistical techniques for the analysis of driven activity has prompted a good many innovative approaches to single unit data analysis, quantitative and qualitative. In the main these have concentrated on patterned visual presentations of the data. There are two reasons for this.

(1) The eye is highly capable of detecting order in the midst of apparent chaos. Visual data inspection often yields rather comprehensive insights into the nature of the response activity.

(2) The computer, while thus far limited in its ability to detect subtle response patterns, is quite adept at generating useful displays of large amounts of data.

These displays can be presented rapidly on cathode ray tubes during the course of an experiment, once the necessary preliminary computations have been made. They can also be preserved for examination after the experiment by a variety of techniques such as oscilloscope photography, plotter drawings, and magnetic tape storage. The visual display permits the observer to obtain a rather comprehensive picture of the results of an experiment and to form judgments as to the way the unit or units are responding to the stimuli. Subtle relationships, inaccessible to expectation density or serial correlogram approaches, may be made apparent. The weak point of a visual display is that the judgments based upon it are in the main qualitative and therefore somewhat unreliable statistically. We describe here one oscilloscopic display technique, the dot display (Wall, 1959). It has been widely useful in interpreting unit activity that is driven by brief, repeated stimuli. It appears to lend itself to the development of associated statistical tests. Hopefully, other display techniques with comparable utility will be

developed to handle the wide variety of stimulus situations that
are not so simply described.

In the dot display (Fig. 6.11) a cathode ray tube screen is

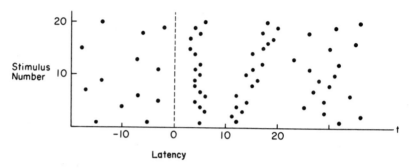

Fig. 6.11. Idealized dot display of single unit activity
before and after stimulus onset at t = 0. The second spike in
the response shows a trend toward increasing latency. The time
between consecutive stimuli exceeds the sweep duration.

scanned at constant speed horizontally from left to right in
raster fashion, the raster starting at the bottom. Each scan is
triggered a fixed time before stimulus onset in order to permit
the display of spontaneous activity prior to the stimulus. The
CRT beam is blanked during the scan except when a response occurs.
Then it is unblanked briefly and delivers a spot of light to the
screen at one point. The scan duration is set to be long enough
to display all the poststimulus responses of interest. If the
CRT has long persistence or is of the storage type, this spot will
be visible long after the response point has been registered.
When a sweep has been completed, the still blanked beam returns to
its leftmost position, slightly above its previous starting point.
A new sweep is started at the same fixed time before the next stimulus is delivered. The associated responses will appear along the
new sweep path as they are recorded. The upward displacement of
the beam with each new stimulus is determined by the number of
stimuli to be delivered and by the resolution capabilities of the
CRT. About 100 sweeps are typical for this type of presentation.

A simple way of recording the data, even on a nonpersistent CRT
screen, is by oscilloscopic photography. The dot presentation can
be generated with rather modest equipment with or without a real-
time computer. As Fig. 6.11 shows, it is quite easy to note when
the first, second, third, etc. responses occur to each of the stimuli and how the responses to each of the stimuli vary as the stimulation sequence proceeds. Furthermore, latency trends are visible.
They would be marked by gradual, orderly displacments of a response
pattern to the left or the right. Fig. 6.11 shows this in the increasing latency of the second spike in the response. Information
such as this is not available in the peristimulus time histogram
because the PSTH is indifferent to the order in which the stimuli
are delivered. The display also clearly indicates when spikes
that tend to have certain latencies are absent. This information
is also impossible to obtain from the ordinary PSTH.

The dot display provides a compact, easily comprehended
presentation of unit activity. Its format suggests the formulation
of tests which can be used for quantifying this activity, e.g.,
detection of trend in the latency between the stimulus and the
kth subsequent response. The dot display in modified form has
also proved to be of value in the study of multiple unit activity,
helping to determine how the activity of two and sometimes three
units are interrelated (Gerstein and Perkel, 1972; Perkel et al.,
1975). The displays of unit activity, called joint impulse configuration scatter diagrams, seem best suited to data analysis
after the completion of an experiment. They are discussed in more
detail in the following chapter.

REFERENCES

Abramowitz, M. and Stegun, I. A., "Handbook of Mathematical
     Functions," Dover, New York, 1965.
Arnett, D. W. and Ellert, B. M., *IEEE Trans. Biomed. Eng. BME*-23,
     65 (1976).
Burešová, O., Marusyeva, A. M., Bureš, J. and Fifková, E.,
     Physiol. Bohemosl. 13, 227 (1964).

Bradley, J. V., "Distribution-Free Statistical Tests," Prentice-Hall, Englewood Cliffs, 1968.

Courant, R., "Differential and Integral Calculus," Interscience, New York, 1937.

Cox, D. R. and Lewis, P. A. W., "The Statistical Analysis of Series of Events," Methuen, London, 1966.

Cramér, H., "Mathematical Methods of Statistics," Princeton Univ. Press, Princeton, 1946.

Davenport, W. B., Jr., and Root, W. L., "An Introduction to the Theory of Random Signals and Noise," McGraw-Hill, New York, 1958.

Ekholm A. and Hyvärinen, J., *Biophys. J.*, 10, 773 (1970).

Firth, D. R., *Biophys. J.*, 6, 201 (1966).

French, A. S. and Holden, A. V., *Kybernetik*, 8, 165 (1971).

French, A. S., Holden, A. V. and Stein, R. B., *Kybernetik*, 11, 15 (1972).

Gerstein, G. L. and Kiang, N. Y. S., *Biophys. J.*, 6, 15 (1960).

Gerstein, G. L. and Perkel, D. H., *Biophys. J.*, 12, 453 (1972).

Green, D. M. and Swets, J. A., "Signal Detection Theory and Psychophysics," Wiley, New York, 1966.

Huggins, W. H., *Proc. I.R.E.*, 45, 74 (1957).

Hyvärinen, J., *Acta Physiol. Scand.*, 68, Suppl. 278 (1966).

Kiang, N. Y. S., "Discharge Patterns of Single Fibers in the Cat's Auditory Nerve," MIT Press, Cambridge, 1965.

Kuffler, S. W., Fitzhugh, R. and Barlow, H. B., *J. Gen. Physiol.* 40, 683 (1957).

Lewis, P. A. W., *J. Sound Vibr.*, 12, 353 (1970).

Lewis, P. A. W., in "Stochastic Point Processes," (P. A. W. Lewis, ed.), p. 1. Wiley, New York, 1972.

McCann, G. D., *J. Neurophysiol.* 37, 869 (1974).

Moran, P. A. P., *Biometrika*, 54, 395 (1967).

Mountcastle, V. B., Davies, P. W., and Berman, A. L., *J. Neurophysiol.*, 20, 374 (1957).

Nakahama, H., Ishii, N. and Yamamoto, M., *Kybernetik*, 11, 61 (1972).

Nakahama, H., Ishii, N., Yamamoto, M. and Fujii, H., *Kybernetik*, 15, 47 (1974).

Nakahama, H., Ishii, N., Yamamoto, M., Fujii, H. and Obata, T., *Biol. Cybernetics*, 18, 191 (1975).

Parzen, E., "Stochastic Processes," Holden-Day, San Francisco, 1962.

Perkel, D. H., Gerstein, G. L. and Moore, G. P., *Biophys. J.*, 7, 391 (1967).

Perkel, D. H., Gerstein, G. L., Smith, M. S. and Tatton, W. G., *Brain Res.* 100, 271 (1975).

Poggio, G. F. and Viernstein, L. J., *J. Neurophysiol.*, 27, 517 (1964).

Smith, D. R. and Smith, G. K., *Biophys. J.*, 5, 47 (1965).

Wall, P. D., *J. Neurophysiol.*, 22, 305 (1959).

Weiss, B., in "The Theory of Reinforcement Schedules,"
    (W. N. Schoenfeld, ed.), p. 277. Appleton-Century-Crofts,
    New York, 1970.
Werner, G., in "Medical Physiology," (V. B. Mountcastle, ed.),
    Vol. 2, p. 551. Mosby, St. Louis, 1974.

Chapter 7

MULTIPLE UNIT ACTIVITY

7.1. INTRODUCTION

The view of neuronal organization provided by the study of single unit activity offers little more than a glimpse of the continual interplay of the excitatory and inhibitory interactions that occur within large populations of neurons. These interactions, however, cannot be deciphered by studying the activity of individually isolated cells, for such studies are essentially only reports of one participant's activity in a multiparty conversation. No matter how many solitary units we explore in this way, the dynamics of the neuronal interactions remain irretrievable. To understand these dynamics, how one neuron influences others and how it is itself influenced by them, it is necessary to study the concurrent activity of numbers of cells, starting with two and going on to as many as can be practically dealt with. In doing this, one encounters problems that are difficult and challenging both in their experimental and analytical facets. The problems of demonstrating the existence of a relationship between stimulus and response now becomes a search for relationships between the stimulus and each of the observed units and amongst the units themselves. The latter may exist even when the stimulus is absent or ineffective. The activity of the units may also differ qualitatively, e.g., some may be spontaneously active and others not. The diversity of experimental situations one may encounter practically guarantees that the analytical procedures adopted must be tailored to suit the different experimental conditions as they arise.

While the observed behavior of neurons during spontaneous activity can reveal something about the manner in which they interact, observations of their interactions assume even greater significance when the units respond to stimulation. During stimulation, the neural networks perform information processing associated with the tasks that evolutionary development has imposed upon them. Since stimulation can bring into use synaptic pathways which were inactive during spontaneous activity, it can expose aspects of the connectivity of the nervous system that spontaneous activity cannot. A stimulus which alters the activity of one or more observed units can do so in one of two ways. First, it can separately drive neurons which are functionally unrelated. In this case, the units' responsiveness to the stimulus may spuriously give them the appearance of being functionally related. Any analysis of concurrent unit activity must be capable of recognizing this situation. Second, the stimulus can act upon the observed neurons via common pathways within which the resultant activity is modulated by the units acting directly upon each other or indirectly via interneurons The two dependency situations for a pair of neurons are illustrated schematically in Fig. 7.1. Although the functional relationships between the units may be inferred from observations of their interactions, there is generally no synaptically stereotyped way by which they are realized. Only detailed physiological and anatomical correlations can reveal which realization the nervous system employs in any particular instance.

How can we analyze multiple unit activity in order to reveal unit interdependency (a) in the absence of a stimulus, and (b) in the presence of a stimulus? The initial step is to identify those pairs (triples, quadruples, etc.) of units whose activity does not conform to the null hypothesis of interdependence in spontaneous activity or during stimulation. Once this is done, we encounter problems of how to describe the dependencies. Here an ample array of possibilities confronts us. For example, we must determine as before whether the individual unit processes are Poisson, renewal, Markov, or even more complex, and whether they are stationary or not. Then we must decide the nature of the units' interactions. Does unit U depend upon unit V or vice versa or both? How does

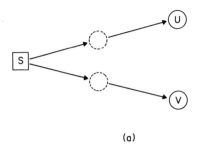

(a)

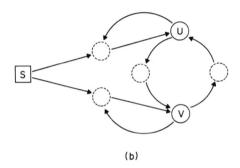

(b)

Fig. 7.1. (a) *Stimulus S acts upon neurons U and V through separate pathways. The arrows indicate synaptic influences that are either excitatory or inhibitory. The dashed circles here and in (b) indicate unobserved interneurons. There are no synaptic pathways between U and V. (b) The stimulus acts upon U and V through pathways influenced in part by the activity of U and V. The two units can also interact by pathways different from those taken by the stimulus.*

the activity of one unit affect the activity of the other and in what ways is this interdependence affected by the various parameters of a stimulus? Few, if any, of these problems are trivial ones. The methods proposed thus far to attack these problems still leave much to be desired in effectiveness and power. Furthermore, they are with few exceptions devoted to the study of pairs of units. While this is certainly a significant step beyond the study of isolated units, it is still unclear as to how fruitfully the techniques can be applied to three or more units. There also arise difficulties, to be discussed later in the chapter, of performing reliable identification of the unit discharges: which spike belongs to which neuron. In addition to this, the time required for data processing itself increases rapidly, perhaps factorially, with the number of concurrently active units. So does the cost. Thus, whether many of the subtleties of unit interactions will succumb to the kinds of data analysis discussed here remains to be seen.

There is no simple experimental recipe as to how to proceed in terms of data acquisition or analysis when dependency between units is suspected. Intuition is certainly the single most important factor in a multiple unit experiment just as it is with single unit work. Adroit manipulation of experimental parameters can make dependencies obvious which would not have been revealed by the most advanced of current data analytical techniques. But the limitations of intuition in real time are very well known, and sooner or later one must fall back upon unhurried data processing in the hopes of finding in the data what was not immediately apparent during the experiment. In this chapter we describe some of the tests and procedures that have been devised for revealing the nature of unit interdependencies.

7.2. CROSS-COVARIANCE METHODS

The analytical tests for unit interdependency that have received the most prominence are those based upon the second-order statistics of the units, with the units considered a pair at a time, unit U and unit V. What is involved are the cross-covariance properties of the units usually expressed in terms of cross-expectation densities (Perkel et al., 1967b; Moore et al., 1970), or cross-interval histograms (Gerstein, 1970). The procedure is to compare either of these with the results that would be expected under the null hypothesis of no unit interaction. If the experimental result is sufficiently different, the conclusion is that

the units do interact in some manner. A more detailed examination
of the same data can then reveal to some extent the nature of the
dependency, excitatory or inhibitory. Four possibilities are immediately apparent: (1) the activity of unit U depends upon that
of unit V or vice versa in a one-way fashion; (2) the activity of
each unit influences the other reciprocally; (3) one or both units
is under the influence of one or more unobserved units or the sti=
mulus itself; (4) some combination of all the foregoing. The different types of temporal interactions that may occur are nearly
endless. Furthermore, dependencies may be revealed only during
stimulation and then only under rather special stimulus conditions.
Many of the manifestations of inhibitory interactions fit this
description: they are not seen except when suitable stimuli are
employed.

Perkel and co-workers have examined the details of neuronal
interactions, availing themselves to a large extent of model simulation studies in which neuronal networks incorporating various
forms of excitatory and inhibitory couplings were synthesized by
computers. The individual elements in the simulated networks are
assigned some reasonable form of spike-generating mechanism and
the network is then activated. The behavior of the units is observed and analyzed by the same techniques used to study real
neuron activity. This procedure makes it possible to see how
different forms of excitatory and inhibitory couplings produce
different kinds of cross correlations or other measures of unit
interaction. Observations of similar behavior in real neurons
would then argue strongly, but not conclusively, that the real
neuronal network has the same properties as the model. Uniqueness
is not assured because it remains to be established that the interaction measures being studied display such behavior only under the
postulated set of circumstances or that alternative possibilities
can be rejected for other reasons. The approach is effective
although it is limited in its applicability mainly to units which

exhibit maintained activity in the presence or absence of stimulation. Even in this case, difficulties in deciding upon dependency
occur when the individual neurons exhibit pacemakerlike activity.
Such activity produces near-periodic rhythmicity in the cross correlation even when the units are independent. Thus, it is not a
simple matter to decide dependency merely on the basis of rhythmicity in the cross correlation. With these points in mind, we describe some cross-covariance analyses of unit interaction that are
based upon the use of the cross-expectation density and the cross-
interval histogram of spontaneously active and stimulated units.

A. CROSS-EXPECTATION DENSITY ANALYSIS

There are four types of intervals that enter into interdependency analyses of unit activity when a stimulus is absent:
$U-U$, $U-V$, $V-U$, $V-V$. A $U-U$ interval is one that starts and terminates with a spike from neuron U. A $U-V$ interval starts with a
spike from neuron U and terminates with a spike from neuron V.
$V-V$ and $V-U$ intervals are interpreted accordingly. The interval
measurements may or may not disregard the occurrence of intervening
events. Later on we specifically consider those intervals which
contain no intervening events. An additional pair of interval
types must be considered when an intermittent stimulus is present:
$S-U$ and $S-V$. The $S-S$ intervals themselves may be of importance
when their lengths are comparable to the other intervals or if
they themselves fluctuate because of some randomized stimulus
delivery schedule. When a repeated, intermittent stimulus is
present, we treat it as a third point process whose events represent the stimulus onset. (In some experiments it may be more
appropriate to let this process represent the times of stimulus
offset or the times of change of a stimulus parameter.)

The cross-expectation density (CED) for two spike processes
is a generalization of the expectation density for a single process. It deals with the times between events in one process and
those in another concurrently observed. The definition of the
CED is

$$m_{uv}(\tau) \ d\tau = \text{prob}\{V \text{ event in } (t + \tau, \ t + \tau + d\tau) \ | \ U \text{ event at } t\}$$

$$(7.1)$$

This is the conditional probability of intervals which start with a reference event in process U and terminate with a target event in process V. The V target event does not have to be the next V event following the U event; it is any V event that occurs with latency τ from the reference event. A corresponding cross-expectation density $m_{vu}(\tau)$ can be defined for intervals which start with a V reference event and terminate with a U target event. Since we can consider a UV interval either as one starting with a U reference event and terminating τ sec later with a V target event, or as one terminating with a V reference event after starting τ sec earlier with a U target event, the following relationship becomes obvious:

$$\nu_u m_{uv}(\tau) = \nu_v m_{vu}(-\tau) \tag{7.2}$$

where ν_u and ν_v are as before the average event rates in the two processes. Thus, the expectation densities m_{uv} and m_{vu} are derivable from each other when both the average firing rates are known.

B. *THE CROSS-EXPECTATION DENSITY DURING SPONTANEOUS ACTIVITY OR CONTINUOUS STIMULATION*

The cross-expectation density $m_{uv}(\tau)$ for two independently active units has a constant value independent of τ during spontaneous activity. Experimentally the CED estimate $\hat{m}_{uv}(\tau)$ is obtained by sorting UV intervals into a histogram whose abscissa represents the time between events. If there are B bins in the histogram each of width Δ, m_{uv} can be estimated by

$$\Delta \cdot \hat{m}_{uv}(b\Delta) = n_{bv} / N_u \Delta \tag{7.3}$$

where n_{bv} is the number of UV intervals falling into the bth bin and N_u is the number of U events triggering the histogram. That this is so can be seen by referring to Eq. (7.1) before the limit is taken. The probability there is estimated by the number of

events in $d\tau$ sec occurring per U event, n_{bv}/N_u. Replacing $d\tau$ by Δ,
Eq. (7.3) follows. Independence of the units is associated with a
constant value for $m_{uv}(\tau)$, and that is what $\hat{m}_{uv}(b\Delta)$ can be tested
for. Some methods for doing this have been described in Chapter 6.

The expectation density makes it possible, to a certain extent, to infer some of the detailed excitatory and inhibitory properties of the neuronal network. These inferences are suggested
by analysis of simulated neural networks that have had incorporated
within them the postulated synaptic connectivities. Unfortunately,
several types of connectivity may give rise to similar types of behavior of the expectation densities, and as a result, a unique
interpretation of the real data is not likely. Nonetheless,
it is possible by studying the expectation density properties of
simulated neural networks to obtain useful insights into the properties of real neural networks investigated by means of the CED.

A detailed study of the uses of the auto- and cross-expectation densities for revealing synaptic interaction has been made
by Moore *et al.* (1970) using both real data from *Aplysia* neurons
and simulated data from computer simulations. It is essential to
study the triad of expectation densities $m_{uv}(\tau)$, $m_{uu}(\tau)$, $m_{vv}(\tau)$
because the behavior of the latter two influences the first and a
valid interpretation of interaction cannot be obtained unless
these influences are known. As Moore *et al.* point out, features
of the presynaptic unit's expectation density show up in the CED
at both positive and negative values of τ, while features of the
postsynaptic unit's expectation density show up only in the positive τ region. Each type of network relationship can be considered
to exhibit a recognizable "signature" in the expectation density
triad. An example is shown in Fig. 7.2 for the case of simple
monosynaptic excitation. Two types of features on the CED have
been described, primary and secondary. The primary effect covers
the peaks and troughs near the origin and reflects the synaptic
potentials associated with mono- or polysynaptic excitatory or
inhibitory connections. The secondary effect covers features

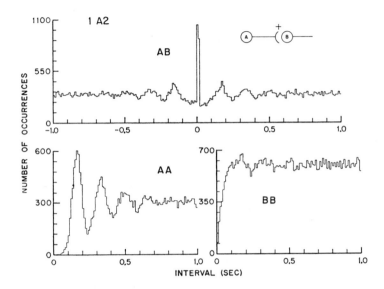

Fig. 7.2. The auto- and cross-expectation density histograms
when unit A excites unit B monosynaptically. The cross-expectation density is above, the expectation densities for A and B individually, below. [Adapted from Moore et al., Biophys. J., 10,
876 (1970). By permission of the publisher.]

occurring at longer time lags and reflects the properties of the
excitation densities of the pre- and postsynaptic units. In
Fig. 7.2 the primary effect is the sharp peak near the origin. It
is interpreted, because of the short delay, as representing a monosynaptic excitatory synapse between units A and B. The secondary
effect is the decaying wave at positive and negative τ which is
interpreted as arising from the rhythmicity of the presynaptic
unit A.

The use of the expectation density as a tool in investigating
synaptic interactions has the advantage of preserving time relationships between neural events. There arises, however, the question of whether spectral techniques might also be appropriate. In
particular, the coherence function discussed in Chapter 3 in connection with continuous processes may be of value here in refining
measures of interaction. Thus far, however, this approach has not
been investigated.

C. THE CROSS-EXPECTATION DENSITY DURING STIMULATION

It is useful to consider three different categories of relationship between the units and an applied stimulus.

(1) Units independent of one another and the stimulus. In this situation, the CED between neuron U and V will be unchanged during the time the stimulus is applied. The PST histograms for each unit will tend to be flat.

(2) Units independent of one another but either or both is driven by the stimulus. Here the PST histogram will depart from flatness for the unit that is influenced by the stimulus. There will also be a change exhibited in the CED between the two units but this change will be produced solely by the effects of the stimulus on the units individually. Perkel *et al* (1967b) have shown that when the stimulus is periodic, the cross-expectation density, $m^{\dagger}_{uv}(\tau)$, is given by the integral

$$m^{\dagger}_{uv}(\tau) = \int_{0}^{T_s} m_{su}(t) m_{sv}(t + \tau)\ dt \qquad (7.5)$$

T_s is the period between stimuli and the background activities have been first subtracted out from m_{su} and m_{sv}. The dagger indicates that a stimulus is present. This stimulus-induced change in the CED arises from the fact that t sec after the stimulus is delivered, there is a probability $m_{su}(t)$ that a spike from unit U will occur and τ sec later, the probability $m_{sv}(t + \tau)$ that a V spike will occur. Either of these probabilities may be different from the spontaneous situation, provided that the stimulus influences at least one of the units. The altered expectation density $m^{\dagger}_{uv}(\tau)$ is then obtained by an integration over all latencies from stimulus onset. If there are changes in the uniform rate of background activity caused by the stimulus, these will be present also in $m^{\dagger}_{uv}(\tau)$ and need to be taken into account. For a more detailed discussion, see Perkel *et al.* (1967b). Because $m^{\dagger}_{uv}(\tau)$ is derived entirely on the assumption that the stimulus affects the activity of U and V separately without regard to interactions between them, it can be used to test for independence of the units during stimulation. To do this we compare the estimate $\hat{m}^{\dagger}_{uv}(\tau)$, the estimated interunit CED histogram, with the convolution of $\hat{m}_{su}(\tau)$ and $\hat{m}_{sv}(\tau)$ as per Eq. (7.5). We accept independence if the difference between the two is not "significant."

An equivalent method of testing for the null hypothesis is to section the data from one of the units, say the V unit, at each of the N_s times of stimulus delivery. We then shuffle the sections randomly and determine a new cross-expectation density from the shuffled V and the unshuffled U sequences. Assuming that the interaction effects between units become negligible at time lags greater than a stimulus period, the shuffling will leave only stimulus-related effects. Shifting one of the unit records an integral number of stimulus periods with respect to the other produces the same effect. The shuffled or shifted CED will therefore exhibit only the effects of the stimulus acting separately on each of the units, essentially Eq. (7.5). Comparison of the shuffled and the unshuffled CEDs will permit judgment of whether the differences are great enough to infer the existence of unit interaction.

(3) Units that are interdependent and driven by the stimulus. In this situation the interunit CED in the absence of stimulation will be significantly different from uniform. When a stimulus is applied, unit activity may be altered because the stimulus has a direct effect upon the interdependency between the units. If interdependency is not affected, and if average unit spontaneous firing rates are unaltered, Perkel *et al.* (1967b) have shown that the interunit CED during stimulation will be just the sum of the unstimulated interunit expectation density and the correlation of the PST densities of the individual units. On the other hand, if the ongoing spontaneous activity of either process is altered during stimulation, this will displace the interunit expectation density upward or downward by an amount equal to the change in

average firing rate. The CED for the two responses during stimulation is $m'_{uv}(\tau)$. If we assume that the stimulus does not affect unit interaction, i.e., that the stimulus simply has an additive effect, we can predict that the CED will be (Perkel *et al.* (1976b).

$$m'_{uv,\text{pred}}(\tau) = m_{uv}(\tau) + \nu'_v + (1/\nu'_u T_s) \; m^\dagger_{uv}(\tau) \tag{7.6}$$

where ν'_u and ν'_v are the average rates of activity during stimulation for unit U and V. $m_{uv}(\tau)$ is the component of the stimulus-free cross-expectation density that remains after the constant background activity component has been subtracted out. $m^\dagger_{uv}(\tau)$ is the convolution of the individual stimulus-unit cross-expectation densities $m_{su}(\tau)$ and $m_{sv}(\tau)$, also with constant background contributions subtracted out. Our null hypothesis is that the stimulus affects the responsiveness of the units in the additive way described above. It implies that the stimulus does not alter the functional interdependency of the units. To test whether or not the stimulus alters the interdependency, we examine the difference $\hat{m}'_{uv}(\tau) - \hat{m}'_{uv,\text{pred}}(\tau)$. If the additivity assumption is valid, the difference can be shown to tend toward

$$\hat{m}'_{uv}(\tau) - \hat{m}'_{uv,\text{pred}}(\tau) = \hat{m}'_{uv}(\tau) - \hat{m}_{uv}(\tau) - \hat{\nu}'_v - (1/\hat{\nu}'_u T_s) \; m^\dagger_{uv}(\tau)$$

$$= \hat{m}'_{uv}(\tau) - \hat{m}_{uv}(\tau) - \nu'_v$$

$$- (1/\nu'_u T_s) \left[\hat{\nu}'_v + m'_{uv,\text{shuf}}(\tau) \right] \tag{7.7}$$

The estimate of $\hat{m}_{uv}(\tau)$ is available from the unit activity in the absence of stimulation while the estimates $\hat{m}'_{uv}(\tau)$ and $m_{uv,\text{shuf}}(\tau)$, $\hat{\nu}'_u$ and $\hat{\nu}'_v$, are taken from the data obtained with the stimulus applied. For conformity with the null hypothesis of no stimulus effect upon interaction, the right hand side of Eq. (7.7) will be small at all values of τ. It is thus possible to see the extent to which the stimulus alters the interdependency of the units. Since we are comparing shapes, we can also note the regions of τ where stimulus influence may be more pronounced.

The information that the CED can yield on unit behavior is limited because it does not preserve the temporal order in the original data either in a given poststimulus period or from one stimulus period to the next. Rather it involves averaging over the entire time of the data segment. When a stimulus is present, the averaging is also performed with respect to the period of stimulus repetition. Thus, the stimulus-related changes in unit activity that occur predominantly near the onset or cessation of the stimulus or over the course of many stimuli tend to be undetectable in the CED. So do slow nonstationary trends that are unrelated to the stimulus. The CED weights equally the activity at all times during and after the stimulus. Activity at poststimulus times where little has changed is combined with activity at other times where much has changed. Still, Perkel et al. (1967b) have pointed out that the ineffectiveness of the cross-expectation density as a detector of trends does not seriously impair its usefulness as an indicator of various forms of synaptic relationships. Consequently, as long as the trends are not severe, the CED can be employed beneficially in this regard. We shall shortly see that scatter diagrams preserve some of the temporal properties of the spike sequences and therefore can reveal details of unit activity that are not accessible by expectation density techniques. What is still needed, however, are more methods which preserve and exploit the temporal properties of unit activity. They have the greatest promise of revealing the connectivity properties of neuronal networks. Though spectral techniques that are related to expectation densities by the Fourier transform seem to be obvious candidates in this regard, they have not proved to be effective and so we do not discuss them.

7.3. INTERSPIKE INTERVAL TESTS FOR UNIT DEPENDENCY

A difficult problem associated with cross-covariance analysis is that we cannot be assured that two units are truly independent

when they exhibit no significant cross covariance even when their
spike sequences are stationary. The reason for this is that the
covariance measures are based upon the second-order properties of
the unit processes. That is, there is no guarantee that when point
processes are uncorrelated they are also independent. This clearly
leaves room for other tests that do consider the higher order properties and that could reveal forms of unit interactions not dis-
closed by cross covariance. Such tests should first be examined
for their utility by applying them to simulated neuronal networks
to see how capable they are of revealing different types of excitatory and inhibitory coupling.

While tests based upon the covariance properties of units do
have demonstrable weaknesses, they are useful and simple to apply.
In one form or another they can reveal some of the different aspects of unit interaction. In this regard, we describe two other
types of second-order statistics which may be useful. They deal
with pairs of units on the basis of the probability densities of
the intervals between neighboring events in the different processes.
These emphasize certain aspects of unit interactions which cross-
expectation densities do not. The first interval statistic to
discuss is the cross-interval histogram (Gerstein, 1970). It is
constructed in the following way for two processes. For each
event in one process, we measure the time to the next succeeding
or preceding event in the other process regardless of how many
other events in the first process have occurred in the interim.
We do this for each event observed in the U and V processes.
There result two histograms, one based upon U events as references
and V events as targets, and the other based upon V events as
references with U events as targets. If the two processes are
independent, each histogram is an estimate of a waiting time distribution, the time measured from an arbitrary origin (the reference event) to the first event of the other (target) process.
The waiting time distribution for the V process is defined (Cox
and Lewis, 1966) as

$$w_v(t) = v_v[1 - F_v(t)] \qquad (7.8)$$

v_v is the average rate of V events and $F_v(t)$ is the cumulative distribution function for intervals in the isolated V process. A way, then, to test for dependence between processes is to compare the two cross-interval histograms with the estimated waiting time distributions as obtained from the individual processes in isolation. Significant differences in either comparison would lead to rejection of the null hypothesis of independence. Figure 7.3 shows an

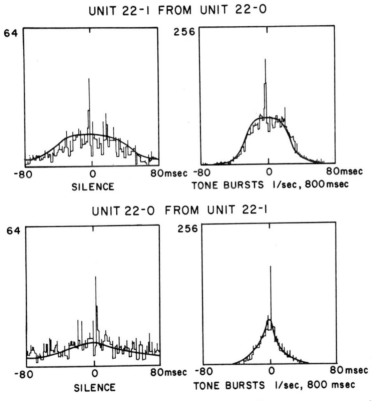

Fig. 7.3. Cross-interval histograms from two neurons in cat cochlear nucleus. The upper records are obtained with respect to leading events from one unit, the lower records are with respect to leading events from the other unit. [Adapted from Gerstein in "The Neurosciences. Second Study Program," (F. O. Schmitt, ed.), p. 648. Rockefeller Univ. Press, New York, 1970. By permission of the publisher.]

an example of cross-interval histograms obtained from a pair of cat cochlear nucleus neurons with stimulus absent and present. The sharp peaks near 3 msec permit two possible interpretations: (a) there is a direct or indirect synaptic connection between the two units such that one tends to fire 3 msec earlier than the other; (b) both units are independent but are separately driven by a third, unseen neuron. The data do not, by themselves, permit resolution of this issue. Note that over large regions of the histogram there is no marked difference between the data and the control situation (assumed independence). This means that tests, such as the chi-squared one, based on overall shape differences will not be adequate to detect departures from the null hypothesis. Instead, a detailed examination of the interval histogram over the entire time axis is required to ascertain regions where there may be marked local differences.

The second method for utilizing interval statistics deals only with the first-order intervals associated with neighboring events. These intervals are somewhat complex to deal with analytically. However, they are easy to measure experimentally and for this reason they offer promise in testing for dependence between pairs of units selected from a large population of observed units. The null hypothesis we are interested in testing is that two units with stationary ongoing activity are independent of one another. The units can be either spontaneously active or observed during a period of continuous stimulation. Under this hypothesis we can predict the probability functions for the four possible types of interunit interspike intervals when we know the properties of each unit's activity by itself. These predicted probability functions can then be compared with the experimental data relating the activity of unit U to unit V. If there is a large enough discrepancy between predicted and experimental values, the units will be said to be dependent. The nature of their dependency then remains to be explored.

The four types of interspike intervals to consider are

(1) *UU* intervals, the intervals between two consecutive *U* events or spikes, *with no intervening V events*. We call these resident intervals.

(2) *UV* intervals, the interval between a *U* event and a *V* event, *with no other events intervening*. We call these transition intervals.

(3) *VV* intervals, defined in the same way as the *UU*.

(4) *VU* intervals, defined in the same way as the *UV*.

For each of these types of intervals, interval histograms are easily obtainable. Also easily obtainable are the ordinary interval histograms for the *U* and *V* units considered individually (in isolation). Let us define a probability function $q_{uu}(t)$ for the resident intervals between consecutive *U* events in the interleaved sequence of *U* and *V* events:

$$q_{uu}(t) \, dt = \text{prob\{next } U \text{ event between } t \text{ and } t + dt \,|$$
$$U \text{ event at } t = 0 \text{ and no intervening } V \text{ events\}}$$

This conditional interval density function (CIDF) requires that the *V* unit be silent between two consecutive *U* spike occurrences. The integral of $q_{uu}(t)$ over all positive values of t is Q_{uu}, the fraction of *UU* intervals in the total population of intervals. It is less than unity, indicating that the CIDF is not a true probability density function. Nonetheless, it is quite useful to us particularly when the *U* and *V* processes are independent. In that situation we can compute $q_{uu}(t)$ by utilizing the waiting time or forward recurrence time probability density for the *V* process in isolation, $w_v(t)$. In the case of interleaved *U* and *V* processes, the arbitrary instant for determining a *V* event waiting time is the time of the leading *U* event. Then in order to have a *UU* resident interval, the *V* process waiting time must exceed t. If $p_u(t)$ is the probability density function for isolated *UU* intervals, i.e., ignoring all *V* events, we find

$$q_{uu}(t) \ dt = p_u(t) \ dt \int_t^\infty w_v(x) \ dx$$

$$= \left[v_v p_u(t) \int_t^\infty \{1 - F_v(x)\} \ dx \right] dt \qquad (7.9)$$

A similar equation can be written for the $q_{vv}(t)$, the CIDF for VV resident intervals:

$$q_{vv}(t) \ dt = \left[v_u p_v(t) \int_t^\infty \{1 - F_u(x)\} \ dx \right] dt \qquad (7.10)$$

We can also define CIDFs for the UV and VU transition intervals:

$q_{uv}(t) \ dt = $ prob{next V event between t and $t + dt|$

U event at $t = 0$ and no intervening U events}

A similar definition holds for the VU transition intervals. The equation for $q_{uv}(t)$ and $q_{vu}(t)$ are somewhat simpler to arrive at. Consider the UV transition intervals; here the waiting time distribution also applies. But now the waiting time to the next V event must be shorter than the time to the next U event. Thus we can write

$$q_{uv}(t) \ dt = w_v \ dt [1 - F_v(t)]$$

$$= v_v [1 - F_v(t)] [1 - F_u(t)] \ dt \qquad (7.11)$$

Interchange of the subscripts in the above equation shows that $q_{uv}(t)$ and $q_{vu}(t)$ are proportional:

$$q_{vu}(t) = v_u [1 - F_v(t)] [1 - F_u(t)] \ dt \qquad (7.12)$$

Therefore, under the condition of independence, the distribution of UV transition intervals has the same shape as that for the VU transition intervals. This can be applicable to the situation in which one is interested in determining whether an individual unit U responds to a randomized stimulus sequence that is represented by the V process. A test based on the similarity in the shapes of the $q_{uv}(t)$ and $q_{vu}(t)$ histograms can help to decide the dependency question regardless of what the shapes of the interval distributions of the V and U processes in isolation may be.

Equations (7.9) to (7.12) provide the opportunity to test units for independence under the stated assumption of stationarity. Estimates of the $p(t)$ and $F(t)$ are available for each unit from the experimental data, and from them estimates of the CIDF that would prevail under independence can be computed. These can then be compared with the actual CIDF. The extent to which these functions are similar in shape determines whether independence is accepted. For this purpose statistics such as the distribution-free Kolmogirov-Smirnov or Cramér-von Mises tests (Cox and Lewis, 1966) or the chi-squared goodness-of-fit test (Cramér, 1946) seem to be applicable to the normalized distribution functions of the $q(t)$, that is, to interval distributions put in the form

$$F_{uu}(t) = \frac{1}{Q_{uu}} \int_0^t q_{uu}(x)\ dx \qquad (7.13)$$

While the CIDF holds for stationary point processes in general, when the processes are renewal and Poisson with average rates ν_u and ν_v, some simplification results. It then becomes possible to compute how much each interval type contributes to the total number of intervals measured. We show this for the intervals that begin and end with a U event. Let the fraction of intervals in the total population that begin with a U event and end with a V event be P_{uu} where

$$
\begin{aligned}
P_{uu} =\ & \text{prob\{first event is a } U \text{ event\}} \\
& \cdot \text{prob\{second event is a } U \text{ event}| \\
& \text{first event is a } U \text{ event\}}
\end{aligned}
\qquad (7.14)
$$

The first probability in the above expression is just $\nu_u/(\nu_u + \nu_v)$ and the second probability is the integral of $q_{uu}(t)$. Thus,

$$P_{uu} = \frac{\nu_u}{\nu_u + \nu_v} \int_0^\infty q_{uu}(t) \; dt \qquad (7.15)$$

When both the U and V processes are Poisson, it is a straightforward matter using Eq. (7.9) in Eq. (7.15) to show that the transition probabilities are

$$P_{uu} = \nu_u^2 / (\nu_u + \nu_v)^2 \qquad (7.16)$$

Similarly,

$$P_{uv} = \nu_u \nu_v / (\nu_u + \nu_v)^2$$

$$P_{vv} = \nu_v^2 / (\nu_u + \nu_v)^2 \qquad (7.17)$$

$$P_{vu} = P_{uv}$$

From this it can be seen that $P_{uu} + P_{uv} + P_{vv} + P_{vu} = 1$ as required. As an example, let the average rate of the V process be twice that of the U. Then $\nu_u = 2\nu_v$ and $P_{uu} = 4/9$, $P_{vv} = 1/9$, $P_{uv} = P_{vu} = 2/9$. The departure of the processes from independence can be tested by measuring the average rate of events in each process and the relative fraction of each type of interval, and then comparing these fractions with those to be expected under the condition of independence. Since the P's may be considered as components of a density function and P_{uv} and P_{vu} are constrained to be equal, a chi-squared test with 2 degrees of freedom is appropriate for this purpose. When the processes are renewal but not Poisson, simple relationships like this do not occur and the probabilities associated with the null hypothesis must be determined from Eqs. (7.8) through (7.11) before the P's can be tested.

The ability of the test to detect dependence has been tested in a simple situation in which the U process was Poisson and the V process a replica of it delayed in time by the average interval between events. This yields transition probabilities of 0.216 for UU and VV intervals, and 0.283 for UV and VU intervals. The transition probabilities would all be 0.25 if U and V were

independent, equal rate Poisson processes. The difference between
the corresponding probabilities is 13.6%. Tests of data sequences
about 1500 transition intervals in length consistently rejected the
null hypothesis of independence at better than a 0.001 confidence
level. The decision to reject the null hypothesis could have been
arrived at by examination of the cross expectation but that technique is computationally more complex.

When a stimulus process S is present, the method may be
applied to see if the stimulus is effective in driving either unit.
One may also test whether the stimulus affects the relationship
between the units by comparing the several types of interspike
interval histograms and transition probabilities obtained in the
presence of the stimulus with those that are found in its absence.
Changes, for example, in the UV and VU intervals would be indicative of a stimulus effect upon unit interactions. Another possible
application is to multiunit analysis when three or more units are
observed. In this situation, the test may make it possible to
identify rapidly those units which are interdependent so as to
permit the investigator to concentrate his attention solely upon
them and disregard the independent units.

The independence proposed here is not based upon expectation
densities or serial correlograms, and so examines a somewhat different aspect of the unit relationships than those described by
Perkel et al. (1967b) and Moore et al. (1970). Such tests look
for independence on the basis of the second-order or covariance
properties of the processes. It is well known that processes can
be dependent and still exhibit lack of covariance. The test described here is in a sense, then, complementary to covariance
tests because it is based upon interval density functions and not
covariances or correlations. Both tests can be used to see if
independence prevails. If either fails, the units are dependent.
But independence is not guaranteed even if both indicate it to be
probable. Also it is not clear how the test might fare with units
which act like pacemakers. As Perkel et al. (1967b) have pointed

out, false attributions of dependence to independent pacemakers can easily occur with tests based upon expectation densities.

The interval densities described here fall far short of describing the full relationship between stationary processes. To do so it would be necessary to consider the distributions of such intervals as, for example, those between one U event and the second one following it with no, one or two, etc., V events intervening. This clearly complicates the analysis drastically. Since we have only considered the intervals between neighboring events, the resulting view of process interdependency is, in a sense, as fragmentary and incomplete as that provided by expectation densities.

7.4. DATA DISPLAYS FOR TWO STIMULATED UNITS-- THE PERISTIMULUS TIME SCATTER DIAGRAM

When stimulation is applied to two or more simultaneously observed units, stationarity assumptions which may have been valid in the absence of stimulation tend to be no longer so. What one needs is a means for conveniently examining both the interactions between the discharging units and their relationship to the stimulus. A promising technique for application to this three-way situation is the peristimulus time (PST) scatter diagram of Gerstein and Perkel (1969). It is a computer-generated dot display of the simultaneous activity of the responsive units in relation to the times of stimulus delivery. The scheme for generating the display is shown in Fig. 7.4. The origin of the display represents the stimulus onset time. The ordinate axis represents the time t_u from stimulus onset to the occurrence of a U spike; the abscissal axis represents the corresponding time t_v to a V spike. Consider that following the delivery of the ith stimulus S_i there occurs a single U spike at latency t_{u1}. This latency is represented as a horizontal line in the diagram. Suppose the same stimulus evoked spikes from the V unit at latencies t_{v1}, t_{v2}, t_{v3}. These latencies are represented as vertical lines. The points of intersection of the horizontal and vertical lines are the UV response pairs contri-

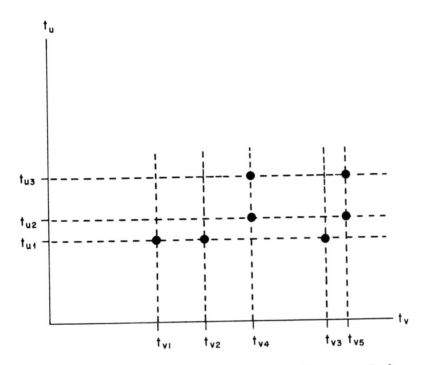

Fig. 7.4. The peristimulus time scatter diagram. Each point represents a pair of responses to a particular stimulus. Here the responses to the first stimulus are t_{u1}; t_{v1}, t_{v2}, t_{v3}. The responses to the second stimulus are t_{u2}, t_{u3}; t_{v4}, t_{v5}.

buting to the scatter diagram. For a single stimulus, the number of points placed in the diagram is the product of the number of U and V events associated with it. The total number of points on the PST diagram is the sum of these products for each individual stimulus. Note that the diagram does not reveal which response pair is associated with which stimulus.

The scatter diagram presents a clear visual indication of how the units may be related to the stimulus and to one another. Should there be qualitative positive indications of dependency, the data used to construct the diagrams can be employed in more quantitative statistical tests. Some of the modes of interaction which the scatter diagram is capable of dealing with are

(1) The stimulus has no effect upon mutually independent units U and V.

(2) The stimulus excites unit U or V or both.

(3) The stimulus inhibits unit U or V or both.

(4) Unit U excites unit V or vice versa.

(5) Unit U inhibits unit V or vice versa.

(6) U and V interaction is modulated by another unit or units controlled by the stimulus.

There may also be combinations of these interactions such as unit U being excited and unit V inhibited by the stimulus. Each of these conditions results in a display whose gross features are characteristic in the manner described below.

(1) Units independent of each other and the stimulus. The points are distributed uniformly at random over the display so that the density of points in any small area tends to be constant and independent of its location.

(2) The stimulus excites one or both units. If only the U unit is excited, the dots in the display tend to cluster in a horizontal band whose distance from the t_v axis is a measure of the latency of the driven activity produced in the U unit. Elsewhere in the display the points will tend to be distributed uniformly and randomly. If it is the V unit that is driven, the band will be vertical and its distance from the t_u axis will be the latency measure. Simultaneous independent excitation of both units produces both vertical and horizontal band clusters. (See Fig. 7.5a.)

(3) Stimulus inhibits unit U or V or both. The inhibitory effect reduces the activity in the U unit for a brief interval of time. This will be visible as a relatively clear horizontal band in the display. The distance of the band from the t_v axis corresponds to the latency measure. V unit inhibition produces equivalent effects along the other axis. If U and V are independent and both inhibited by the stimulus, there will be clear vertical and horizontal bands in the display (Fig. 7.5b).

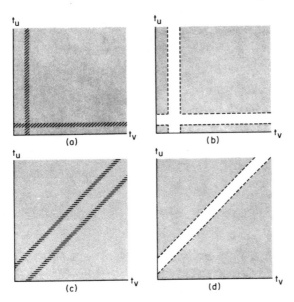

Fig. 7.5. Schematized representation of the PST scatter diagram for four different situations: (a) both units are independent and excited by the stimulus; (b) both units are independent and inhibited by the stimulus; (c) the units are excited by each other and not driven by the stimulus; (d) V inhibits U and neither is affected by the stimulus. The gray background indicates a low density uniform distribution of points.

(4) Unit U excites unit V. Each discharge of the U unit produces a marked increase in the firing probability of the V unit for a brief period of time afterward. The synaptic linkage may in fact be strong enough to produce an almost certain firing of the V unit at a fixed latency after the U unit discharge. In this situation, the dependency of V firings upon U activity will be marked by a narrow band of dots at a 45° angle slightly to the right of or below the diagonal through the origin. The breadth of the band is a measure of the time period after the U discharge during which V firing probability is enhanced. If the V unit drives the U, the band is to the left of and above the 45° diagonal. If there is mutual facilitation wherein each unit's activity

enhances the firing of the other, the band will tend to fall on both sides of the diagonal (Fig. 7.5c).

(5) Unit U inhibits unit V. The presence of inhibitory interaction is marked by a diagonal band relatively free of dots in the same location where excitation had produced a high clustering of dots. That is, when the U unit inhibits the V, the clear band will be below or to the right of the main diagonal. Inhibition of U by V moves the band to the other side of the diagonal (Fig. 7.5d).

(6) U and V interaction is modulated by other units controlled by the stimulus. This is a situation in which the U and V units interact even in the absence of a stimulus. Dark or clear bands are seen along the diagonal during spontaneous activity (stimulus intensity of zero). If, when a stimulus is applied, a change in the band density is observed which is time-locked to the stimulus, that is, a density change is found at certain latencies, it can be inferred that unobserved neural units are altering the firing probabilities of either cell. One such possibility is that there is one or more interneurons interposed between the dependent cells and that their activity is affected by the presence of the stimulus. Another possibility is that the driving neuron, either U or V, is affected by other neurons which are themselves driven by the stimulus. A third possibility is that the driven neuron, either V or U, is affected by other stimulus-related neurons which alter its ability to respond to the driving cell. All these situations may coexist in greater or less degree in any particular situation. It can be seen that the interpretation of the scatter diagram requires care and can be of great value. Further discussion is given by Moore et al. (1970).

The scatter diagram approach may be extended to the study of three interacting units with the construction of a three-dimensional scatter diagram first employed by Kristan and Gerstein (1970). Gerstein and Perkel (1972) have applied quantitative techniques to the scatter diagram. These include the use of a control scatter diagram derived from the original data by a shuffling technique. The control diagram forms the basis for testing various hypotheses about unit interactions. They have also discussed use of the diagram to study three or more interacting neurons, with and without a stimulus.

A limitation of the scatter diagram is its inability to preserve information regarding trendlike changes in response patterns related either to time or stimulus number. A possible remedy to this defect is to use a three-dimensional scatter diagram in which the third axis represents the order of the stimulus. The other two axes represent the U and V latencies as before. For a given stimulus in a sequence, the U-V activity plane contains only the corresponding activity of U and V responses. A view of the entire three-dimensional diagram may then demonstrate trends in unit interactions.

It is worth pointing out that while the scatter diagrams have provided us with an increased ability to discern different kinds of dependencies, the statistical reliability of these findings is less than that attainable from the PST histograms and cross-expectation densities that are derived from the same data. This is because the latter are marginal distributions of the scatter diagrams. They collapse the two-dimensional data onto a single dimension, thereby bringing about a decrease in the variance of the estimates. To obtain comparably low variance estimates from scatter diagrams requires that we use a substantially longer length of data--by a factor dependent upon the bin width. For a variety of experimental reasons this is often impractical and so we should view scatter diagrams not as replacing the other less penetrating interaction measures but as supplementing them. It is best to use our measures (and the controls that accompany them) in order to maximize the reliability of our interpretations of neuronal interactions. This is likely to apply equally well to newer methods of analysis as they are developed.

7.5. DATA DISPLAYS FOR THREE UNITS--
THE SNOWFLAKE DIAGRAM

The dot display technique developed first for the stimulated single unit and then extended to pairs of stimulated units has been extended to cover three unstimulated (or continuously stimulated) units by Perkel *et al.* (1975). The three unit display is formally called a joint interval configuration scatter diagram and more succinctly a "snowflake" diagram because of its hexagonal appearance. In it, individual points represent the three-way time intervals between spike events in one process and those in the other processes. It is intended principally for off-line classification and description of unit interactions in terms of the neuronal circuitry. This is done by detailed examination of the pattern of points in the display. The display's principle of construction is shown in Fig. 7.6a. The three units are here labeled *A, B, C.* Intervals between *A* and *B* spikes are measured along the *AB* axis. A positive distance means that the *B* spike occurs later than the *A* spike, i.e., $t_B - t_A > 0$. A negative distance means the opposite. The same is true for the other two axes: Positive distances along the *BC* and *CA* axes mean, respectively, that $t_C - t_B > 0$ and $t_A - t_C > 0$. Any triad of spikes, one from each unit, will be characterized by the times between them: $t_B - t_A$, $t_C - t_B$, $t_A - t_C$. If any two are known, the other is uniquely determined. This follows from the obvious identity

$$(t_B - t_A) + (t_C - t_B) + (t_A - t_C) = 0 \qquad (7.19)$$

The point corresponding to a particular event triad is plotted by laying off the appropriate times along any two of the axes. Perpendicular lines drawn from the end points of these vectors intersect in the desired point *P*. A perpendicular dropped from this point to the third point will yield the third interevent interval. This can be proved by elementary geometry. The point *P* thus uniquely defines the triad of spike intervals. It falls into different regions of the diagram according to the order of spike

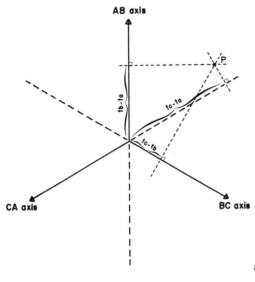

a

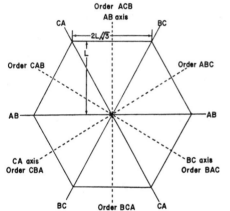

b

Fig. 7.6. Above, how a point in the snow-flake diagram is uniquely determined from the time intervals between any two of a set of three events. The AB axis measures time from A to B events and similarly for the axes. Below, in the sector "order ACB" the sequence of events is ACB, and similarly for the other sectors. L is the maximum interval plotted for any event triad. [From Perkel et al., Brain Res., 100, 271 (1975). By permission of the publisher.]

precedence. For example, any point above the horizontal axis represents a triad in which the B event occurs after the A event. The order of occurrence can be specified more precisely according to the 60° sector of the diagram P falls into. In the upper sector centered on the AB axis, Fig. 7.6b, it can be deduced that the temporal order of spikes is ACB. Each pie-shaped sector has its own spike order which is indicated in the illustration. The lines labeled AB, BC, and CA are the loci where the corresponding event times coincide. That is, along the BC "coincidence" line $t_B = t_C$.

Additional properties of the snowflake diagram may be found in Perkel *et al.* (1975).

We construct the snowflake diagram from a T sec record of the three units, by considering all event triads whose length between extreme events does not exceed L. Each triad is plotted as a point. The same event can be a member of many triads and contribute to the location of many points. To see approximately how many, assume the three processes are independent and random with rates v_A, v_B, and v_C. If a diagram is constructed with maximum event separation L, there will be about $3v_A v_B v_C L^2 T$ points in it. In time T, about $(v_A + v_B + v_C)T$ events will have occurred. This means that each event will contribute about $3[v_A v_B v_C/(v_A + v_B + v_C)]L^2$ points to the display. It is this participation of an event in many points which gives the snowflake plot the ability to expose discharge patterns and help identify interneuronal relationships. The patterns are similar in some respects to those described in the PST scatter diagram but, because a third unit participates, the snowflake diagram can reveal additional complexities of synaptic interaction. A fuller description of interaction patterns may be found in the reference. Here we summarize several of them briefly in terms of the display feature and the associated property of the neurons.

(1) Uniform distribution of points--no interaction.

(2) A straight line or zone of increased point density normal to the *AB* axis--excitatory synaptic relation between neurons *A* and *B*. If the line intersects the positive part of the *AB* axis, *A* is presynaptic to *B*.

(3) A straight line or zone of decreased point density normal to the *AB* axis--an inhibitory synaptic relation between neurons *A* and *B*. The presynaptic neuron is identified as in (2).

(4) A localized winglike or chevron pattern of increased point density--a coincidence detecting circuit in which the postsynaptic neuron fires only if the presynaptic neurons are nearly simultaneously active.

(5) Intersecting lines or zones of increased point density--
excitatory relations between the three cells. These may be in
the form of a chain of converging or diverging paths.

The patterns of (5) are illustrated in Fig. 7.7a-c, which presents

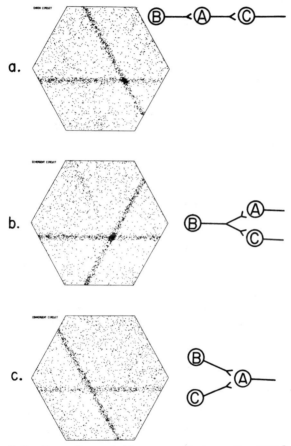

Fig. 7.7. Examples of three excitatory neuronal networks
and their snowflake diagrams. The top is a chain circuit, the
middle a divergent, and the bottom a convergent circuit. All
the networks involve only two active connections. Since B always
excites C, each diagram shows a dark horizontal line below the
origin. [From Perkel et al., Brain Res., 100, 271 (1975). By
permission of the publisher.]

the snowflake patterns along with the model network giving rise
to them. The location of the bands permits inference of connec-

tivity. In (a), the dark horizontal line below the origin, negative $t_B - t_A$, means that unit B fires at a nearly constant time before unit A and so may be inferred to be presynaptic to it. The inclined line to the right of the origin, negative $t_A - t_C$, indicates that unit A fires at a nearly constant time before unit C and should be presynaptic to it. The coordinates of the intersection of these two lines give the preferred sequence of spike activity. Analysis of the location and the density of the lines in patterns (b) and (c) permits us to distinguish between the convergent and divergent circuits that give rise to them. Careful analysis of the different snowflake patterns obtained from networks with unknown connectivity can reveal a good many properties of the underlying neural circuits. In some instances these patterns reveal functional relationships that cannot be seen with a set of the three cross-expectation densities obtained from the same data.

A principal application suggested for the snowflake diagram is to assemble from computer simulations a catalog of neuronal networks and their activity patterns as exhibited by the snowflake diagram. This might be particularly useful for dealing with *intrinsic* circuits, those in which the connectivity involves only the three observed neurons. Even for these relatively simple circuits, Perkel *et al.* (1975) have partially enumerated 728 circuits involving combinations of inhibition and excitation. The catalog might also be of use in studying the far greater population of *extrinsic* circuits, those in which the connectivity involves, besides the three units recorded from, other, unobserved neurons. With such a catalog, the activity of trios of real neurons can be correlated with that of the model networks in order to arrive at a hypothesis about their underlying connectivity. In some circumstances a unique association might be possible; in others, several networks might be candidates and the unique one can only be decided on by further experimentation. Nonetheless, the catalog method of identification could secure a considerable refinement in the range of connectivity description.

The snowflake display has been developed particularly for studying activity that is ongoing or that occurs during continuous stimulation, not activity that is a response to repetitive stimuli. In this sense it differs from the PST scatter diagram in that the latter deals with responses of two or three units to periodic stimuli whose event times are represented by the origin of the diagram. It is possible in the snowflake diagram to consider one of the axes as being associated with a stimulus that is delivered to two units. This might offer some advantages over the PST scatter diagram when the stimulus has a randomized delivery time. It can then be considered as a third unit, but one upon which the other two can exert no excitatory or inhibitory influence.

Like the expectation density, the snowflake diagram does not lend itself toward detecting temporal trends since it does not preserve the absolute time from the start of a trial. This probably does not weaken its ability to reveal neuronal connectivity as long as the trends are not pronounced, but the limitation must be kept in mind. It is possible to conceive of refinements to the display that would help in trend detection. In these, the display might present only the activity occurring within the most recent T_r sec. Trends might then be observed as progressive alterations in the display pattern.

The computations necessary for the snowflake display can be done on a laboratory-size computer. The display itself is the critical component of the method. Techniques using oscilloscope photography and mechanical plotting devices have been employed with success. In neither case, however, is the display compatible with real-time usage.

7.6. SEPARATION OF ACTIVITY OF CONCURRENTLY DISCHARGING UNITS

Any discussion of methods of data analysis for neurons whose activity is observed concurrently must ultimately depend upon the efficacy of techniques for separating the spikes of one neuron from those of another. Only if the spikes are properly identified can an interaction analysis have any meaning. This problem of spike train separation is particularly important whenever the activity of several neurons is observed in the record of a single electrode. Most studies of unit dependencies are based upon such data since the units observed are likely to be neighbors and synaptically related. The spike sorting problem has two aspects: (1) the identification and measurement of those spike waveform parameters that make the spikes of different neurons distinguishable from one another in a noisy background; and (2) the determination of how the errors in the sorting process affect the reliability of the analyses of interunit dependency. Spike sorting generally becomes more difficult as the number of simultaneously observed units increases, since the more units observed, the greater is the likelihood of sorting errors. It is not difficult to see why. As the number of units in the data increases, the "signature" differences between the spikes of different neurons decrease. Given the existence of noise and a certain amount of intrinsic fluctuation in the waveforms of the spikes, there exists a nonzero probability of making incorrect identification. This error probability increases with the noise level, the waveform fluctuations and the number of units observed. At some error level, difficult to specify, it becomes imprudent to attempt any analysis of unit interactions. The difficulty arises because each type of interaction analysis has its own sensitivity to identification error and this is best evaluated empirically. The probability of identification error itself depends upon the separation techniques employed and upon the particular spike parameters encountered in a specific record. We present here a brief discussion of some of the methods thus far employed to identify and separate unit activity. [For a more complete review, see Glaser (1970).] We also present an introductory discussion of how identification errors affect analyses of unit activity.

A basic assumption underlying all waveform separation methods is that it is possible to represent any waveform by a set of unique values of independent parameters, hopefully, whose values uniquely determine it. If we assume a one-to-one correspondence between the waveform and its neuronal source, measurement of these parameters thereby uniquely determines that source. To get at the parameters, the waveforms must be passed through filters, not necessarily linear, whose outputs provide the desired estimates.

A. USE OF SALIENT WAVEFORM PARAMETERS: AMPLITUDE, WIDTH, SLOPE

The simplest waveform parameter capable of providing some reliability in separation is spike amplitude. It is often used on extracellular microelectrode data because the spikes of the observed neurons frequently have markedly different amplitudes. These amplitude differences are likely to be caused by such factors as differing distances of the neurons to the electrode, variations in their size, and morphology. Spike amplitude separation is performed by use of an amplitude filter or window. In its simplest form the window produces an output pulse only when a spike has a peak amplitude between the selected upper and lower window levels. The necessity for the filter to wait until the peak of the spike has passed before generating a possible output pulse means that there is a certain intrinsic delay built into the filter, a delay which may vary according to the width of the kinds of spikes to be separated. This is not usually a serious performance deficit, and in fact the delay is sometimes a useful separation parameter.

A limitation to the performance of the amplitude filter is that in most experimental situations the spike being filtered is immersed in noise, and because of this its apparent peak amplitude can fluctuate appreciably from spike to spike. Occasionally the observed spike amplitude will be so elevated or depressed as to fall outside the window set for it, and occasionally there will be a noise spike of sufficient amplitude to masquerade as a true neural spike. The amplitude measurement is also sensitive to fluctuations in the spike amplitude that may be due to small movements of the electrode or to slight changes in the spike-generating

407

mechanisms within the cell. Some degree of compensation for this can be achieved by broadening the discrimination window so as to permit most of the fluctuating amplitudes to fall within the window. For spikes from a single well-isolated neuron, performance of the amplitude filter is usually adequate as long as the average spike amplitude is more than three times larger than the rms noise level.

When the spikes from several concurrently active neurons are to be separated, the situation becomes more difficult. Because each spike must be substantially greater than the noise in order that it can be reliable distinguished from the noise, this often means that the spike amplitude ranges of the different neurons will overlap one another. Confusion in spike identification then results, and analysis of unit interactions becomes meaningless. In a multiunit recording situation, the amplitude filter is usable only if the windows set for the units individually do not overlap. The greater the number of units to be separated, the higher is the likelihood that there will be overlap in the individual spike amplitude distributions. It is likely that the practical limit to the amplitude filter occurs when there are three units, since usable extracellular spikes tend to range between about 50 and 300 microvolts and the noise level is of the order of tens of microvolts.

An obvious extension of the amplitude filtering technique is to couple its use with other parameters of the waveform that are subject to variation in spikes emitted by different neurons. Some candidates for this are: the width of the spike at a chosen amplitude level, the slope of the spike at particular points on its rising or falling edge, and amplitudes at particular times after spike onset. Since the spikes are usually not fixed waveforms varying in amplitude only, there is certain to be a variety of waveform parameters that vary among the spikes of different neurons. Each of these can be examined to see if the interunit variation is large enough to make it help serve as a reliable basis for spike separation. It is difficult to find waveform parameters that are totally independent. Spike width and peak amplitude, for example, clearly are not independent, since a change in electrode location that causes the received spike amplitude to increase will also cause an increase in the spike width at a fixed voltage level. Those parameters that are most useful for spike separation are ones that behave independently so that a change in one has no effect upon a change in another. When satisfactory spike separation parameters have been found, they are best used in some joint fashion. Thus, if amplitude and width are taken to be the two separating parameters, a spike identified as coming from unit U if its amplitude falls between levels A_1 and A_2 and its width between W_1 and W_2--these being the criterion levels decided upon after examination of the data representing the activity of unit U and other units. The decision based upon the use of both parameters will be better than that based upon one, say amplitude, if the second parameter measures a facet of the waveform that is not entirely dependent upon the first and if there is reasonably large signal-to-noise ratio in the second parameter. The determination of signal-to-noise ratio depends upon the particular waveform parameter chosen and can be difficult to specify in theoretical terms. In any event, resort to a second waveform parameter should be made only if the performance of the spike separation system is markedly greater with its use. An illustration here is useful. Figure 7.8a shows two waveforms which are to be separated on the basis of amplitude and width between half-amplitude points. In Fig. 7.8b are the probability density functions for amplitudes only in a background of noise. A threshold level θ_A is shown, below which spike amplitudes are associated with unit U, and above with unit V. The level is chosen so that there is minimum probability of making an error when each spike is equally likely to occur. In Fig. 7.8c is shown the decision boundary θ_{AW} corresponding to the use of both amplitude and width. These are superimposed upon curves representing equiprobability density contours for each spike. The decision boundary provides the minimum probability of

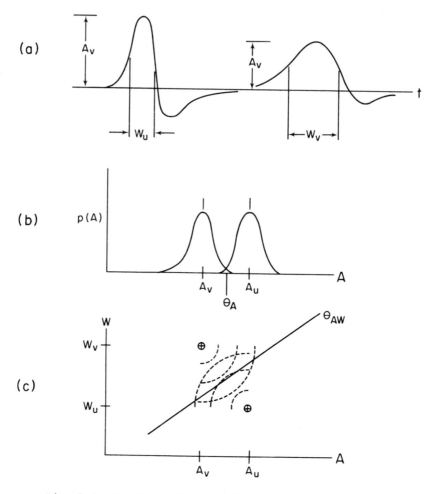

Fig. 7.8. (a) Two spike waveforms generated by neurons U
and V. (b) Probability densities for the amplitude of each spike
when they are observed in background noise. The decision threshold
is θ_A. (c) Straight-line decision contour based upon both spike
amplitude and width of each waveform. Waveform U is decided when
a measurement falls below and to the right of θ_{AW}; waveform V,
otherwise.

incorrect spike identification and is determined by the probability

densities for the two units. Assuming that the noise is Gaussian

and has an additive effect upon both the amplitude and width esti-

mates of the invariant spike waveforms, the boundary will be a

straight line (Van Trees, 1968). The straight line boundary θ_{AW}
is represented by $W - mA = b$. m is the slope of the line and b is
its intercept on the W axis. This means that whenever a particular
pair of measurements A_i and W_i is such that $W_i - mA_i \geq b$, the decision is that the spike belongs to unit V; otherwise, it is assigned
to U. Should θ_{AW} turn out to be a vertical line, the decision rule
is the same as that used for amplitude separation alone and there
will have been no improvement obtained by using the width parameter.

The situation considered above is the simplest one in that the
waveforms themselves are constant from spike to spike. But the
basic notion holds even when there are waveform variations due
either to electrode movement or to intrinsic variations in the
unit's spike-generating mechanism.

As stated above, spike width and other waveform measures such
as its slope at a fixed latency following onset or at a given amplitude tend not to be independent parameters. Their estimators
when the spikes are in noise also tend to be correlated and to have
non-Gaussian statistics. The result is that it is analytically
difficult to predict or evaluate the performance of separation
systems using them. However, a separation procedure that is based
upon nonindependent parameters will not be as good as one which is,
i.e., which employs the same number of measurements on independent
waveform parameters. Nonetheless, spike-separating schemes based
upon a few salient waveform properties have been employed with some
success. Two of note afford the investigator the option of selecting the salient waveform features which appear capable of yielding
the greatest discriminability. The methods are those of Simon
(1965) and Calvin (1972). Simon's method is of additional interest
because it represents the waveform as a vector in a two-dimensional
space and permits the investigator to select decision regions in
this space. Calvin's technique looks only for a single point along
the spike waveform where the spikes from different neurons are most
dissimilar, hence it is basically a one-dimensional technique in
which the time point used for separation is chosen by the observer.

411

There are advantages and disadvantages to placing the choice
of separation criteria in the hands of the experimenter. The advantages are that the instrumentation tends to be relatively simple
and that the experimenter has the ability to exercise his judgment
in difficult situations. The disadvantages are that the procedures
required can be time consuming and tedious. In many cases these
procedures may be performed more effectively by an automated procedure. The choice of the approach to use depends upon the problem
being studied.

B. USE OF THE ENTIRE SPIKE WAVEFORM

The limitations of separation techniques based on amplitude,
width, and so on, make it desirable to seek others with greater
performance capabilities. A more generalized approach is one which
considers a waveform to be constructed from a set of independent
and orthogonal constituent waveforms. When these waveforms or
components are properly weighted and summed, they reconstitute the
original waveform. This approach is quite closely related to the
Fourier series representation of repetitive waveforms. In contrast
to the Fourier series representation, however, the waveform need
not be periodic and the constituent waveforms will usually not be
sinewaves. They are in fact determined by the waveforms being
analyzed. The motivation behind such a decomposition approach to
neural spikes is that it is specifically directed toward arriving
at measures which are independent. These measures are the amplitudes of the constituent or component waveforms. It also happens
that by using this approach, the background noises interfering
with the measurement of the individual component amplitudes turn
out to be independent. As we have seen in discussions of evoked
responses in Chapter 5, not all orthogonal decompositions of waveforms lead to components which are independent. This is true as
well for spike separation. What is sought here is a waveform expansion specifically tailored to the spikes present in any given
record of data, an expansion that will, using the minimum number

of waveforms possible, perform waveform separation to a desired criterion level.

Once again we consider a waveform as a vector in a signal space. In the case of spike waveforms, each spike of constant shape will be represented by a point in the signal space. When noise is present in the record, each received spike will deviate randomly from its expected location according to the strength of the interfering noise. When the noise is strong enough, waveforms generated by one neuron will often fall close enough to the expected location of waveforms produced by another to be identified as waveforms generated by that other neuron. The separation procedure establishes boundaries in the signal space such that a received waveform is identified according to the region it falls into. Errors, while generally unavoidable, will be minimized. It is also worth noting that here, as in all presently conceived separation schemes, waveforms are considered as they occur, one at a time and with no consideration given to their relative frequency. Clearly, factors such as this ought to be taken into account in separation systems. Thus if a waveform occurs that seems to have slightly greater likelihood based upon its shape that it was generated by neuron U rather than V, it will be so identified even if neuron V is discharging considerably more often than U.

It is useful to introduce the principles associated with this spike separation method by first describing a waveform separation technique (Gerstein and Clark, 1964) which decomposes spikes into basic waveforms and uses them to classify the spikes according to shape differences. The Gerstein and Clark method represents the spike waveform by means of 32 equally spaced amplitude samples straddling the spike in time. The spikes can thus be conceived of as vectors in a 32-dimensional space. Because the instantaneous spike amplitude changes slowly in the time between consecutive samples, neighboring samples will tend to be closely related, not independent. Even when noise is present, the correlation between neighboring samples is likely to be large. We point this out

because it implies there is some redundancy in the waveform information conveyed by these amplitude samples and that there exist, as we
shall see, more compact and efficient means of representing the entire spike waveform without loss of information.

A useful method of measuring waveform differences or dissimilarities is by the distance D between vectors. Vectors which are
sufficiently close together are judged to differ from one another
only because of noise contributions to the spike vector (or intra-
neuronal fluctuations that alter spike shape), and therefore to
originate from the same neuron. To separate spikes, one searches
the data for compact, well-isolated clusters of spike vectors and
then assigns a neuron source label to each.

The separation procedure can start in several ways. One
reasonable choice is to pick a representative from the largest
waveforms present and call it the reference vector. The dissimilarity numbers, the distances of all other waveforms in the record
from the reference vector, are then calculated and plotted in histogram fashion--the number of waveforms versus dissimilarity number.
If the technique is successful, one sees several peaks in the D
histogram, the first near 0 and others at higher values of D.
These peaks may or may not be completely resolvable. The situation
is illustrated in Fig. 7.9. The peak near the origin (stage 1)
can be removed from the mixed sequence by culling from the data all
the spikes with D values below the criterion value (indicated by
the arrow), and choosing a new reference vector based upon the
spikes remaining. A new dissimilarity histogram is constructed
(stage 2) and new separable clusters are looked for. If found,
the one nearest the origin is removed and the process continued
until all clusters appear to have been isolated (stage 3). At the
end one can discard waveforms whose dissimilarity numbers are not
close to any of the clusters. These discarded waveforms may be
random noise peaks, overlapping spikes from simultaneously discharging neurons, atypical spikes from the neurons observed or
perhaps occasional spikes from other infrequently discharging
neurons near the recording site.

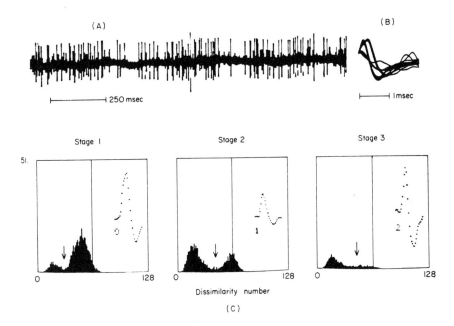

Fig. 7.9. Some spike waveforms and the results of their separation using the dissimilarity number technique. (A) Approximately 1.5 sec of interleaved action potentials. (B) Superimposed oscilloscope sweeps showing three distinguishable spike waveforms. (C) Population as a function of dissimilarity number during successive stages of separation. [From Gerstein and Clark, from Science, 143, 1325 (1964). Copyright 1964 by The American Association for the Advancement of Science. Reproduced by permission.]

It is easy to see that the success of this separation method depends upon whether the waveforms segregate sufficiently well into isolated clusters so that each cluster can be assigned to a particular neuron with a high degree of confidence. If the clusters are not so well resolved, the probability for incorrect identification of a waveform is high. Just how waveform assignment errors affect interaction analyses is poorly understood. However, the reliability of these analyses can be expected to diminish as the degree of error in waveform assignment increases.

Consideration of the spike waveform in toto means that waveforms with the same peak amplitude but different shapes may differ from one another by rather large dissimilarity numbers. On the other hand, the waveforms must be sufficiently large compared to the noise and to their own intrinsic fluctuations as to make the clusters associated with them resolvable. It is also possible that when using the distance or dissimilarity measure, two or more different waveforms can be mistakenly identified as one. The reason for this is that the dissimilarity number is a measure of distance only. It ignores the direction of vectors in the waveform space, i.e., the nature of its waveform difference. The result is that all waveforms approximately equidistant from the reference waveform will tend to fall into one unresolvable cluster along the dissimilarity number axis. Hopefully, when a confused waveform is used as a new reference waveform, the ambiguity would be resolved.

While the Gerstein and Clark separation technique processes all the waveform samples similarly, it should be evident that not all of them may be of equal importance in resolving the shape of a neural spike. The samples near the tails of the spikes tend to contribute little, since the strength of the spike relative to the noise is small in these regions. The question then arises as to just how many and which waveform samples are necessary to perform adequate spike separation. The answer will depend upon the shapes of the spikes being dealt with, and will therefore vary from experiment to experiment. Finally, the Gerstein and Clark technique is an automated one up to the point of selecting reference waveforms and cluster boundaries, a matter left solely to the discretion of the experimenter.

More completely automated approaches to spike separation have been developed with varying degrees of success. One of them (Glaser and Marks, 1966) is decomposition of the spike waveforms. This technique is similar in most respects to the principal component analyses performed on evoked responses. Spike waveforms are represented in terms of orthogonal component waveforms whose shapes are determined solely by the spikes observed in a particular experiment. The principal components technique characterizes a spike waveform by a set of independent parameters, the amplitudes of the individual components. Only those component amplitudes whose signal-to-noise ratio is high enough to contribute to the reliability of identification are utilized. These are identifiable in the separation procedure.

The principal component technique is based upon diagonalizing a covariance matrix derived from the original set of spike waveforms observed in the data. The dimensions of this covariance matrix depend directly upon the number of samples used to represent the spikes. Diagonalization of the covariance matrix yields a set of orthogonal vectors, the eigenvectors into which each spike waveform can be resolved. That is, each waveform $s(t)$ is to be decomposed into a set of components according to

$$s(t) = \sum_{i=1}^{\infty} a_i \phi_i(t) \qquad (7.19)$$

where the $\phi_i(t)$ are the eigenvectors, the basic waveforms, and the a_i are their coefficients or principal component values. The decomposition of the spike waveforms can then proceed, usually by reanalyzing the data by employing either digital or analog filters so as to obtain the vector representation of each waveform in the space of the basic waveforms describing the spikes. One way to examine the decomposed waveforms is by means of a multidimensional scatter diagram. An example of this derived from some experimental data on optic nerve spikes is shown in Fig. 7.10.

A considerable amount of spike separation can be achieved if only the first two principal components are employed. A display of the scatter diagram will reveal clusters of points around which it is necessary to establish the decision boundaries for assignment of a spike to a neuron. If the spike waveforms vary only because of the background noise and if the average rate of discharge of each neuron is nearly the same, the decision boundaries will be straight lines in the two-dimensional space, planes in three-space,

417

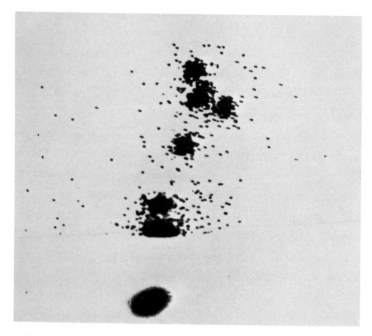

Fig. 7.10. Clusters of waveform points obtained from a two-dimensional principal component decomposition of limulus optic nerve spikes. The display, obtained by time exposure, represents approximately a three-minute observation of the nerve activity. [From Glaser and Marks, in "Data Acquisition and Processing in Biology and Medicine, Vol. 5," (K. Enslein, ed.), p. 137. Pergamon Press, New York, 1968. By permission of the publisher.]

and hyperplanes when more than three components are used for discrimination. The decision rule is to associate the spike in question with the center of the cluster of waveform vectors that it is nearest to (Nilsson, 1965). The decision rule is a linear one (it depends upon sums of the principal components) and is applied to each waveform, assigning it to a particular neuron on the basis of its location with respect to the decision boundaries. A set of linear algebraic computations is performed on each spike waveform. When the waveform fluctuations are different for different neurons and when their average rates of firing are different, the decision rule is altered somewhat. This is a matter beyond the scope of this book. An excellent discussion may be found in Nilsson (1965).

The advantages of the principal component technique are that it permits the spike waveforms to be expressed in a compact, efficient manner which extracts close to the maximum amount of usable information from the waveforms. This part of the procedure is carried out free of user intervention. Two passes on the data are required, the first to determine the eigenvectors and the second to extract the principal components, estimate cluster centers, establish decision boundaries and assign the waveforms to the (hopefully) proper neuron source. Cluster center estimation itself is performed with operator intervention using a display of the waveform points to establish the coordinates of the centers. In a two-dimensional resolution of the waveforms, only one display is needed. Multidimensional resolution can be obtained from a sequence of two-dimensional displays, one following the other to uniquely locate the cluster centers. The decision boundaries may be set up as hyperplanes or hyperspheres surrounding the cluster centers. The latter is a "reasonable proximity" rule which assigns a waveform to a given neuron only if it is close enough. It rejects other large waveforms as artifacts or perhaps as intrusive spikes produced by rarely active neurons. The hypersphere boundary (a circle in two-dimensional space) does not provide minimum probability of error as does the hyperplane when the neuron sources are all identified and fluctuations are only due to noise, but it clearly has advantages meriting its application (Gerstein and Clark, 1964). Other decision boundaries have been employed as well, usually on the basis of simplicity of instrumentation. Mishelevich (1970), for example, has used rectangles in his spike separation procedures.

The techniques described above utilize the data available from a single electrode located within the neural tissue. They are applicable to the many situations in which there is no opportunity to view the concurrently active units from more than one electrode. This is because the neurons are small and their activity can only be seen at distances of less than several hundred microns. Thus it is not usually possible to position more than one electrode close enough to them so as to be able to see the simultaneous activity of more than one or two units. There are opportunities, however, when it is possible to use an array of electrodes to view the concurrent activity of six or more units, such as when recording from ganglionic or efferent nerve trunks. In such situations, Roberts and Hartline (1975) have shown that it is possible to separate the activity of up to six units with a high degree of reliability. The technique they employ is based upon the matched filter concept as applied to the data arising from the electrode array. The data the electrodes furnish can be considered to be a K-dimensional time-varying vector where K is the number of electrodes in use. They synthesized by digital techniques a bank of filters, one for each unit to be separated. Each filter in the bank is designed to have unity output when the normalized spike waveform it is "tuned" to is present and to have minimal output when the ongoing noise or the spikes generated by the other observed units are present. The matched filter for each unit represents a spatial (with respect to the electrodes) and temporal weighting of the observed activity. Using such a bank of filters, Roberts and Hartline reported that highly reliable separation is possible when the number of electrodes equals or exceeds the number of units to be separated. This is true even when there is simultaneity between spikes from different units. Synthesis of the filter responses requires that there be available a sample of the activity of each of the units to be separated. And, in common with the other separation techniques discussed, performance suffers when spike waveforms vary during the acquisition of data or when there is nonlinear summation of waveforms of different units. Nonetheless, the parallel usage of the data from the electrode array markedly improves the ability to separate the activity of neighboring units and permits the detailed analysis of their interactions.

Summarizing, separation procedures can be broken down into four steps:

(1) Detection of the presence of spike activity;

(2) Estimation of the shapes of the various spike waveforms;

(3) Establishment of decision criteria based upon the differences of these shapes;

(4) Testing of each waveform to determine the neuronal group it belongs to.

Of the various techniques now used in the second step, those based upon matched filter concepts or linear decomposition of waveforms have some theoretical justification for superiority. They utilize the structure of the entire waveform in the waveform identification but tend to be instrumentally complex. The simpler shape estimation techniques are based upon what are best referred to as local properties of the waveforms; e.g., the amplitude of peaks, slopes, the times between different parts of the waveform, and so on. They have the advantage of relative simplicity in instrumentation and have demonstrated a measure of success in waveform separation. The reliance upon local features rather than on the waveform as an entity makes it certain that such techniques can never be as effective as ones using the entire waveform.

C. IDENTIFICATION ERRORS AND THE ANALYSIS OF UNIT INTERACTIONS

The ultimate goal of spike waveform separation is the ability to describe the functional dependencies between concurrently active units, i.e., their connectivity and excitatory or inhibitory influences. The descriptions will depend entirely upon analyses of the temporal relationships between the spikes. A crucial question that arises is, how reliable can such analyses be if the data they are based upon is faulty? Faulty data here means that some of the spikes have been attributed to the wrong neurons and some spikes have been erroneously dismissed by simply not being detected. Then what is judged to be the overall spike activity of one neuron can in fact contain an assortment of spikes from other neurons, occasional noise spikes, and in addition, may not contain all of its own spike activity. It is easy to see that the spike separation methods described here will be error-free and exhibit nonoverlapping clusters of spikes only under relatively rare circumstances where the spikes are strong compared to the noise and free from intrinsic fluctuations. More commonly, the clusters will overlap to an extent that depends upon the similarity of the waveforms of the spikes and how much noise there is in the records. In these circumstances spike identification errors are bound to occur. We then find ourselves analyzing contaminated representations of neuron spike sequences. It would be useful under these circumstances to know to what degree such contamination affects the reliability of interdependency analyses. We could then put a reliability measure on a judgment, say, that neuron U receives an excitatory input from neuron V. How reliable is this judgment when 10% of the spike assignments to each neuron are in error? 5%? 1%? Unfortunately, very little is known about this at present. Some work has been done on the effects of decision errors (false alarms and false dismissals) on the serial correlogram of just a single unit (Shiavi and Negin, 1973). In a computer simulation of unit activity they found that error rates in excess of .5% could cause serious misinterpretations of the unit's activity. This kind of work needs to be extended to other statistical measures of unit activity and to interactions of two or more units. The kinds of decision errors that are possible increase with the number of units under observation and so it seems likely that the requirements for accurate spike separation will accordingly become more stringent. To combat the assignment errors, an increasingly large amount of data would have to be available. This may very well put a limit to the number of concurrently active units that can be usefully analyzed if data are derived from a single electrode. The details of this problem remain to be explored.

7.7. MULTIUNIT ACTIVITY AS AN ENTITY

Our previous discussions approached the analysis of multi-unit activity in terms of resolving that activity into spike sequences generated by individual neurons. They proceeded from the notion that a microelectrode records from a limited population of cells and that with careful control the electrode could be positioned so that the active neurons can be individually identified and analyzed. This conception of multiunit activity analysis fails in a number of experimental situations where, at least with current experimental techniques, there seems to be no practical way of satisfactorily isolating individual neurons. In these situations it would seem that the neurons are small compared to the exposed tip of the microelectrode or so tightly clustered together that no amount of adroit manipulation of the electrode's position or variation of the stimulus parameters can resolve the individual units. What is observed in these cases is a barrage of spikes whose peaks have a relatively small amplitude range and tend to overlap one another in time. But inability to resolve these spikes does not mean that they should be discarded from further study. As Verzeano (1973) and Buchwald *et al.* (1973) have pointed out, there is a significant amount of retrievable information contained in multi-unit records. For example, under certain circumstances the activity can be identified as arising from several physiologically different classes of neurons. Multiunit records can thus be profitably analyzed by paying attention to the behavior of a class of neurons rather than to the individual members.

Verzeano (1973) correlated the activity of the different spike amplitude classes of neurons with the temporal features of the slow wave activity observed from the same locality of the brain, i.e., the peaks and rising and falling fronts of these waves. He showed that correlation differed with amplitude class. (See Fig. 7.11.) He also demonstrated that the different spike amplitude classes of neurons are affected differently by drugs

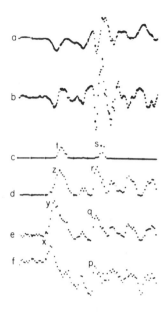

Fig. 7.11. Electrical activity in the visual cortex of paralyzed cat. (a) The average gross response and (b) its first derivative. (c), (d), (e), (f) are histograms of unit activity from, respectively, spikes whose amplitudes are in the ranges > 320, 100-140, 60-100, 30-60 microvolts. The peaks x, y, z, t and p, q, r, s represent the progressively increasing latencies of activity in units showing higher spike amplitudes. Note that peak x in trace f corresponds to the early negative peak in the first derivative of the gross response. (From Verzeano, in "Bioelectric Recording Techniques, Part A," (R. F. Thompson and M. M. Patterson, eds.), p. 243. Academic Press, New York, 1973. By permission of the publisher.]

and therefore represent different physiological classes. Buchwald *et al.*, (1973) analyzed multiunit activity by measurement of spike rate counts as a function of time, starting from the onset of a stimulus. A threshold level is adopted which noise spikes are unlikely to exceed. The number of spikes occurring in a small interval of time is a measure of the average spike activity in that time interval. It indicates how the responsiveness of the multiunit population varies over the poststimulus time epoch. The rate measurements need not be restricted to activity in the presence of a stimulus but can also be compared with other ongoing indications of brain activity, such as the EEG.

The notion of identifying classes of neurons by their range
of spike amplitudes is not without problems. Extremely vigorous
activity can cause spikes to overlap to such an extent that small
units will sum together to be identified as large ones. This
could also occur in the not entirely unlikely situation of nearly
exact synchrony of unit firings during stimulation. Thus small,
spontaneously active units can become time-locked during stimulation and interpreted as a class of large units which are silent
in the absence of a stimulus. It remains to be seen whether more
refined experimental procedures or data analysis techniques can
surmount such difficulties.

REFERENCES

Buchwald, J. S., Holstein, S. B., and Weber, D. S., in "Bioelectric
    Recording Techniques, Part A," (R. F. Thompson and M. M.
    Patterson, eds.), p. 201. Academic Press, New York, 1973.
Calvin, W. H., *Electroenceph. Clin. Neurophysiol.*, 34, 94 (1973).
Cox, D. R. and Lewis, P. A. W., "The Statistical Analysis of
    Series of Events," Methuen, London, 1966.
Gerstein, G. L. and Clark, W. A., *Science*, 143, 1325 (1964).
Gerstein, G. L. and Perkel, D. H., *Science*, 164, 828 (1969).
Gerstein, G. L., in "The Neurosciences. Second Study Program,"
    (F. O. Schmitt, ed.), p. 648. Rockefeller Univ. Press,
    New York, 1970.
Gerstein, G. L. and Perkel, D. H., *Biophys. J.*, 12, 453 (1972).
Glaser, E. M. and Marks, W. B., in "Data Acquisition and Pro-
    cessing in Biology and Medicine, Vol. 5," (K. Enslein, ed.),
    p. 137. Pergamon Press, New York, 1968.
Glaser, E. M., in "Advances in Biological and Medical Engineer-
    ing, Vol. 1," (S. Fine and R. M. Kenedi, eds.), p. 77.
    Academic Press, New York, 1970.
Kristan, W. B., Jr., and Gerstein, G. L., *Science*, 169, 1336
    (1970).
Mishelevich, D. J., *IEEE Trans. Biomed. Eng.*, BME-17, 147 (1970).
Nilsson, N. J., "Learning Machines," McGraw-Hill, New York, 1965.
Moore, G. P., Segundo, J. P., Perkel, D. H., and Levitan, H.,
    Biophys. J., 10, 876 (1970).
Perkel, D. H., Gerstein, G. L., and Moore, G. P., *Biophys. J.*,
    7, 391 (1967).
Perkel, D. H., Gerstein, G. L. and Moore, G. P., *Biophys. J.*,
    7, 419 (1967).
Perkel, D. H., Gerstein, G. L., Smith, M. S., and Tatton, W. G.,
    Brain Res., 100, 271 (1975).

Roberts, W. M. and Hartline, D. K., *Brain Res.*, 94, 141 (1975).
Shiavi, R. and Negin, M., *IEEE Trans. Biomed. Eng.*, BME-20, 374 (1973).
Simon, W., *Electroenceph. Clin. Neurophysiol.*, 18, 192 (1965).
Van Trees, H. L., "Detection, Estimation, and Modulation Theory, Part I," Wiley, New York, 1968.
Verzeano, M., in "Bioelectric Recording Techniques, Part A," (R. F. Thompson and M. M. Patterson, eds.), p. 243. Academic Press, New York, 1973.

Chapter 8

RELATIONS BETWEEN SLOW WAVE
AND UNIT ACTIVITY

8.1. INTRODUCTION

Up to now we have investigated the analytical methods for
dealing separately with continuous wave type of activity of the
nervous system and with the spike activity of its individual
neurons. We largely ignored the possibility that there might be
interactions between them. We also tended to simplify the study
of stimulus-response interactions by restricting our attention to
continuous stimuli or to brief ones such as clicks, light flashes,
or shocks delivered at more or less regular intervals. This is a
particularly confining point of view and it is appropriate that we
now broaden our discussion to cover interactions between continuous and point processes. We undertake this for two reasons. First,
it is important to deal with single unit activity in conjunction
with continuous processes representing either stimuli or the responses to them. In the former case, time-varying stimuli provide
more powerful probes of nervous system activity and they resemble
more closely the stimuli that animals cope with in normal life.
The investigation of neuronal responses to such continuous stimuli
will hopefully lead us to more fertile mathematical models of nervous system function. The continuous processes may also represent
organismic responses to single unit activity, such as the tension
produced by muscles or the movement of joints that are driven by
the spike activity of motoneurons. Body temperature change produced by hypothalamic unit activity is another example of continuous and point process interaction wherein stimulus-response analysis of the two types of processes can lead to useful models of
system function. It can be seen from these illustrations that a
continuous process can drive a point process or vice versa.

The second reason for studying the interactions between the two types of processes is that it permits us to deal with the slow wave and unit activity that always coexist in the brain even in the absence of external stimuli. The relationships between these forms of electrical activity, though obscure, are likely to be of fundamental importance in understanding nervous system function. To unravel these relationships, we must employ analysis techniques suited to both continuous and point processes. In this chapter we describe some such techniques, principally linear ones. As we shall see, they represent but a first step in the description of relationships that are basically nonlinear. Our methods cover only the situation in which there is a fixed time-invariant relationship between the two kinds of processes. This, it will be realized, is also quite restrictive but the ability to do more than this remains beyond our grasp. Also, although it is of great importance to understand the neural responses to simultaneously applied stimuli, we confine ourselves to stimulus-response analysis involving but a single stimulus. The analytical problems posed by the use of multiple stimuli such as those used in the study of the mechanisms of sensory inhibition are difficult ones. This is especially so inasmuch as the underlying neuronal mechanisms involved are by and large nonlinear ones. The analysis methods described in this chapter may be of some value here but, unquestionably, more powerful techniques need yet to be developed.

8.2. SOME GENERAL CONSIDERATIONS ON COVARIANCE AND SPECTRAL ANALYSIS

The currently predominant methods for studying process interactions, whether they be continuous or point, are based upon the linear approaches of covariance and spectral analysis. The two are closely interrelated by way of the Fourier transform as has already been pointed out. When the point process is the driving one, it is possible for the relationship between it and the driven continuous process to be linear and therefore characterized by an intervening

system whose impulse response is $h(\tau)$ and whose transfer function
is $H(f)$. In this case covariance or spectral analysis will be thoroughly adequate to describe the relationship. If there are nonlinearities, such an analysis will be less rewarding for it will
be incapable of describing the nonlinearities. It may, however,
still provide useful information about the linear component of the
system. When the continuous process is the driving one, we are
confronted with the fact that any relationship between the two
processes must be essentially nonlinear, although it may have a
linear component. The reason for this is that there is no purely
linear means by which a continuous function of time can be transformed into a discontinuous point process. At the least there are
threshold operations involved in the relationship. As a result,
any analysis of these kinds of process interaction that is based
upon covariance and cross spectrum notions will be handicapped by
its weakness in coping with nonlinear relationships.

To point this up, let us consider the zero-crossing detector,
the classic example of a driving continuous and driven point process
which generates an impulse whenever its continuous input process
passes through 0. We are concerned here with determining how the
statistical properties of the point process representing the impulses are related to the statistical properties of the continuous
process (Rice, 1944). Even when the continuous process is stationary, Gaussian noise with arbitrary spectral properties, there has as
yet been no completely adequate solution that fully describes the
statistics of the zero crossing intervals. The same is true when,
instead of zero crossings, the crossings of an arbitrary threshold
level are involved. This is a problem of some relevance to neurobiology since a neuron's fluctuating intracellular potential (including the PSPs) and its spike-generating threshold correspond
approximately to the continuous process and its threshold level.
Our inability thus far to find an adequate solution to this simple-
appearing problem should alert us to exercise great care in analyzing and interpreting systemic relationships between a driving con-

tinuous and a driven point process. When the techniques employed
are based upon covariance and spectral analysis methods, we must
always be aware that these analyses may obscure some of the vital
aspects of the processes.

One way of circumventing the nonlinear relationship between
a driving continuous process and a driven point process is by investigating a particular parameter of the point process that we
believe is adequate to represent the information-bearing message.
We may, for example, be reasonably convinced on empirical grounds
that the average spike rate is the neural code for stimulus information. In assuming this to be so, we effectively consider the
spike activity to be, in communication theory terms, a modulated
carrier of information. The modulation is the average spike rate.
Once we make this assumption we have converted our problem into
an analysis of two simultaneous continuous processes because, subsequent to the spike activity, we have inserted some operationally
defined demodulator which converts the point process back into a
continuous one. One possible definition (among many) for the average rate is the number of spikes occurring in the last T sec. The
demodulator is then defined by a linear circuit whose impulse response $d(\tau)$ is given by

$$d(\tau) = \begin{cases} 1/T, & 0 < \tau \leq T \\ 0, & \tau > T \end{cases} \tag{8.1}$$

and whose transfer function $D(f)$ is given by

$$D(f) = \left[\frac{\sin \pi f T}{\pi f T}\right]\exp(-j\pi f T) \tag{8.2}$$

The output of the demodulator will be a sequence of discontinuous
steps, each representing the spike rate by the number of spikes
that have occurred in the last T sec. To smooth these steps out
to a continuously varying output, a subsequent low-pass filter
$G(f)$ is needed. It eliminates aliasing when we deal with sampled
representations of the average rate. We have thus converted the

the sequence of spikes $r(t)$ into a continuous response $q(t)$
$= r(t)*d(t)*g(t)$, where $g(t)$ is the weighting function or impulse
response of the low pass filter. Our linear analysis of the system
is then based upon the covariance and/or spectral analysis of $s(t)$
and $q(t)$. Whatever coherence existed originally between $s(t)$ and
$r(t)$ is preserved in the relationship between $s(t)$ and $q(t)$ since
the latter is purely a linear transformation of $r(t)$. This also
means that an estimate of the transfer function between processes
S and Q is an estimate of the product $H(f) \cdot D(f) \cdot G(f)$. Because
$D(f)$ and $G(f)$ are known, we have the means for estimating $H(f)$.
$H(f)$ is the transfer function between S and R. This approach of
dealing with a continuous linear transformation of the point process., here its average rate, can be a useful approach. It preserves in principle the dependencies between the processes because
the linear transformations do not destroy information contained
within the frequency band of interest. However, the filtering
operations can in practice suppress information content in the
higher frequencies of the point process, and this may be of some
importance in the analysis of nonlinear interrelationships.

Though continuous point process relationships may be divided
into the two dependency classes we have described, it is not generally true, given an initial uncertainty about which is the driver
and which the driven, that a covariance or spectral analysis of
the activity of the two processes can unmistakably tell which class
of dependency is involved. What the analysis will reveal is that
there is some kind of linear connection between the processes,
measured in covariance or cross-spectral terms. If there is a
clear case of driving, it will usually be known at the outset of
the experiment. In that situation the outcome of the data analysis
is a more quantitative detailed description of the relationship.
If there is no secure knowledge of the direction of the dependency,
as when we are dealing with spikes and slow waves, it is doubtful
that the analysis will entirely resolve the situation. They may
be jointly dependent. Or it may be true, for example, that both

431

the continuous and the point process are being driven by a third, unseen process and that neither is directly related to the other. This kind of interrelationship is similar to that discussed in Chapter 6 in connection with the spike activity of a pair of units driven by some unobserved third unit. Although covariance-spectral analysis may not directly settle the issue of process dependency, hopefully it will lead to the design of other more revealing physiological investigations which would be able to do so.

8.3. ESTIMATION OF THE LINEAR COMPONENT OF PROCESS INTERACTIONS

In the following linear analysis of process interactions, we make no sharp distinction between continuous and point processes since we deal mainly with covariance functions and spectra and these are well defined for both types of processes. If the response process R is linearly related to the stimulus process S, we have

$$r(t) = \int_{-\infty}^{\infty} h(\tau)s(t - \tau)\, d\tau \tag{8.3}$$

where $h(\tau)$ is the impulse response describing the system connecting the two processes. Taking the Fourier transform of this equation gives

$$R(f) = H(f)S(f) \tag{8.4}$$

When the processes R and S are random, we can also speak of the relationships between their covariance functions and their spectra, as we have already done in Chapters 2 and 3. These relationships are

$$c_{sr}(\tau) = \int_{-\infty}^{\infty} h(u)c_{ss}(\tau - u)\, du, \quad \text{all } \tau \tag{8.5}$$

$$C_{sr}(f) = H(f)C_{ss}(f) \tag{8.6}$$

They are valid when either or both of the processes is a point process. There is an interpretational difficulty, however, when

S is a continuous process and R is a point process. This occurs in the meaning to assign to $h(t)$. As we have mentioned previously, a linear relationship cannot fully describe such a situation. Therefore, if we find there is a linear correlation between a driving continuous process and a driven point process, the $h(t)$ and $H(f)$ must be recognized as just the linear component of the overall nonlinear relationship. Provided that a nonlinear system does not vary with time and has a finite memory, it is possible to describe its nonlinearities using an extension of correlation and spectral analysis first described by Wiener and developed for more practical application to biological problems by Marmarelis and McCann (1973), Marmarelis and Naka (1974), and McCann (1974). These techniques can also be applied when more than one stimulus is applied simultaneously, but they are beyond the scope of this presentation.

Since the continuous and point process data that we deal with experimentally usually are measured in a background of unrelated, noiselike processes, our analysis techniques must be able to surmount these obstacles. Let us consider a generalized situation in which the measurements of what we consider to be the stimulus and response processes are corrupted by independent noise processes. This is illustrated in Fig. 8.1. (See also Bendat and Piersol, 1971.) $s(t)$ is regarded as the driving process. As a particular example, $s(t)$ may be a component of a continuous slow wave process giving rise to single unit spike activity $r(t)$. The relationship between the two is represented in part by $h(\tau)$, a linear transfer function. $z(t)$ is unrelated slow waves or spikes that are observed along with $s(t)$ from the same recording electrode. $v(t)$ represents that part of the unit's activity which is driven by sources unrelated to $s(t)$ or which may be intrinsic to the neuron. Then $x(t)$ and $y(t)$ are our observations of both processes. Adopting for greatest simplicity a linear approach to the mixing of these processes, we have

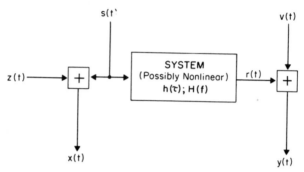

Fig. 8.1. A possibly nonlinear system relates response r(t) to stimulus s(t). Measurements of these data may be corrupted by unrelated noise sources v(t) and z(t) to yield the observations y(t) and x(t).

$$x(t) = s(t) + z(t) \qquad (8.7a)$$

$$y(t) = r(t) + v(t) \qquad (8.7b)$$

If we consider the expected value of the products $x(t)x(t + \tau)$ and $y(t)y(t + \tau)$, it is a simple matter to show that

$$c_{xy}(\tau) = c_{sr}(\tau) \qquad (8.8)$$

Our previous experience with covariance function estimation indicates that temporal averaging of the product of $x(t)$ and $y(t + \tau)$ will lead to a good estimate of $c_{sr}(\tau)$. If, furthermore, the stimulus is chosen properly, it will also lead to an estimate of the linear impulse response relating the two processes. This will be discussed in the next section.

The spectral approach to analyzing process interrelationships is perhaps more attractive than covariance analysis because of the ease with which Fourier transforms may now be obtained. We have seen in Chapter 3 that the coherence function provides a measure of linear dependency between two processes at frequency f.

$$\kappa^2_{xy}(f) = \frac{C^2_{xy}(f)}{C_{xx}(f)\, C_{yy}(f)} \qquad (8.9)$$

The nearer the coherency is to unity, the greater is the linear association between processes x and y. If the coherency is small, there is either (a) little linear association between the processes because a large component of either or both is due to noise, (b) a dependency of one or both processes upon other processes not measured, or (c) a nonlinear dependency between the processes. As long as the coherence is significantly greater than 0, the linear component of dependency between the processes can be estimated with accuracy. We defer further consideration of spectral analysis until Section 7.

8.4. ESTIMATION OF CROSS COVARIANCE BETWEEN A CONTINUOUS AND A POINT PROCESS

The fundmental cross-covariance relationship between the specimen functions of two processes is (see Section 1.11)

$$c_{sr}(\tau) = c_{rs}(-\tau) \tag{8.10}$$

This indicates that it is mathematically unimportant as to which of the two processes is considered the input or driving process, and which is the output or driven process. One cross-covariance function uniquely determines the other. Experimentally the situation is different in terms of estimating the covariance functions. However, some consideration of the nature of the data will indicate that for estimation purposes it is more convenient to regard the point process as the driving process. Only at those time instants in the point process where an event occurs will the value of its specimen function be different from zero and be capable of contributing to the raw cross-covariance estimate. Hence it is best to obtain the cross-covariance estimate by waiting for an event to occur and then measuring the amplitude of the continuous specimen function τ sec later. When recorded data are available or when there is short-term storage of the continuous specimen function in a real-time data processor, τ can be chosen to be negative as well as positive. Averaging the value of the continuous function at each time lag of interest for each of the N events in a sequence generated by the point process yields a function $f(\tau)$ proportional to the raw estimate of the cross-covariance function, $\hat{c}_{sr}(\tau)$:

$$f(\tau) = \frac{1}{N} \sum_{i=1}^{N} r(t_i + \tau) \tag{8.11}$$

t_i is the time of occurrence of the ith event in the point process and $r(\tau)$ is the continuous process. This can be seen to correspond to the time domain definition of the cross-covariance function estimator,

$$\hat{c}_{sr}(\tau) = \frac{1}{T} \int_0^T s(t) r(t + \tau) \, dt \tag{8.12}$$

$s(t)$ is here a specimen function from the point process and is a sequence of delta functions, N of which occur within the T sec of interest. $r(t)$ is defined to be 0 outside of $0 \leq t \leq T$. Under these conditions, Eq. (8.12) becomes

$$\hat{c}_{sr}(\tau) = \frac{1}{T} \sum_{i=1}^{N} r(t_i + \tau), \quad -T \leq \tau \leq T \tag{8.13}$$

If the average rate of occurrence of events is ν, in T sec there will be $N \simeq \nu$ events.

$$\hat{c}_{sr}(\tau) \simeq \frac{\nu}{N} \sum_{i=1}^{N} r(t_i + \tau) = \nu f(\tau) \tag{8.14}$$

Thus one obtains the estimate of the cross-covariance function by computing $f(\tau)$, the average response of $r(t)$ to each event in the point process, and then multiplying that average by the mean rate of occurrence of events. For large N, Eq. (8.14) is a good approximation to Eq. (8.12). This method of estimating the cross-covariance function between a continuous and a point process was employed by Frost and Gol (1966). An example of some of their data analyzed in this way is shown in Fig. 8.2. Note that the cross-covariance function need not be symmetrical about $\tau = 0$. This

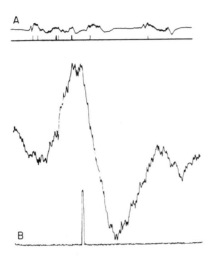

*Fig. 8.2. (A) Spike train and concurrent EEG in the same
area of isolated cerebral cortex. (B) Average EEG obtained by
averaging the EEG over a 2 sec interval whose beginning is time-
locked to each spike occurrence. The location of the spike is
shown in the lower trace. [From Frost and Gol, Exp. Neurol., 14,
506 (1966). By permission of the publisher.]*

means the average response should be determined for negative and

positive τ, a requirement that is not particularly difficult to

fulfill. The alternative method for estimating the cross-covari-

ance function between point and continuous processes is to consi-

der the continuous process as the driving process. This approach

appears to be less useful both conceptually and experimentally

since it involves dealing with both the cross-expectation density

of point process events (measured from a reference time in the

continuous process) and the amplitude distribution of the continu-

ous process. Fortunately, because of Eq. (8.10) we are assured

that the ccvf yielded by considering the point process as the

driving process is a satisfactory one.

The interpretation of the ccvf as the average response of

the continuous process to individual events in the point process

is of interest in itself. It suggests that much of the methodo-

logy developed for average response determination can be applied to cross-covariance estimation. For example, under circumstances in which artifacts contaminate the continuous process data, it may be desirable to estimate the ccvf by the median response rather than by the average response, techniques that have been described in Chapter 4. When spurious events occur within the point process data, the estimate will be plagued by average responses to non-events. It is possible that these effects may also be moderated by use of the median response although this must be evaluated carefully. One may also wish to consider how the variance of the covariance function estimate behaves as a function of τ, and to test the continuous process for conformity with the hypothesis that it is a combination of a response component driven by the point process and a noiselike background component. The latter component is commonly taken to be Gaussian, stationary and additive to the driven component. If this hypothesis is valid, the variance about the estimated ccvf would tend to be a constant independent of τ.

The estimation of the ccvf has been considered in terms of the average response (at both negative and positive time lags) to an event in the point process. Since other events occur prior and subsequent to the ones triggering the averager, their effects on the response must be present in the average. The result is that the average response does not necessarily tend to approach the response to an *isolated* event. In fact, the contribution of the other events depends upon the acvf $c_{ss}(\tau)$ of the point process. Let us assume, for simplicity, that the continuous process is composed partly of the sum of responses to individual events in the point process and partly of uncorrelated background activity. If we denote the continuous process response to a single event in S by $h(t)$, then the output of the cross-covariance computer can be determined using Eq. (8.5). If $h(t)$ is not 0 for negative t, it would signify that responses can occur prior to the events that elicit them. In the present situation, we consider this not to be the case and that the response only follows the causative event and so $h(t)$ must be 0 for negative t. Thus,

$$c_{sr}(\tau) = \int_0^\infty h(t)c_{ss}(\tau - t) \, dt, \quad \text{all } \tau \qquad (8.15)$$

The acvf of the point process S here involves negative values of
time. Previously, the expectation density from which it was derived was defined in Chapter 6 as a conditional probability of an
event occurring subsequent to one at $t = 0$. It was then extended
to negative times without difficulty so that the two-sided expectation density is symmetrical about 0. That is, given an event at
$t = 0$, the probability that another event preceded it τ sec earlier
is just the same as the probability that another event will follow
it τ sec later. Thus the acvf is also symmetrical about 0 as is
proper. $c_{sr}(\tau)$ is defined, it will be noticed, for negative as
well as positive values of τ. This is because the average response to the events consists in part of the residue of the responses to events occurring before 0. This residue will exist at
negative values of τ and Eq. (8.15) holds for this situation.
When, in practice, the averaging is performed over the responses
to all the N events in a T sec observation time, the resulting
average response output is an estimate of the ccvf. It should be
clear then that averaging the continuous wave preceding and following the occurrence of each event gives an estimate of the true
ccvf and not the response to an isolated event, except when the
responses do not overlap. Emphasis must also be placed on the
fact that Eq. (8.15) holds only when the relationship between the
processes is a linear one and the continuous responses to individual events have no suppressive or facilitatory effect upon each
other. Equation (8.15) also provides a guide to the development
of procedures for extracting the putative response to an individual
event from the ccvf when $c_{ss}(\tau)$ is known. As stated, these procedures are most sensible when there is good evidence that the point
process events are responsible for the continuous process activity
and not vice versa. When the estimates of the ccvf and the expectation density are available, it is possible to estimate $h(\tau)$

by deconvolution or spectral analysis techniques (Oppenheim and Schafer, 1975). If the results indicate that $h(\tau)$ is significantly different from 0 for negative values of τ, one could conclude that the point process is not driving the continuous one via some linear transfer function. Rather, the existence of an anticipatory component to $h(\tau)$ would tend to indicate that the dependency relationship between the processes is bidirectional or directed from the continuous process to the point process.

We can allow for an anticipatory response by making the lower limit in Eq. (8.15) minus infinity. We can also replace $c_{ss}(\tau - t)$ in the same equation by expressing it in terms of its corresponding expectation density $m(\tau - t)$ and mean rate of events ν. It will be remembered that as τ becomes large, $m(\tau)$ approaches ν. We then have

$$c_{sr}(\tau) = \int_{-\infty}^{\infty} \nu h(t) \left[\delta(\tau - t) + m(\tau - t) - \nu \right] dt \qquad (8.16)$$

This can be simplified to

$$c_{sr}(\tau) = \nu h(\tau) + \nu \int_{-\infty}^{\infty} h(t) \left[m(\tau - t) - \nu \right] dt \qquad (8.17)$$

It can be seen from this that the ccvf consists of two components, the first being proportional to the response to an individual event $h(\tau)$, while the second is proportional to the convolution of that response with $m(\tau) - \nu$, the deviation of the expectation density from the average rate of events. Whether $h(\tau)$ is anticipatory or not, the second term indicates that $c_{sr}(\tau)$ can exist for negative τ according to how the expectation density depends upon time. If the point process is Poisson, $m(\tau) = \nu$, and the second term vanishes. Then the ccvf will be proportional to the response to an isolated event regardless of the average rate of events. It must be remembered that this result depends entirely upon the assumed linear relationship of the continuous process to individual events in the point process (which implies freedom from response interactions within the continuous process).

8.5. SOME DANGERS IN CROSS-COVARIANCE ESTIMATION
BY AN AVERAGE RESPONSE COMPUTER

The foregoing discussion dwelled upon the relationship between the ccvf and the average response of a continuous process to
an event in the point process. It is worth pursuing this a little
further in order to reveal some difficulties that are encountered
if the notion is pursued uncritically. A common technique for
estimating the ccvf between a point process and a continuous response suspected to be related to it is to obtain the average of
the continuous response before and after the occurrence of the
delivery of point process events. It has also been employed
(de Boer and Kuyper, 1968) when the roles of the processes were
reversed: the continuous process serving as the stimulus (a white
acoustic noise) and the point process as the response (single unit
firings in the acoustic nerve). In this case the event-locked
averaging of the continuous stimulus was over the time intervals
preceding the single unit events. We can consider the point process to be the stimulating or driving one without loss of generality. As long as the continuous response dissipates completely before the next event occurs, it is certain that the average response
obtained is an accurate estimate of the ccvf under the conditions
of the experiment. If the point process is known to be undriven
by the continuous one, there is assurance that the ccvf will approach 0 for all negative values of τ. This may not be true if
the continuous process is the driving one.

Suppose we consider the situation in which individual,
externally applied stimuli occur at random such that one of them
occasionally occurs before the response evoked by its predecessors
has disappeared. Or, suppose we are concurrently observing the
spontaneous firings of a neuron and the associated slow wave potentials within which there may be overlapping components related to
the spike activity. In either case we have seen in Eq. (8.5) how
the ccvf between the two processes is related to the acvf of the
driving process. Let us try to estimate the ccvf by what appears

to be a straightforward extension of the average response technique. We cause an average response computer to be triggered by an initial event of the point process. It samples the continuous process for the next T sec and then remains off until another event occurs. At that time it is retriggered and operates on the continuous response, again for T sec. This procedure continues until N triggering events have occurred and their associated responses averaged. The question posed here is: How good an estimate of the ccvf can be obtained from the resulting average response?

The answer can be arrived at by utilizing the fact that the events which trigger the averager are a subpopulation of the parent point process and constitute a new point process that we call the triggering process. Its event times are easy to define. The interval between successive events is T plus the waiting time to the next subsequent event in the parent process. (This assumes there is no special relationship between T and event times in the parent process.) From this it can be seen that the expectation density $m'(\tau)$ for the triggering process will be different from that of the parent process $m(\tau)$, whenever events in the parent process can occur more frequently than T sec apart. $m'(\tau)$ must be 0 for $\tau \leq T$ and its exact form for $\tau > T$ will depend upon the parent process. The triggering process can never be Poisson although it can approach this when $T \ll 1/\nu$. A detailed analysis of the difference between the ccvf associated with the parent process and with the triggered process has been made (Glaser, 1974). It applies to the situation in which the continuous process consists in part of linearly summing waveforms $h(\tau)$ associated with each event in the point process. The analysis shows that the two ccvfs can be significantly different under a broad variety of circumstances. However, if the point process is close to Poisson and if $h(\tau)$ is oscillatory with average value close to zero, the difference between the two ccvfs will be small. Also, if $h(\tau) = 0$ for $\tau > T$ and the minimum interval between events in the parent process exceeds T, then the output of the triggered averaging procedure

442

tends toward the true ccvf. This, of course, is just the situation encountered in the routine use of the average response computer. Unfortunately, in the general situation we can never be certain beforehand of the degree to which these special conditions hold. The use of triggered averaging for estimating the ccvf is to be discouraged because the procedure ignores the presence of the non-triggering events while observing their consequences upon the continuous process. It attributes these consequences to the triggering events. It also discards a significant amount of the available data by simply ignoring the relationship of the continuous process to events that are not the triggering ones.

8.6. CROSS-EXPECTATION RELATIONS BETWEEN A POINT PROCESS AND LOCAL FEATURES OF A CONTINUOUS PROCESS

It is useful to recall some aspects of the ccvf between the events generated by a zero-memory (nonlinear) threshold crossing detector and the continuous wave it operates upon. Since in a threshold detector the events are dependent only upon the amplitude of the continuous wave at a particular time, $c_{yr}(\tau)$ need not be different from 0 except at $\tau = 0$, and it may be 0 even there. For example, the ccvf between a continuous Gaussian process and the spikes occurring at its zero crossings will be 0 for all τ. This is because we are considering both positive- and negative-going zero crossings. If the threshold level of the detector is different from 0, $c_{yr}(\tau)$ will be equal to the threshold level when $\tau = 0$ and will gradually subside to 0 as the magnitude of τ increases. But in this case the ccvf reflects more the properties of the acvf of the continuous process than the single-instant dependency of the point process upon the continuous process. This is one of the shortcomings of the cross-covariance analysis between continuous and point processes, that it is a linear attempt to detect process interactions which are usually intrinsically nonlinear. Though the weakness is serious, it does not mean that all attempts to analyze process interactions by methods based upon cross-covariance concepts should be abandoned. Some such methods can be helpful if they are designed to bring out aspects of process interactions that the straightforward ccvf does not.

An interesting method, based upon ccvf ideas, for examining the interdependency of continuous and point process is by means of the cross-expectation density between some local feature of the continuous process, say negative peaks, and the events in the point process. There can be considerable value to this approach as has been demonstrated by the study of Creutzfeldt *et al.* (1966) of the EEG and concurrent cortical single unit activity. What we do is to select, by a priori insight or guess, some local characteristic or feature of the EEG wave which is to be examined for its correlational properties with the point process. Each occurrence of this characteristic then can be used to trigger an event of a derived intermediate point process. Representative continuous process features might be an amplitude maximum, a slope maximum, a threshold crossing, etc. The definition of a wave feature can be further broadened to include more complex constellations of waveform features, such as a particularly shaped wavelet, but the principle is the same: Each occurrence of the EEG feature is considered to generate a fiduciary event in synchrony with it.

The next step is to obtain the ccvf estimate of the two point processes, one derived from the continuous waveform, the other representing the actual spikes. It matters little which of the two is considered input and output, since in either case the procedures involved are the same. Creutzfeldt *et al.* (1966) chose to consider, in effect, the EEG process as the driver of spike activity in the cortical region being observed (see Fig. 8.3). They aligned salient negative waves at their peaks or onsets and examined the concurrent spike activity with respect to these reference events. They were able to show that the probability of spike events, as represented by peaks in the PST histogram,

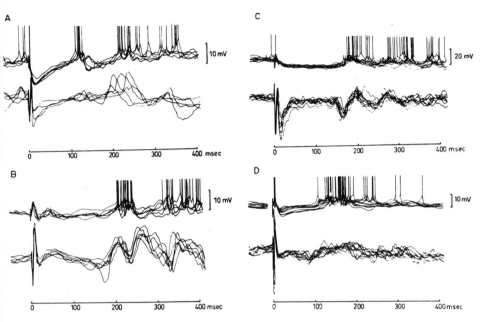

Fig. 8.3. Superimposed traces of EEG waves and spike activity recorded from the same region of cerebral cortex during the same time interval. The EEG waves are aligned along the vertical dotted lines at negative (upward) peaks. The spike trains accompanying each EEG trace are translated accordingly. [From Creutzfeldt et al., Electroenceph. Clin. Neurophysiol., 20, 19 (1966). By permission of the publisher.]

depended upon the separation between them and these EEG features. The ccvf function between the EEG features and the single unit process U can be expressed in terms of a conditional expectation density $m_{fu}(\tau)$ linking the spikes to the feature-related point process F arising from the EEG waveform.

$$m_{fu}(\tau) = \lim_{\tau \to 0} \frac{\text{prob}\{U \text{ event in } \tau, \tau + \Delta\tau \mid \text{EEG feature } F \text{ at } \tau = 0\}}{\Delta\tau}$$
(8.18)

$m_{fu}(\tau)$ is the cross-expectation density for a U event given an F event at $\tau = 0$. The ccvf $c_{fu}(\tau)$ is derivable from it and the mean rates of occurrences ν_u and ν_f of the two processes:

$$c_{fu}(\tau) = \nu_f [m_{fu}(\tau) - \nu_u]$$
(8.19)

This relation is obtained in a way that is similar to that used in Chapter 6 for deriving the acvf of a single point process. The two processes are considered as differential counting processes, ΔF_τ and ΔU_τ. Note the absence of the delta function at $\tau = 0$. The equation also indicates that an estimate of the ccvf between the feature and spike processes is obtainable from the histogram of spike activity formed by using the F events of the EEG process as the time origin.

The acvf estimates $c_{uu}(\tau)$ and $c_{ff}(\tau)$ of the spike and feature processes can then be used to determine the degree of correlation between the U and F processes. It can be seen that this procedure for relating continuous and point processes is an indirect one since the neural spike process is being examined for its correlation with respect to a particular feature of the continuous process and not with the continuous process itself. If different features were selected for correlation, it could be expected that there would be differences in the correlations, differences which would depend upon how the various features of the continuous process are correlated among themselves. Thus if the continuous process is a combination of two independent processes, perhaps one containing predominantly high frequencies and the other predominantly low ones, it is possible that the feature selection based upon frequency related features, e.g., sharp peaks as compared to broad ones, may produce gross differences in covariance functions. There may be other waveform features not so obviously based upon frequency that will also exhibit significantly different interprocess covariances. But nothing in the analysis technique itself can serve as a reliable guide for selecting what these might be. The most reliable guides are the experience and judgment of the investigator. Finally, it might be true that the occurrence of single unit activity is related to the occasional near-synchrony of a peculiar combination of relatively independent EEG features. In this situation no choice of simple individual waveform feature will be capable of revealing this dual dependency. But this is only another kind of limitation inherent in the cross-covariance analysis of processes.

8.7. CROSS-SPECTRAL ANALYSIS

We turn now to cross-spectral analysis as an alternative method for studying the extent of linearity in the relationship between a point and a continuous process and as a means of estimating the linear transfer function between them.

The coherence function of Eq. (8.9) is a measure of how much two processes are linearly interrelated at frequency f. The two extreme cases are $\kappa^2(f) = 1$ or 0. If the coherence is unity, then at that frequency, all the variance in one process is linearly attributable to the variance in the other process. If there is no coherence, none of the variance of one process is linearly attributable to the other. If the coherence is somewhere between 0 and 1, the variance of the individual processes arises from some combination of either their own intrinsic variability, their dependence upon other unobserved processes, or from a nonlinear relationship between the two processes.

The first step in searching for a linear relationship between two processes is to estimate the coherence function over the frequency range of interest. Let us return to the situation illustrated in Fig. 8.1. If there are substantial contributions of the independent noise processes Z and V to the two observed processes X and Y, the coherence between X and Y will be less than the coherence between the underlying processes of interest S and R. The measured coherence function between processes X and Y can be shown (Bendat and Piersol, 1971) to be related to $\kappa_{sr}^2(f)$ by

$$\kappa_{xy}^2(f) = \frac{\kappa_{sr}^2(f)}{1 + \dfrac{C_{zz}}{C_{ss}} + \dfrac{C_{vv}}{C_{rr}} + \dfrac{C_{zz}}{C_{ss}}\dfrac{C_{vv}}{C_{rr}}} \qquad (8.20)$$

where for convenience we have suppressed the functional dependence of the spectra upon f. This means that, as we might have expected, background noise makes the problem of detecting and estimating coherence between two processes more difficult.

The estimator for the coherence function between processes S and R is

$$\kappa^2_{sr}(f) = \frac{\left|\hat{C}_{sr}(f)\right|^2}{\hat{C}_{ss}(f)\hat{C}_{rr}(f)} \tag{8.21}$$

where the spectral estimates are spectrally smoothed ones with d.f. degrees of freedom. Here we have ignored the background noise processes Z and V spoken of in Section 8.3. In effect, we are admitting that we have no way of separating them from the S and R processes of interest.

Estimation of the auto- and cross-spectra of the point process can be done in several ways. One way is to deal directly with the spectrum of the pulse train as obtained by employing the sampling technique of French and Holden (1971). This technique consists of two steps. First, the delta function spike train is filtered by a low-pass rectangular filter with gain $1/2F$ up to the cutoff at F, the highest frequency of interest. The impulse response of this filter is $(\sin 2\pi Ft)/2\pi Ft$. It is clearly physically unrealizable, having tails that extend out to plus and minus infinity; but it can be well approximated by digital methods when real-time operation is not a requirement. The approximation involves simulation of the impulse response over only a finite range of time and "dejittering" the input spike train, that is, considering the spikes to occur only at computer-clock intervals. The filtered output is then sampled at the Nyquist rate $2F$. As long as this rate is low compared to the clock rate, the effects produced by dejittering are not serious. The resulting sampled output is in no way different from that obtained from any band-limited

continuous process. Its average value is subtracted out to eliminate bias effects near 0 frequency in the subsequent spectral
computations.

Another method of estimating the point process spectra is to
obtain the spectral estimates by Fourier transformation of the
auto- and cross-expectation densities. The two methods are equivalent. If the latter method is chosen, it should be remembered that
the cross-expectation density is required over positive and negative values of τ in order to permit computation of the estimated
cross-spectrum. Smoothed spectral estimates are obtained by use
of a lag window with each of the expectation densities.

The considerations that apply to the estimation of the coherence function of continuous processes (See Section 3.19) apply as
well to point processes. In addition, one must take into consideration the special properties of the smoothed estimates of auto- and
cross-spectra of point processes. The average rate of events in
the point process will be the determining factor in the amount of
smoothing that can be obtained from a given sample of data. This
applies to the estimates of the power spectrum of the point process
and the cross-spectrum.

Another important property of the unsmoothed spectral estimator of a point process is that its estimates at two different
frequencies are not uncorrelated. For a Poisson process, the
correlation between the estimates at any two frequencies that are
multiples of the observation interval tends to the value $1/(1 + N)$
where N is the number of events in the T sec data observation
(Lewis, 1970). Note that this correlation is independent of the
frequency separation of the estimates. If N is small, which it is
not in most experimental situations, the correlation between estimates in the point process periodogram can be high. This is different from the situation encountered with continuous processes
where the analog of a Poisson point process is white Gaussian

noise. For such noise, there is 0 correlation between spectral estimators at the harmonic frequencies n/T (Jenkins and Watts, 1968). It is also true that the unsmoothed spectral estimator has a significant bias term at 0 frequency that is proportional to $\hat{\nu}$ or $\hat{\nu}^2 T$. The bias arises from the average value of the N spikes during the T sec period of observation. The bias can be removed by subtracting each segment's average spike rate from the data before taking its Fourier transform.

Finally, in any comprehensive analysis of the coherence between two processes observed over extensive lengths of time, there are bound to be certain fractions of the estimates that indicate significant coherence. As Elul (1972) points out, careful analysis needs to be made to see that these coherences are not spurious ones.

Stein et al. (1972) and Mannard and Stein (1973) have employed linear coherence functions to study the relationship between the continuous states of muscle contraction and motor nerve spike activity produced by stimulation at different average rates. They have shown that under some conditions there are significant coherences at frequencies up to 30 Hz. French, Holden, and Stein (1972) have employed the same techniques to study the relationship between a continuous stimulating force on a mechanoreceptor and the point process representing its output spikes. They observed a coherence that was near 0 for frequencies less than 5 Hz and increased gradually to 0.4 as the frequency increased to 50 Hz. These results point to the fact that there can be a significant linear component to the transfer function between the continuous and point processes associated with nervous system activity.

8.8. TRANSFER FUNCTION ESTIMATION

Once we have established a statistically significant coherence between two processes, we can then proceed to estimate the linear transfer function $H(f)$ from T sec segments of their data.

Let us assume for simplicity that the noise processes Z and V shown in Fig. 8.1 are negligible. Then the estimator of the transfer function is defined as

$$\hat{H}(f) = \frac{\hat{C}_{sr}(f)}{\hat{C}_{ss}(f)} = |\hat{H}(f)| \exp[-j\hat{\phi}(f)] \qquad (8.22)$$

How good an estimate of the transfer function is depends upon the estimated coherence obtained from the same data and the degrees of freedom used in the spectral smoothing. Bendat and Piersol (1971) have shown that at a confidence level α, the confidence interval $\hat{r}(f)$ for the magnitude of $H(f)$ is given by

$$\hat{r}^2(f) = \frac{2}{d.f.-2} F_{2,d.f.-2;\alpha} \left[1 - \hat{\kappa}^2_{sr}(f)\right] \frac{\hat{C}_{rr}(f)}{\hat{C}_{ss}(f)} \qquad (8.23)$$

$d.f.$ is the number of degrees of freedom of the spectral estimates and $F_{2,d.f.-2;\alpha}$ refers to the 100 α percentage point of an F distribution with 2 and $d.f. - 2$ degrees of freedom (Abramowitz and Stegun, 1965). The corresponding confidence interval for the phase angle of $H(f)$ is

$$\Delta\hat{\phi}(f) = \arcsin[\hat{r}(f)/|\hat{H}(f)|] \qquad (8.24)$$

These results were derived from continuous processes but they can be applied to point processes provided that adequate consideration is given to the special properties of point process spectra that were discussed previously. If the input noise source $z(t)$ shown in Fig. 8.1 is not small, there will be additional errors in the estimate of $H(f)$ because the input spectrum is now $C_{ss}(f) + C_{zz}(f)$ and this will exert a biasing effect on $\hat{H}(f)$. Note, however, that an uncorrelated noise $v(t)$ at the output will not produce a biasing effect since it only contributes to $C_{xy}(f)$ and and $C_{xy}(f) = C_{sr}(f)$.

If one of the two processes we are studying is a stimulus we generate, we can, by proper stimulus design, facilitate the

PRINCIPLES OF NEUROBIOLOGICAL SIGNAL ANALYSIS

estimation of the transfer function. If the stimulus is a point process, as when we might stimulate the axon of a motor nerve, then a stimulus with Poisson properties is highly useful. This was pointed out earlier in Section 8.4. The acvf of such a process is $\nu\delta(\tau)$ and its power spectrum is flat; the ccvf between it and the response process is just the impulse response of the system, as Eq. (8.17) indicates. This means we can estimate the impulse response by response averaging techniques. Alternatively, spectral analysis can be employed and the transfer function estimated. Stein *et al.* (1972) and Mannard and Stein (1973) tested motor function by using random stimulation of ventral root fibers. They did not, however, employ Poisson stimulus sequences. If the system is purely linear, variation of the average rate ν of a Poisson stimulus would not alter the impulse response or the transfer function. In a nonlinear system such an alteration might occur, and so a random, preferably Poisson pulse train of variable average rate can be an effective probe of system nonlinearity. An alternative to random stimulation is stimulation at a sequence of fixed rates covering the range of stimulus frequencies to which the preparation is responsive. This is the classical procedure for system response determination. It permits a frequency-by-frequency measurement of the gain and phase properties of the transfer function. But the experimental time required is long and the data are therefore subject to trend variations and to other hazards associated with long experimental trials. Because the frequency-by-frequency test applies only one frequency at a time to the preparation, it is inherently a less effective probe than the random stimulus in which all stimulus frequencies are simultaneously present.

Now let us consider situations in which the stimulus is a continuous process. This would be the case, for example, in experiments involving the sensory system. A highly useful stimulus to employ here is white noise, and essentially for the same reasons associated with a Poisson point process: Its acvf is a delta funtion $\sigma^2\delta(\tau)$ and its power spectrum is flat. Suppose we apply such a stimulus to a linear system with an impulse response $h(\tau)$. The ccvf between the input and output is given by

$$c_{sr}(\tau) = \int_{-\infty}^{\infty} h(t) c_{ss}(t - \tau)\, dt = h(\tau) \tag{8.25}$$

This means that we can determine $h(\tau)$ by measuring $c_{sr}(\tau)$. In the frequency domain, we have

$$C_{sr}(f) = H(f)\, C_{ss}(f) \tag{8.26}$$

and, since $C_{ss}(f)$ is a constant, the transfer function is proportional to the cross spectrum. An estimate of the latter is then an estimate of $H(f)$. This means that a white noise stimulus provides us with a simple method for estimating the linear component of the responding biological system. Of course, since the noise stimulus is random, we must still perform the standard spectral smoothing procedures on it as well as on the output in order to arrive at the proper coherence function and transfer function estimates.

Further simplifications in coherence function and transfer function estimation occur if we employ instead of a truly random noise a so-called pseudorandom noise. This is a synthetically generated noiselike signal which is actually deterministic and periodic. It has been used by Møller (1973, 1974) to describe response properties of neurons in the auditory system to time-varying stimuli. The period of the pseudorandom noise is generally taken to be long compared with the period of possible periodicities or response times of the system under study. Its spectrum is synthesized to be nearly flat and rectangular from 0 frequency to a maximum frequency somewhat higher than the highest frequency observed in the biological response. This means that if the repetition period of the noise is T, its spectrum will consist of lines $1/T$ Hz apart up to the band limit. If this stimulus $s(t°\Delta)$, which we characterize now by its sample values, is applied repetitively to the biological preparation, and if the observed unit's responses are then used to compile a PST histogram whose duration is equal to the repetition period, we obtain an average unit response $\hat{r}(t°\Delta)$. It is then a simple matter to compute the ccvf between the stimulus and the averaged response, $\hat{c}_{sr}(t°\Delta)$; it is in fact a circular ccvf. From this we obtain by Fourier transformation the raw cross spectrum $P_{sr}(f)$. We also compute the response periodogram $P_{rr}(f)$ from the PST. We now smooth these spectra and, in conjunction with $C_{ss}(f)$, the known spectrum of the stimulus, estimate the coherence and transfer functions of the system. It can be seen that pseudorandom noise is an attractive stimulus to use in that, while it simulates noise, it is exactly known.

8.9. CONDITIONAL PROBABILITY DESCRIPTIONS

The cross-covariance function of two processes provides a description of one aspect of their average behavior. When one of the processes is a point process, the ccvf is the average amplitude of the continuous process delayed τ sec from an event in the point process. Because the ccvf describes only average behavior, it is seriously limited in its ability to reveal dependency relationships between continuous and point processes. Thus, we have already seen that it fails to reveal the connection between a continuous Gaussian process and the point process representing its zero crossings. The ccvf in this case is identically 0 for all τ. Let us, instead of estimating the ccvf for this pair of processes, compile a set of histograms of the amplitudes of the continuous process at different values of delay from events in the point process (Frost and Elazar, 1968). We would in this case see at $\tau = 0$ an amplitude histogram with only a sharp spike at 0 amplitude. As the value of τ departs from 0, this spike will broaden gradually until at large values of τ it becomes a normal density function centered at 0 with a variance equal to the variance of the continuous process. The behavior of the set of histograms would make it apparent that the events occur only when the amplitude of the continuous process is 0. If the events were generated at the crossing of a non-zero threshold, this would also be revealed by the location and shape of the amplitude histograms obtained at different time delays. This example points out the important fact that conditional amplitude probability densities contain substantially more information about the process than the ccvf, and can be of considerable help in revealing the relationships between the processes. Let us now examine a slightly different version of the zero crossing problem to demonstrate this, one in which events are generated only at positive-going zero crossings. A conditional probability density at $\tau = 0$ will again exhibit a sharp peak at 0 amplitude. The conditional probability amplitude density obtained at a value of τ different from 0 will indicate that it tends to be negative before and positive after a zero crossing. To establish more strongly the hypothesis that events occur only at positive-going zero crossings, we could then determine the conditional probability density of the slope of the continuous wave. It would reveal that events occur only when the slope is positive.

8.10. CONTINUOUS PROCESS PROBABILITIES CONDITIONED BY POINT PROCESS EVENTS

A formalization of the definitions of conditional amplitude densities is of some value here. Let each event in the point process U serve as a fiducial event for determining a conditional probability density. For an amplitude density of the continuous process R, we have

$$P_{ur}(x;\tau)\ dx = \text{prob}\{x < r(t + \tau) \le x + dx \,|\, U \text{ event at } \tau = 0\}$$

$$(8.27)$$

Similar conditional probability densities can be defined for the slopes and higher time derivatives of the continuous process. A two-dimensional conditional amplitude density can be defined in terms of the amplitude and slope of $r(t)$:

$$P_{ur\dot{r}}(x,y;\tau) \; dx \; dy = \text{prob}\{x < r(t + \tau) \leq x + dx,$$

$$y < \dot{r}(t + \tau) \leq y + dy \,|\, U \text{ event at } \tau = 0\}$$

$$(8.28)$$

and so on for higher-order conditional densities. Here $\dot{r}(t)$ is
the time derivative of $r(t)$. The conditional density as defined
is determined only with reference to a U event at $\tau = 0$. Nothing
is said about other events that can also have occurred between
that initial one and the time at which the density is being considered. This is the definition followed by Frost and Elazar
(1968). It is well to be aware of the possibility that events both
before and after the event at $\tau = 0$ may exert their own effects
upon the continuous process and that the defined conditional probability does not represent a probabilistic response to a single
event.

A conditional density for a single event can also be defined

$$P_{ur,1}(x;\tau) \; dx = \text{prob}\{x < r(t + \tau) \leq x + dx \,|\, U \text{ event at } \tau = 0$$

$$\text{and none subsequently}\} \tag{8.29}$$

One difficulty with this type of definition is that at large values
of τ, there are comparatively few events to be drawn upon in constructing estimates of the density. It also disregards the effects
of other units prior to $\tau = 0$. Conditional densities for one, two,
or more intervening events can also be defined. Each can reveal
some interesting attributes of the processes. One example is a
nonlinear dependency of the continuous process upon the point
process, such as a response that tends to occur only at brief
bursts of events and not at individual events.

An example of a set of conditional amplitude probability
histograms, 128 of them, derived from simultaneous EEG and single
unit data is shown in Fig. 8.4. The histograms, besides being
available for visual inspection, can be used to obtain a variety
of EEG response measures as a function of time lag. Some of the
measures are shown, among them the mean, median, and variance of

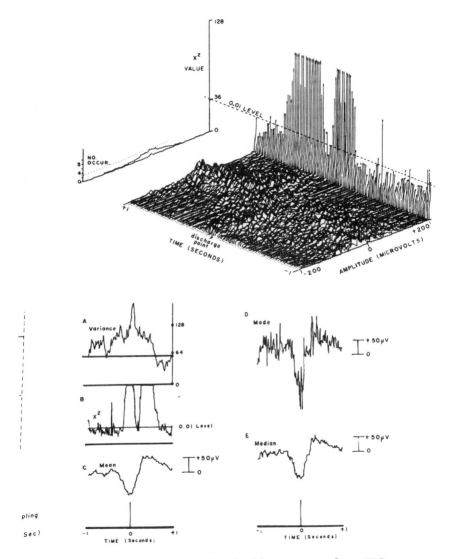

*Fig. 8.4. Above, 128 amplitude histograms of an EEG.
These are obtained by sampling the EEG at times that are locked
to the occurrence of the spikes of a concurrently active neuron.
The histograms are spaced at 16 msec intervals before and after
the spike epoch (discharge point). At the left is shown the
histogram of the EEG obtained by random sampling unrelated to
the spike times. Below, the variance (A), chi-squared (B),
mean (C), mode (D) and median (E) computations from the above
histograms. The horizontal line through the variance (A) is*

the EEG. Also shown is a chi-squared measure of the difference between each amplitude histogram and a reference amplitude histogram obtained by sampling the EEG at random times with respect to the spike occurrences. The high value of the chi-squared measure in two regions along the time axis reflects a significant departure of the spike-locked amplitude histograms from the random sample amplitude histogram. The variance computation shows that the EEG variance tends to be greater at times near the spike occurrences than it is at randomly selected times. Another measure of some interest would be a chi-squared computation in which the mean of the spike-locked histogram was first subtracted out. This would give additional information about how the spike-locked histograms differ from the random one.

What we have attempted to demonstrate is that amplitude probability densities conditioned by time delay from an event in a concurrent point process contain a substantial amount of information about the relationships between the processes. Still more information about process dependencies might be revealed by increasing the dimensionality of the conditional probability densities. But in going to the estimation of second- and higher-order conditional densities, we start to encounter practical limitations in the form of analysis, time, and cost. It is difficult to say, therefore, just how far this avenue should be followed.

8.11. RELATIONS BETWEEN PROCESSES DURING STIMULATION-- COMPARISON OF AEPs AND PSTs

When both continuous and point processes are driven by an externally applied stimulus, the task of relating their activities

---

that of the random histogram. The chi-squared computation is made with reference to the random histogram. [From Frost and Elazar, Electroenceph. Clin. Neurophysiol., 25, 499 (1968). By permission of the publisher.]

encounters a familiar complication: There are three processes to consider instead of two. The stimulus process can seriously interfere with the stationarity or near-stationarity that was so useful to assume in dealing with the continuous and point processes of ongoing brain activity. The techniques that were developed for the study of such activity have to be modified so as to be useful when a stimulus is delivered. Other techniques must also be developed. Fig. 8.5 shows how a stimulus process may act upon

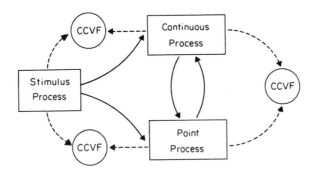

Fig. 8.5. The direction of dependency relations among stimulus and response processes and their relationship to the cross-covariance functions (ccvf) used to discern them.

the ongoing continuous and point processes. The solid lines indicate the effect of one process upon another. Interrelationship judgments are obtained from computations performed upon the observations (dashed lines) of the activity of the processes. These computations are indicated as cross-covariance estimates although they need not be so restricted. To establish with more confidence the relationship between a point and a continuous process, it is necessary that we deal directly with the interaction between the two as they respond to the stimulus process.

For continuous stimulation the procedures could be substantially the same as those employed with ongoing activity. When sequences of brief stimuli or continuous time-varying stimuli are involved, the situation becomes far more complex, and covariance-spectral analyses could not be expected to provide more than a partial description of the interrelationships. However, more fruitful techniques remain to be described.

A useful procedure in relating stimulus-driven single unit activity to evoked potentials is to compare the shape of the PST histogram to that of the AEP. The degree of similarity between the two can provide some index of the strength of their interrelationship. Such a comparison has been made by Fox and O'Brien (1965) who have shown that in several brain locations there are obvious similarities between the two response measures. They found that the higher the amplitude of the AEP at a given latency, the larger the corresponding peak in the PST tends to be. They did not measure the individual EPs and the spikes simultaneously. It is not possible on the basis of this type of averaged data to say whether the spike activity is responsible for the evoked potential activity or vice versa, or whether both reflect different aspects of the same underlying physiological process. In the last situation neither the point nor the continuous process could be deemed the "driving" one. If one of the processes is a driving one, a variety of data interpretations is possible. For example, the similarity of PST and AEP could indicate that the evoked potential is the driving one and that the probability of a spike depends only upon the current amplitude of the evoked potential. This is a spike-generating dependency that involves no memory. However, it seems unlikely to expect that such a simple mechanism can generally explain much of the interaction between evoked potentials and single unit activity. In any case, it must be appreciated that comparisons of PSTs and AEPs are comparisons of average behavior. How the two kinds of response behave with respect to individual stimuli cannot be discerned from averaged data. Furthermore, in more complex situations where there are residue effects associated with previous stimuli or earlier response states, there is no assurance that they will affect both types of response to the same degree. Thus, there can be similarity in isolated responses but obscuring differences brought about by residual responses to earlier stimuli. Yet the foremost fact is that comparisons of ccvfs of continuous and spike responses with respect to a stimulus process are not equivalent to a ccvf analysis between the response processes. Even if the stimulus-related covariance functions $c_{su}(\tau)$ and $c_{sr}(\tau)$ were proportional, there is no complete assurance that the ccvf between response processes $c_{ru}(\tau)$ will be different from 0 during stimulation. Nor is there assurance that one could detect a significant stimulus-evoked alteration in the continuous process amplitude density that is conditioned by the time lag from a single unit event. Such statements must be based upon direct measurement of the interactions between the two types of responses.

8.12. CHANGES OF STATE IN POINT AND CONTINUOUS PROCESSES

The previous discussion of process interrelations has been conducted under the assumption that individual events in the point process were related in some quasistationary way to certain features of the stationary continuous process. This ignores the possibility that the properties of the point process itself, not just individual events within it, can from time to time be affected in some dramatic way by what occurs within the continuous process. The reverse, that the properties of the continuous process can be altered by some special sequence of events within the point process, may also be true. And there exists the possibility that something in the stimulus process may bring about changes in either or both response processes. A particularly familiar example of the latter is the alteration in the rate of single unit activity that occurs briefly in sensory neurons following the delivery of a single stimulus. The resulting activity is often characterized not only by an alteration in average spike rate but also by changes in the distributions of interspike intervals. Bursting activity or some degree of inhibition of spontaneous activity in suitable preparations can be observed. In such cases it is useful to describe what happens in terms of changes of state of the point process and to look for explicit characterizing relationships linking the stimulus to the events following it. One could make a statement about the response process to the effect that at τ_1 sec following the delivery of a stimulus, there is probability $p(\tau_1)$ that the response process will change from state U_1 to state U_2. It remains in this latter state for u sec with probability $p(u)$. During state U_1 there is one rule that describes the generation of spikes, while during state U_2 another rule is in effect. Note that to describe what happens to the response point process as an abrupt transition between discrete states can itself be an oversimplification of a smooth transition from a spontaneous state of activity through a continuum of driven states and back. Similar considerations would apply to a continuous response and its states following the delivery of a stimulus. Thus the switching of responses from one state to another is a special case of nonstationarity. Explanations of single unit activity based upon such considerations have been attempted (Smith and Smith, 1965; Ekholm and Hyvärinen, 1970). We have avoided going into specific details because this type of analysis of process interaction is not well advanced and the merits of any particular approach over another have not been demonstrated.

REFERENCES

Abramowitz, M. and Stegun, I. A., "Handbook of Mathematical Functions," Dover, New York, 1965.

Bendat, J. S. and Piersol, E. G., "Measurement and Analysis of Random Data," 2nd ed., Wiley, New York, 1971.

Creutzfeldt, O. D., Watanabe, S. and Lux, H. D., *Electroenceph.- Clin. Neurophysiol.*, 20, 19 (1966).

de Boer, E. and Kuyper, P., *IEEE Trans. Biomed. Eng.*, BME-15, 169 (1968).

Ekholm, A. and Hyvärinen, J., *Biophys. J.*, 10, 773 (1970).

Elul, R., in "International Review of Neurobiology," (C. C. Pfeiffer and J. R. Smythies, eds.), Vol. 15, p. 227. Academic Press, New York, 1972.

Fox, S. S. and O'Brien, J. H., *Science*, 147, 888 (1965).

French, A. S. and Holden, A. V., *Kybernetik*, 8, 165 (1971).

French, A. S., Holden, A. V. and Stein, R. B., *Kybernetik*, 11, 15 (1972).

Frost, J. D., Jr. and Gol, A., *Exp. Neurol.*, 14, 506 (1966).

Frost, J. D., Jr. and Elazar, Z., *Electroenceph. Clin. Neurophysiol.*, 25, 499 (1968).

Glaser, E. M., *Ann. Biomed. Eng.*, 2, 413 (1974).

Jenkins, G. M. and Watts, D. G., "Spectral Analysis and its Applications," Holden-Day, San Francisco, 1968.

Lewis, P. A. W., *J. Sound Vibr.*, 12, 353 (1970).

Mannard, A. and Stein, R. B., *J. Physiol.*, 229, 275 (1973).

Marmarelis, P. Z. and McCann, G. D., *Kybernetik*, 12, 74 (1973).

Marmarelis, P. Z. and Naka, K.-I., *Kybernetik*, 15, 11 (1974).

McCann, G. D., *J. Neurophysiol.*, 37, 869 (1974).

Møller, A. R., *Brain Res.*, 57, 443 (1973).

Møller, A. R., *Scand. J. Rehab. Med.*, Suppl. 3, 37 (1974).

Oppenheim, A. V. and Schafer, R. W., "Digital Signal Processing," Prentice-Hall, Englewood Cliffs, 1975.

Rice, S. O., *Bell System Tech. J.*, 23, 282 (1944).

Smith, D. R. and Smith, G. K., *Biophys. J.*, 5, 47 (1965).

Stein, R. B., French, A. S., Mannard, A. and Yemm, R., *Brain Res.*, 40, 187 (1972).

SUBJECT INDEX

A 6
B 7
C 8
D 9
E 0
F 1
G 2
H 3
I 4
J 5